Well-Child
ASSESSMENT FOR PRIMARY CARE PROVIDERS

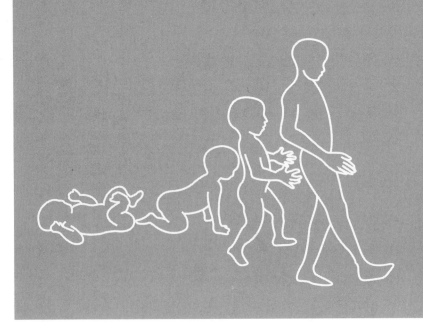

Well-Child
ASSESSMENT FOR PRIMARY CARE PROVIDERS

Margaret R. Colyar
DSN, ARPN, C-FNP/C-PNP
Assistant Professor
University of Utah
Salt Lake City, UT

F. A. DAVIS COMPANY
Philadelphia

F. A. Davis Company
1915 Arch Street
Philadelphia, PA 19103
www.fadavis.com

Printed in the United States of America

Last digit indicates print number: 10 9 8

Acquisitions Editor: Joanne Patzek DaCunha, RN, MSN
Developmental Editor: Marilyn Kochman
Cover Designer: Louis Forgione

As new scientific information becomes available through basic and clinical research, recommended treatments and drug therapies undergo changes. The author(s) and publisher have done everything possible to make this book accurate, up to date, and in accord with accepted standards at the time of publication. The author(s), editors, and publisher are not responsible for errors or omissions or for consequences from application of the book, and make no warranty, expressed or implied, in regard to the contents of the book. Any practice described in this book should be applied by the reader in accordance with professional standards of care used in regard to the unique circumstances that may apply in each situation. The reader is advised always to check product information (package inserts) for changes and new information regarding dose and contraindications before administering any drug. Caution is especially urged when using new or infrequently ordered drugs.

Library of Congress Cataloging-in-Publication Data

Colyar, Margaret R., 1948-
  Well-child assessment for primary care providers / Margaret R. Colyar.

      p. cm.
Includes bibliographical references and index.
   ISBN 10: 0-8036-1005-X   ISBN 13: 978-0-8036-1005-7
   1. Children–Medical examinations. 2. Children–Diseases–Diagnosis. 3.
Pediatrics–Psychological aspects. I. Title.
   RJ50 . C657 2002
   618.92'0075–dc21

                           2002041338

Preface

The idea for this book emerged because well-child assessment texts used for advanced practice were becoming outdated and no new texts were known to be forthcoming. Students have had to purchase several texts to learn the basics of well-child assessment. Health care providers engaged in primary care have also had to rely on two or more references to find basic information to properly assess a child's health and to evaluate anomalies. In response to this need for an advanced well-child health assessment book focused on primary care, I enlisted several health care providers experienced in well-child health assessment to share their expertise and help me to develop a new, up-to-date text.

The major theme of the book is the application of clinical knowledge and skills. The aim is to give both the new and the experienced provider a clear understanding of the components of well-child assessment. Because no two children are exactly alike, overall norms along with normal deviations are included.

A thorough well-child assessment, conducted by a knowledgeable provider, is necessary to ensure the proper growth and development of a healthy child. The three sections in this text cover well-child assessment by body systems (Chapters 1 through 16), well-child assessment by age group (Chapters 17 through 26), and laboratory and diagnostic procedures commonly used with children (Chapters 27 through 39). Each section includes special features to increase the effectiveness of the provider in caring for the child.

Section I includes an overview, basic techniques, and screening, along with a pediatric focus on techniques used to assess each body system. Special features include SOAP charting basics, interviewing and history-taking techniques, and chapters on assessment of the surgical abdomen and assessment of congenital anomalies.

Section II focuses on well-child assessment by age group. Along with the expected information on newborn, infant, toddler, preschool, school-age, and adolescent assessment techniques and findings, this section places special emphasis on assessment of premature infants, sports physical examinations, special issues of international adoptees, and cultural assessment.

Section III is a combination of common laboratory and diagnostic testing and of procedures used with the pediatric population in the primary care setting. Special features include tools for assessing attention-deficit hyperactivity disorder and procedures for removing foreign bodies from the eyes and for performing circumcision and lumbar puncture.

The chapters in this book will not make the provider an expert in any technique or procedure. Instruction and experience with knowledgeable providers are strongly recommended. However, I hope this book will be a good learning tool and a great resource in your practice.

MARGARET R. COLYAR

Acknowledgments

The assistance by providers who have expertise in well-child assessment and procedures has been invaluable. Comments, time, support, and input from editors and reviewers have helped to shape this book. Thanks to all. You are greatly appreciated.

Contributors

TRACY CALL-SCHMIDT, MS, C-FNP
Pain Management Specialist and
Assistant Professor
University of Utah

MARGARET R. COLYAR, DSN, APRN,
C-FNP/C-PNP
Associate Professor
University of Utah

TERRY GESULGA, MS, APRN, C-PNP
Instructor
College of Marin, California

JOANNE HAEFFELE, MS, AORN, C-FNP
Assistant Professor
University of Utah

GEETA MAHARAJ, MSN, APRN, C-PNP
Instructor (Clinical)
University of Utah

GILLIAN TUFTS, MS, APRN, C-FNP
Instructor (Clinical)
University of Utah

WENDY WHITNEY, MS, APRN, C-FNP
Instructor (Clinical)
University of Utah

Reviewers

JANET ALLEN, RN, PHN, MSN
Full-Time Administrator of Hospice and
Palliative Care Program
Kaiser Permanente
Downey, California

PAT ARANGIE, RN, MSN, PhD
Assistant Professor
Arkansas State University
State University, Arkansas

MAUREEN BUMBA, RN, MSN, FNP
Assistant Professor and Coordinator
FNP Program
Medical College of Georgia
Augusta, Georgia

PAT CHICHON, RN, APN-C, MSN
Private Practice Pediatric/Adult NP
The Chrysalis Center, Inc
Lambertville, New Jersey

AMY SEDLACEK COOPER, RN, MSN
Research Nurse Practitioner
Women & Infants' Hospital,
Division of Research
Providence, Rhode Island

ELIZABETH DOMINSKI, RN, MSN,
ARNP, FNP, CRRN
Assistant Professor
College of Nursing, Harding University
Searcy, Arkansas

KELLI S. DUNHAM, RN, BSN
Nurse-Home Visitor in the Nurse Family
Partnership Collaborative
MCP-Hahnemann University
Philadelphia, PA

DIANA GALLER, RN, CS, MSN, FNP
Family Nurse Practitioner
Private Practice
Artesia, New Mexico

HARRIETT GESTELAND, RN, APRN,
C-PNP
Adjunct Assistant Clinical Professor of
Nursing, College of Nursing
Department of Pediatrics,
School of Medicine
University of Utah
Salt Lake City, Utah

MARSHA HEIMS, RN, EdD
Associate Professor
School of Nursing, Oregon Health &
Science University
Portland, Oregon

VICTORIA M. HELMANDOLLAR,
RN, MSN, FNP
University of California Los Angeles
Lancaster, California

WENDY HOBSON, MD
Pediatrician, Community Health
Centers, Inc
Salt Lake City, Utah
Clinical Instructor in Family and
Preventive Medicine,
Clinical Assistant Professor of Pediatrics,
and Master Teacher Fellow
University of Utah
Salt Lake City, Utah
Community Health Centers, Inc, and
University of Utah

CAROLYN HOFFMAN, RN, MSN, CPN
Assistant Professor
University of Louisville
Louisville, Kentucky

BRENDA WALTERS HOLLOWAY, RN,
MSN, C-FNP
Clinical Assistant Professor of Nursing
College of Nursing, University of
Southern Alabama
Mobile, Alabama

LINDA J. KEILMAN, RN, CS, MSN
Assistant Professor, Health Programs
Michigan State University
East Lansing, Michigan

KATHLEEN KELLINGER, RN, MSN,
CRNP, PhD
Chairperson, Department of Nursing
Slippery Rock University
Slippery Rock, Pennsylvania

MARY KNUDTSON, MSN, FNP, PNP,
APRN, BC
Director of FNP Program and Associate
Clinical Professor
University of California Irvine
Irvine, California

KRISTY MARTYN, RN, CS, C-PNP, PhD
Assistant Professor, FNP and PNP Track
Co-Coordinator
University of Michigan
School of Nursing
Ann Arbor, Michigan

HEATHER MCKNIGHT, RN, MSN
Pediatric Nurse Practitioner
Children's Hospital of Philadelphia
Philadelphia, Pennsylvania

CLARETTA MUNGER, RN, MSN,
C-PNP, APRN
Pediatric Nurse Practitioner
Private Practice: Handprints and
Housecalls

KATHRYN MURPHY, RN, MSN, C-PNP
Faculty and Nurse Practitioner at Ottawa
County Health
Muskegon Community College
Nursing Department
Muskegon, Michigan

MICHELLE PARRETT, MSN, RN, C-PNP
Pediatric Nurse Practitioner
The Children's Hospital & Academy
Park Pediatrics
Denver, Colorado

Contents

xiii

SECTION III
PROCEDURES AND DIAGNOSTIC TESTING   433

SECTION I

Techniques, Screening, and Assessment by Body System

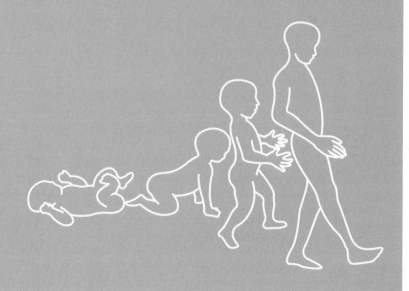

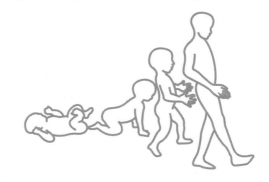

Overview of the Well-Child Examination

MARGARET R. COLYAR

OBJECTIVES
- *Become familiar with the components of a complete well-child examination.*
- *Differentiate between examination of new and established clients.*
- *Determine techniques to gain the cooperation of children during physical examinations.*
- *Analyze age-specific examination requirements by using a periodicity table.*

INTRODUCTION

It is important to distinguish between outpatient encounters that require a complete history and physical examination and those that require an interval history, focused examination, or both. Children are seen in ambulatory care settings for a variety of reasons, including well-child examinations, health problems, and referrals. They may be new to the practice or established clients. Knowing if a particular child is a new or established client helps providers focus questioning during examinations. The child's parents may also have multiple concerns that may change the focus of the examination.

- Establish a trusting and two-way working relationship
- Medical history
  - General state of health
  - Birth history
  - Previous illnesses, injuries
  - Allergies: Food, drugs, environmental
  - Current medications
  - Immunizations
- Surgical history
- Growth and development
  - Nutrition
  - Sleep
  - Motor skills
  - Language skills
  - Personal and social skills
  - School and day care
- Family history
  - Chronic illnesses: Develop a genogram, if possible
  - Family structure and living arrangements
  - Support systems
  - Current resources
- Screening
  - Growth measurements
  - Hematocrit
  - Vital signs
  - Vision
  - Hearing
  - Dental
  - Lead
- Review of systems
- Physical examination
- Diagnoses
- Anticipatory guidance
  - Growth and development
  - Dental care: Fluoride
  - Nutrition
  - Parenting
  - Safety
- Referrals

 # NEW CLIENT EXAMINATION

A complete physical examination is required for all pediatric clients, whether they are seen for well-child care, complicated problems, or second opinions. For an episodic problem, a brief history should be taken and a focused examination performed.

The components of a well-child visit (Table 1–1) include establishing a trusting relationship; taking a history of physical and cognitive development; and performing a physical examination that includes growth and development, appropriate screening tests, immunization status, anticipatory guidance, and therapeutic interventions. Physical examination of new clients should be fairly complete and should include all body systems (see Chapters 5 through 16, which discuss assessment of these systems).

ESTABLISHED CLIENT EXAMINATION

For an established client, review the child's chart before entering the examination room. Review previous well-child visit records, previous problems, the problem list, immunization status, growth charts, medications taken, allergy history, and family and social history. Determine if the visit is for a well-child checkup or an episodic or problem visit.

WELL-CHILD VISIT

In addition to the chart review, check the age-appropriate flow sheet (also known as the periodicity table) to guide the history taking, screening, and examination.

EPISODIC OR PROBLEM VISIT

For episodic or problem visits, review the chart as discussed and check previous diagnoses and therapeutic interventions. With the parent or child, review the chief complaint, determine the history of the present illness (see Chapter 4), and do a review of systems (ROS).

 REVIEW OF SYSTEMS

The review of systems is the subjective information the parent or child provides about problems or changes in specific body systems since the last visit (for established clients) or over the past year (for new clients). ROS data can serve as important indications of the items that should be focused on during the physical examination. A review of all body systems (i.e., head, eyes, ears, nose, and throat [HEENT], respiratory, gastrointestinal, neuromuscular, cardiovascular, genitourinary, integumentary, and endocrine) should be included.

Do not expect the parent or child to remember immediately all the past problems the child has had with a particular body system. Ask specific questions about each body system to cue the parent or child. For example, when asking about the ears, ask, "Have you (or your child) had any ear infections in the past year?" "Any episodes of swimmer's ear?" "Any ringing?" "Any drainage?" "Any decrease in hearing?" Table 1–2 provides a list of suggested questions for each body system.

 PHYSICAL EXAMINATION

Both well-child visits and complicated problems require a fairly complete physical examination. For episodic problem visits, the extent of the physical examination is determined by the reason for the visit. For example, for chief

TABLE 1–2. REVIEW OF SYSTEMS: POTENTIAL QUESTIONS TO ASK

System	Questions to Ask
Head	Have you (or has your child) had:
	Any sores, lumps, bumps on head?
	Head pain or injury?
	Concussion?
Eyes	Drainage from or pain in the eyes?
	Change in vision: Double, blurred, loss?
	Crossed eyes?
	Need to sit closer to TV?
Ears	Any ear infections in the past year?
	Any episodes of swimmer's ear?
	Any ringing in the ears?
	Any decrease in hearing? Not answering when called?
	Drainage from or pain in the ears?
Nose	Runny nose? Stuffy nose?
Throat	Sore throat? Strep throat?
	Abscessed teeth?
	Lumps in neck? Stiff neck?
Respiratory	Shortness of breath?
	Wheezing?
	Croup?
	Cough?
Gastrointestinal	Diarrhea? Constipation?
	Abdominal pain?
	Pain on eating?
	Nausea or vomiting?
	Weight gain or loss?
Neuromuscular	Problems with joints?
	Bone pain?
	Fractures?
	Change in balance or gait?
	Dizziness?
Cardiovascular	Fainting?
	Chest pain?
	Swelling of hands or feet?
	Cyanosis?
Genitourinary	Urinary tract infections?
	Girls: Menstrual problems?
	Pain in genital area?
	Boys: Testicular pain or lumps? Penis pain?
Integument	Suspicious moles or lesions?
	Any rashes?
Endocrine	Excessive thirst, urination, or hunger?
	Intolerance to heat or cold?
	Hair loss or unusual hair growth?

complaints of cold symptoms and cough, examine the ears, nose, throat, sinus, neck, lymph nodes, chest, and lungs. For an ingrown toenail, examine the nailbed and the skin around it and the sensation, warmth, and circulation in the affected foot.

HINTS

During well-child examinations, do what is necessary, but always remember what is important to the parents:

- A healthcare provider who takes enough time
- A healthcare provider who listens
- A healthcare provider who seems to care

These elements are conveyed when you sit down, face the parents and child, and touch the child. A gentle approach with a younger child is less threatening to the child and is appreciated by the parent. The simple act of sitting down conveys the message of "I have time for you. You are important. I want to listen to what you have to say." Find out what is important to the parents and the child and be sure to focus on these items. Do not hesitate to indicate your understanding, clarify anything you do not understand, and indicate empathy and support.

There are different techniques for obtaining a thorough history (see Chapter 4), performing a thorough physical examination (see Chapters 5 through 16), and getting pediatric clients to cooperate. The sections on age-focused examination, including premature infants through adolescents (see Chapters 17 through 23), focus on techniques that help gain cooperation and age-specific examination and issues. A list of techniques is shown in Table 1–3. Age-specific examinations are shown in Table 1–4.

TEST YOUR KNOWLEDGE OF CHAPTER 1

1. When should a provider do a focused examination?
2. What are the components of a complete well-child examination?
3. List three techniques for gaining cooperation for each age group.
4. What components are similar and different between the different age groups?

BIBLIOGRAPHY

Algranati, P. S. (1992). *The pediatric client: An approach to history and physical examination*. Baltimore: Williams & Wilkins.
Coulehan, J. L., & Block, M. R. (2001). *The medical interview*. Philadelphia: F. A. Davis.
Goldbloom, R. B. (1997). *Pediatric clinical skills*. Philadelphia: Churchill Livingstone.

TABLE 1–3. TECHNIQUES TO ACHIEVE COOPERATION	
Age	Technique
Newborn	Use pacifier, gloved finger in mouth.
	Change diaper if necessary.
	Use soothing voice.
Infant	Approach slowly.
	Begin with nonintrusive components of examination.
	Plan distractions based on developmental stage.
	Do not separate infant from parents.
	Do a lap examination or have a parent hold the child.
Toddler	Emphasize observations and use of distraction.
	Encourage physical and verbal activity.
	Slowly acquaint child with yourself.
	Explain equipment and procedures.
	Use toys as icebreakers and for developmental assessment.
	Allow the child to move around the room and explore.
	Do not separate the child from the parent; have the parent put the child on lap for examination.
	Be flexible; expect active resistance rather than cooperation.
Preschooler	3-year-old children: Parent may hold child on lap.
	4-year-old children: Usually feel comfortable on the examination table by themselves.
	Encourage the child to be an active participant.
	Respect the child's privacy and modesty.
	Gain cooperation by seeking the child's help.
	Allow the child to make choices.
	Allow the child to feel a sense of control.
	Use a slow, deliberate approach.
	Use short, simple explanations.
	Talk to the child and explain the steps of examination.
	Do not allow choice when there is none.
	Allow the child to play with equipment to reduce fears.
	Use games (e.g., "blow out the light").
	Give feedback on what you find during the examination.
	Compliment the child on his or her cooperation.
School age	Begin visit by establishing an agenda with the parent or parents.
	Ask child simple social questions to enhance rapport.
	Expand questions if the child is eager to participate.
	If the child does not participate, go back to interviewing the parent or parents.
	Tell the child what you are going to do next and why.
	Teach the child about the body as you go along.
	Set limits.
	Demonstrate how to use equipment.
Adolescent	Interview separately from parents.
	Create an accepting atmosphere.
	Ask open-ended questions.
	Remain objective; do not assume the role of the adolescent's parent.
	Reflect and summarize.
	Maintain privacy.

TABLE 1–4. AGE-SPECIFIC EXAMINATIONS: PERIODICITY TABLE

Months Newborn 2 6 9 12 15 18	Years 2 3 4 5 6 7 8 9 10 11 12
History	At each examination, do interim history update.
Measurements:	
● Height and weight	At each examination, plot on growth chart.
● Head circumference	Newborn through 18 months.
● Blood pressure	Newborn, ages 2 years through 12 years.
Sensory screening:	
● Vision	At all examinations, age specific.
● Hearing	At all examinations, age specific.
Development	At all examinations, age specific.
Behavioral assessment	At all examinations, age specific.
Physical examination	Complete head-to-toe examination at all visits.
PKU	Newborn.
Immunizations	As recommended by CDC.
TB testing	Between ages 12 and 15 years old.
Hct/Hgb	Perform at least once between ages 1 and 2 months and once between ages 15 months and 5 years.
Urinalysis	Perform at least once between ages 1 and 2 months and once between ages 15 months and 5 years.
Blood lead level	Perform if child is at risk (lives in older home or remodeling being done in home) or has symptoms of lead poisoning.
Sickle cell anemia	If a child has been properly tested once for sickle cell disease, the test does not need to be repeated.
Anticipatory guidance	At all examinations, age specific.

CDC = Centers for Disease Control and Prevention; Hct = hematocrit; Hgb = hemoglobin; PKU = phenylketonuria.

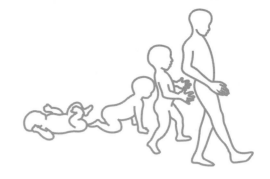

Assessment Techniques

M<small>ARGARET</small> R. C<small>OLYAR</small>

> **OBJECTIVES**
> * *Review basic physical examination techniques.*
> * *Describe age-specific measurement techniques.*
> * *Outline documentation and interpretation of growth charts.*

✋ INTRODUCTION

This chapter reviews the four basic physical assessment techniques of inspection, auscultation, palpation, and percussion, which are used for children as well as adults. The chapter also discusses measurement requirements and techniques for assessing children.

✋ FOUR BASIC PHYSICAL ASSESSMENT TECHNIQUES

INSPECTION (OBSERVATION)

Use your eyes and nose as tools to gather information. Observe the child's gait, stance, and ease of getting on the examination table. This information helps you to evaluate the child's neurologic and musculoskeletal systems. Noting if eye contact is made, how the child interacts with the caregiver and with you, and if the child's clothing is appropriate for the weather give you initial clues about the emotional and mental status of the child. To determine underlying disease processes, observe the color and condition of the client's skin during the examination.

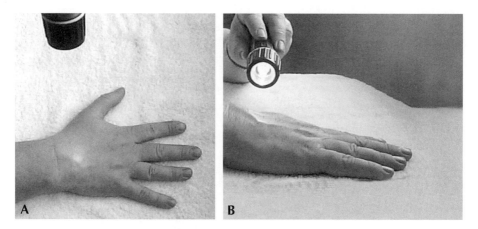

FIG. 2–1. (*A*) Direct lighting. Shine light directly on the surface to be observed. (*B*) Tangential lighting. Shine light horizontally across the surface to be observed.

Observation should be unhurried. Pay attention to detail and take time when looking at each area of the child's body to avoid missing important details. If in doubt, observe the problem area repeatedly until you are able to accurately document the discrepancy.

Lighting is very important when observing clients. You must have adequate lighting to observe with, and the lighting must be without shadows (Fig. 2–1). Two types of lighting are used when observing clients. Direct light is obtained by shining a light directly at the area in question and observing the characteristics at a perpendicular angle. Tangential lighting should be used to cast shadows by shining the light directed across the body part. Use tangential lighting to observe body contours and variations in the body surface and to determine if the surface is elevated or collapsed.

AUSCULTATION

Auscultation is the process of listening for sound produced by the body. It is generally done after observation. Auscultation requires a stethoscope to augment sound. A good stethoscope with short tubes (e.g., 18 inches) is necessary to accurately determine sounds. In addition, the stethoscope must have the appropriate size bell and diaphragm to ensure adequate assessment of sounds (Fig. 2–2). The bell is best for low-pitched sounds and the diaphragm is best for high-pitched sounds. The following hints can assist you in interpreting sounds:

- Be sure that the environment is quiet.
- *Always* place the stethoscope on bare skin.
- Listen for the presence, intensity, pitch, duration, and quality of the sounds.
- Listen intently for nuances.
- Close your eyes for better focus.

FIG. 2–2. Use the correct size stethoscope and blood pressure cuff for the child.

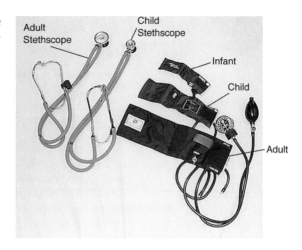

- Concentrate on one sound at a time.
- Recheck several times if you are unsure.
- Perform the technique in an unhurried way.
- Use both the bell and the diaphragm to hear certain sounds (e.g, heart sounds).

A discussion of the auscultatory sounds of the lungs, heart, and abdomen are found in Chapters 7, 8, and 9, respectively.

PALPATION

Palpation uses the hands and fingers to gather information (Table 2–1). Warm the hands before placing them on a child. Short fingernails help you to avoid discomfort or injury to the client. Use gloves if open skin is to be palpated, if the child has a rash, or if a genital or rectal examination is to be performed.

The palmar surface of the hand is more sensitive than the fingertips. Use the palmar surface to determine position, texture, size, consistency, masses, fluid, and crepitus. The ulnar surface is more sensitive for determining vibration. The dorsal surface is best for estimating temperature, including temperature differences on various parts of the body (Table 2–2).

TABLE 2–1. PALPATION HINTS	
Hints	Technique
Hands	Warm by rubbing together
	Use a gentle touch
Fingernails	Short
Gloves	For open skin, rashes, or genital or rectal examination

TABLE 2–2. PALPATION IDENTIFICATION

Hand Surface	Used to Determine
Palm	Position
	Texture
	Size
	Consistency
	Masses
	Fluid
	Crepitus
Ulnar surface	Vibration
Dorsal surface	Temperature estimation
	Temperature differences in various parts of the body

Palpation should be done gently with warm hands. It can be light or deep, depending on the amount of pressure needed. Light palpation is to the depth of 1 cm, and deep palpation is to the depth of 4 cm. Do light palpation before deep palpation so as not to elicit tenderness or disrupt tissue or fluid.

PERCUSSION

Percussion involves striking one object against another to produce vibration and subsequent sound waves, which arise from vibrations 4 to 6 cm deep within the body tissue. Sounds differ according to the density of the tissue the sound wave travels through. The more dense the tissue, the quieter the tone. The tone is loud over air, softer over fluid, and even softer over solid sounds. The five classifications of percussion tones (Table 2–3) are tympany, hyperresonance, resonance, dullness, and flatness.

Percuss one location several times to interpret the tone. Closing your eyes is helpful in interpreting tones. The three basic techniques for percussion (Fig. 2–3) are striking one finger with another finger, striking one finger with a reflex hammer, and striking the flat hand with the fist of the other hand.

TABLE 2–3. PERCUSSION TONES

Tone	Location Where Heard
Tympany (loudest)	Gastric bubble
Hyperresonance	Air-filled lungs (emphysema)
Resonance	Normal lungs
Dullness	Organs (e.g., liver, spleen, kidneys)
Flatness (quietest)	Muscles

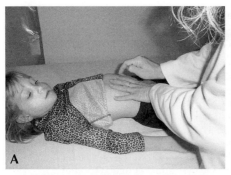
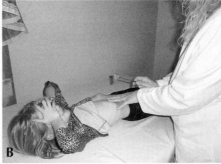
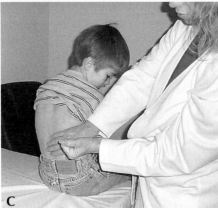

FIG. 2–3. Percussion techniques. (*A*) Place one finger on the child and strike the finger with a finger on the other hand. Snap the wrist. (*B*) Place one finger on the child. Strike the finger with a reflex hammer. (*C*) Place one hand (palm down) on the child. Strike the flat hand with the fist of the opposite hand.

For the first technique (i.e., striking one finger with another finger), put one finger to the body part in question and strike the distal portion of the finger above the nail with a finger on the opposite hand. Then snap the wrist of the tapping finger downward and tap twice. The taps should be rapid and sharp. The tapping finger should not be pointed down because it will dampen the sound; the tapping arm should be held still, and the tapping should be done by snapping the wrist.

Another technique is to place one finger on the body part and strike the finger with a reflex hammer. This technique helps to magnify the sounds.

The third technique is used over dense organs. Place the flat hand palm down over the organ and tap it with the ulnar side of the fist of the other hand. This is used mostly over the kidneys, but can also be used over the liver and gallbladder.

✿ MEASUREMENT

HEIGHT AND LENGTH

Height and length measurement is age specific (Table 2–4). Length should be measured for newborns, infants, and toddlers up to age 2 to 3 years or until

TABLE 2–4. AVERAGE GROWTH PATTERN: LENGTH AND HEIGHT BY AGE

Age	Growth
Newborns and infants	1 inch per month for the first 6 months
	0.5 inches per month up to age 1 year
Toddlers	Growth slows in the second year
	13–24 months: Average of 5 inches
	25–36 months: Average of 4 inches
Preschoolers	2.5: 3 inches per year
School-age children	2 inches per year
	● Girls: Growth spurt at age 9.5 years
	● Boys: Growth spurt at age 10.5 years:
Adolescents	Girls: Growth spurt at age 11–12 years
	Boys: Growth spurt at age 12–14 years

they are able to stand erect. The length is measured with the child supine on the examination table. Measure the distance between the top of the head (i.e., the vertex) and the soles of the feet. Using an examination table with a length-measuring scale is the best and most accurate way to measure length. This type of table has a board at one end, against which you place the top of the child's head, and a board that slides, which should be placed at the bottom of the child's foot. Be sure to straighten the child's leg and dorsiflex the foot to ensure accurate measurements.

If an examination table with a length-measuring scale is not available in your office, use the regular examination table (Fig. 2–4). Place a mark at the top of the child's head on the examination paper. Straighten the child's legs, dorsiflex the foot, and place a mark at the end of the sole of the foot. Then measure and document the distance between the two measurements.

When the child is able to stand upright, a height measurement using a wall poster or an examination scale may be used. Have the child remove his or her shoes; stand upright with the head, buttocks, and heels against the wall; and look straight ahead.

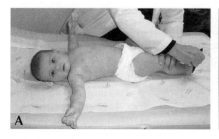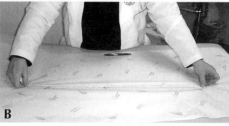

FIG. 2–4. Measuring length on an examination table. (*A*) Mark on the table paper at the top of the infant's head. Straighten the leg and dorsiflex the foot. Place another mark at the sole of the foot. (*B*) Measure between the two marks.

WEIGHT AND GROWTH PATTERNS

There are expected patterns of weight and height increase in children of every age (check *www.cdc.gov/growthcharts* for ranges of height and weight by age and gender). Newborns should be expected to gain 2.2 pounds per month or 1 ounce per day for the first 6 months. After age 6 months, they should gain 1 pound per month up to 1 year of age. By age 3 to 4 months, infants should have doubled their birth weight, and by 12 months of age, tripled their birth weight. Average children quadruple their birth weight by age 2 years.

Weigh newborns and infants with a dry diaper lying on the infant scale. When the child is able to stand, a platform scale may be used. Be sure that the child is not holding onto the scale or the wall to maintain balance because this will alter the result. The normal percentiles are also outlined on the age- and gender-specific growth charts.

Another measurement source to determine if the child is overweight or underweight is body mass. Body mass is calculated by dividing the child's weight by his or her height squared. It is dependent on age and gender. In addition, body fat in boys and girls differs as they mature. Body mass index calculations by age and gender can be found on Web site of the Centers for Disease Control and Prevention (CDC) at *www.cdc.gov/nchs/about/major/ nhanes/growthcharts*.

OCCIPITAL-FRONTAL CIRCUMFERENCE AND CHEST CIRCUMFERENCE

The occipital-frontal circumference (OFC) (Fig. 2–5) should be measured in clients who are 2 years old and younger. The expected growth pattern is between 32 and 37 cm for boys and 31.5 and 36.5 cm for girls at birth. At age 2 years, boys should be between 46 and 52 cm tall, and girls should be between 45.5 and 51 cm tall. To measure the OFC, place a flexible tape measure around the largest part of the cranium just above the eyebrows and ears. Use paper tape if it is available because plastic tape tends to stretch. Take the measurement three times and record the average of the three measurements. Plot your measurement on the growth chart and note the growth pattern.

Chest circumference is slightly less than the OFC at birth. Between the ages of 6 and 24 months, the OFC should equal the chest circumference. After the OFC and chest circumference measurements become equal, the chest grows at a faster rate than the head and should always be larger than the OFC. Although not plotted on the growth chart, the chest circumference measurement also gives you a good indication of how the child's growth is progressing. To measure the chest circumference, place a tape measure around the chest over the nipple line. Take the measurement three times and average the measurements (Fig. 2–6).

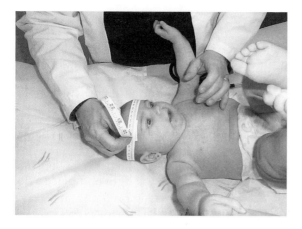

FIG. 2–5. Occipital frontal circumference measurement.

CHARTING ON GROWTH CHARTS

Some basic principles to remember when examining children are:

- Every child progresses at his or her own unique rate.
- Compare a child's measurements with those of his or her peers.
- Evaluate a child's growth over time (normal growth rates progress along a certain percentile).
- Evaluate the parents. Short parents tend to have short children; tall, thin parents tend to have tall, thin children.

Estimated norms of height and weight growth are determined through research on large groups of children. These estimates can be used to evaluate a child in comparison with peers of the same age. Growth charts have been developed and updated by the CDC for tracking height and weight and the OFC for infants and height and weight only for older children. They are available on the CDC's Web site at *www.cdc.gov/growthcharts*.

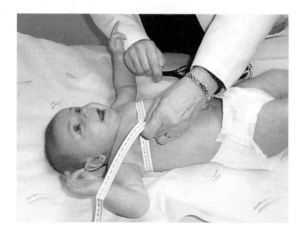

FIG. 2–6. Chest circumference measurement.

Each measurement plotted on the growth chart indicates a cross-section of data plotted at one point in time. The growth charts are age and gender specific.

Growth charts should be updated at each well-child visit and, if time permits, at episodic or problem visits. Many offices now use computer software that automatically updates children's growth charts.

To plot a measurement accurately, determine the child's age across the horizontal axis at the bottom of the chart. Draw an imaginary line upward. Then determine the child's measurement on the vertical axis at the left side of the chart. Draw an imaginary line horizontally to the right and place a dot on the chart where the two points intersect (Fig. 2–7).

Because growth charts are legal documents and become legal parts of the medical record, they should contain identifying information. Therefore, *do not* forget to chart the child's name, date of birth, and measurement data on the growth chart in the appropriate spaces.

INTERPRETATION OF GROWTH CHART INFORMATION

Interpretation of the measurements plotted is very important. Look where the dot falls on the chart; it should correspond with a certain percentile marking. For example, if an 18-month-old boy weighs 28 pounds, he is on the 75th percentile. This indicates that 25% of American boys 18 months of age are heavier and 75% are lighter.

NORMAL GROWTH

Normal growth should continue along the same percentile. When you obtain several of a child's measurements, look at the pattern of growth over time. The child should follow the same percentile curve, which indicates normal growth. Be aware that, for a child who is following a growth curve, whether it is the fifth percentile or the 75th percentile, both are normal. Neither growth curve is better or worse than the other.

ABNORMAL GROWTH PATTERNS AND PROBLEMS

Abnormal growth patterns or problems are indicated when the plotted growth pattern changes from the beginning percentile to a lower one. This is known as "falling off the curve," and it represents an abnormal growth pattern. Abnormal growth patterns indicate the need for further evaluation to determine the problem.

VITAL SIGNS

Vital signs (Table 2–5) should be measured at each visit. This usually includes temperature, heart rate, and respiratory rate. If there is concern about circulation problems, blood pressure (BP) and oxygen saturation

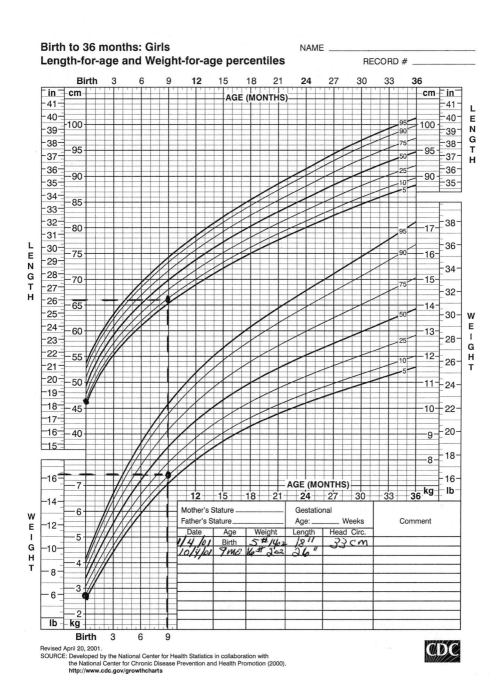

Birth to 36 months: Girls
Length-for-age and Weight-for-age percentiles

NAME _____

RECORD # _____

Revised April 20, 2001.
SOURCE: Developed by the National Center for Health Statistics in collaboration with
the National Center for Chronic Disease Prevention and Health Promotion (2000).
http://www.cdc.gov/growthcharts

FIG. 2–7. Plotting on a growth chart.

19

TABLE 2–5. VITAL SIGNS: NORMS BY AGE

Age	Heart Rate Range, bpm	Respiratory Rate Range, breaths/min	BP Range (5th–95th percentile), systolic/diastolic
Newborn	93–154	28–42	(60–90)/(40–60)
1–11 months	90–170	24–36	(75–100)/(50–70)
1–2 years	89–151	22–30	(72–110)/(38–71)
3–4 years	73–137	21–27	(72–110)/(40–73)
5–7 years	65–133	18–24	(75–116)/(40–75)
8–11 years	62–130	18–22	(80–123)/(43–81)
12–15 years	60–119	14–20	(88–130)/(49–86)
>15 years	60–100	14–20	(93–130)/(49–84)

should also be measured. Likewise, respiratory problems require measuring the client's oxygen saturation level. Vital signs vary with age and gender similar to height and weight.

Temperature measurement in newborns and infants is most accurate when done rectally. Other techniques (e.g., tympanic, forehead strip) are not as accurate because ambient temperature may alter the result. Of course, glass thermometers should be kept out of the child's mouth to prevent injury if the thermometer is broken because of biting.

Heart rate and respiratory rate must be taken for 1 full minute to get an accurate measurement. Heart rate and respiratory rate in newborns are normally irregular. Take an apical heart rate in children.

The BP must be taken with a properly sized cuff (see Fig. 2–2). If the cuff size is too small, the BP measurement will be elevated. If the cuff size is too large, the BP measurement will be lower than the actual value. The stethoscope should have a pediatric diaphragm, tubing approximately 18 inches in length, with no sharp edges and with an appropriately sized bell or diaphragm. Place the earpieces angled toward the tympanic membrane to get better sound.

The measurement of oxygen saturation takes less than 5 seconds when the child is cooperative. Always measure the oxygen saturation level when cardiovascular and respiratory problems are suspected. There are special attachments (earlobe and toe) for newborns and infants to allow a more accurate result. Oxygen saturation should be between 85% and 90% in newborns and between 95% and 99% in all other age groups.

TEST YOUR KNOWLEDGE OF CHAPTER 2

1. How and why are OFC and chest circumference measured?
2. List the components of accurately measuring height in an older child.
3. What are the two types of lighting needed to evaluate a child, and when should each be used?
4. What is the difference between light and deep palpation?

5. Describe the use of different hand surfaces for palpation.
6. What tones can be heard on percussion? Describe them.
7. What are the three percussion techniques? Where on the body are they used?
8. What vital signs should be measured in pediatric clients?
9. Which vital signs should be measured if cardiovascular or respiratory problems are suspected?
10. What are the expected growth patterns of the different age groups?
11. Why is body mass index important?
12. How are height, weight, and OFC documented on growth charts?
13. What does the percentile indicate on growth charts?
14. What considerations are there when evaluating growth chart measurements?

 BIBLIOGRAPHY

Algranati, P. S. (1992). *The pediatric patient: An approach to history and physical examination*. Baltimore: Williams & Wilkins.

Goldbloom, R. B. (1997). *Pediatric clinical skills*. Philadelphia: Churchill Livingstone.

Jarvis, C. (2000). *Physical examination and health assessment*. Philadelphia: W. B. Saunders.

Siberry, G. K., & Iannone, R. (2000). *The Johns Hopkins Hospital. The Harriet Lane handbook*. St. Louis: Mosby.

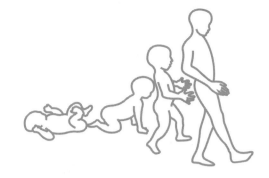

CHAPTER 3

Screening

MARGARET R. COLYAR

OBJECTIVES
- *Determine the components of screening for well-child visits.*
- *Determine the components of screening for cognitive and ego development.*
- *Understand six screening tools: Denver Development, Lead, Tanner, Glasgow, Concussion, and Apgar.*
- *Ascertain which screening tools are used periodically.*

🏐 INTRODUCTION

Screening is done at all well-child visits to determine vital signs, height, weight, head circumference (newborn and infant only), dental, vision, hearing, developmental milestones (i.e., fine motor, gross motor, social, and language), ego development, cognitive development, and nutrition. Screening that is done at selected visits includes measuring hematocrit (Hct) level, lead level, and sexual development. Other screening tools are used only when abnormalities occur.

🏐 SCREENING DONE AT EVERY WELL-CHILD VISIT

VITAL SIGNS

Vital signs should be obtained at every well-child visit. They include temperature, heart rate, respiratory rate, and blood pressure (usually after age

3 years). Normal values and tips for measuring vital signs for each age group are discussed in Chapter 2.

HEIGHT AND WEIGHT

Height and weight are measured at each well-child visit to determine if a child is growing at an appropriate rate. Growth charts provide a scale to determine children's growth patterns and to screen for problems (see Chapter 2).

HEAD CIRCUMFERENCE (OCCIPITAL-FRONTAL CIRCUMFERENCE)

Occipital-frontal circumference (OFC) is measured until age 2 years, when brain growth is maximal. Also, head circumference should be measured if there are concerns about growth or neurologic status.

DENTAL

At each visit, note the number of the client's teeth and the condition of the teeth and gums. The first dental visit should be at age 3 years, as recommended by the American Academy of Pediatrics (see Tables 5–4 and 5–5 for teeth development by age).

VISION

Vision should be examined at each visit. Note the red reflex, pupillary reaction, and accommodation (newborns cannot accommodate). Check for corneal light reflex, extraocular movement, and strabismus (cover and uncover test) in all children (see Table 6–4 for age-related eye screening examinations).

HEARING

Newborns are tested before leaving the hospital. At subsequent visits in the ambulatory care setting, response to sound should be done using the whisper test. Tympanometry and audiometry should be done before a child starts school or when a hearing deficit is suspected.

DEVELOPMENTAL MILESTONES

The Denver Development II Test is a standardized screening tool used to screen development and to detect subtle delays for children from birth to age 6 years. It helps providers know what is expected of children as they age. It tests 125 activities, which are divided into four parts: fine motor/adaptive, gross motor, personal/social, and language development. The test kit is composed of red yarn pompons, a rattle, a bell, a tennis ball, a red pencil, raisins, a small bottle, and a doll with a bottle. Assess the child in all four areas to determine appropriate development.

Directions for Using the Denver Development II Test

Draw a vertical line on the child's age on the test form. To be accurate, calculate the child's age by subtracting the child's date of birth from the year, month, and date of the test.

Ex:	Year	Month	Day	
	90	5	10	(date of test)
	−90	1	4	(child's date of birth)
		4 mo	6 days	(calculated age)

If the child is younger than age 2 years, determine if the child was born prematurely. If he or she was 2 or more weeks premature, divide the number or weeks premature into months and days. Use 4 weeks to a month and 7 days to a week. Subtract the number of weeks early from the calculated age.

Ex:	Year	Month	Day	
	90	10	20	(date of test)
	−89	1	4	(child's date of birth)
	1 yr	9 mo	16 days	(chronological age)
	−	1 mo	14 days	(6 weeks premature)
	1 yr	8 mo	2 days	(adjusted age)

Draw the age line accurately. If the calculated age is adjusted, mark the number of weeks premature at the top of the form.

Each item is specified on a bar, which indicates that 25%, 50%, 75%, and 90% of children tested were able to the perform the item. The "R" on the left end of the bar indicates that the item can be understood without special instructions. A number refers to instructions on the back of the form, which must be followed.

Scoring

Begin with three items to the left of the age line to increase parents' confidence and pleasure. Score at the 50% mark. A score of "P" indicates that the child was able to complete the task, "F" indicates that the child was unable to complete the task, and "R" indicates that the child refused to perform the task. "No" indicates that there was no opportunity to perform the task. To determine if a child is developmentally delayed, do three items before the child's age range, three in the age range, and then three after the age range.

Interpretation

Interpret the test as follows:

- Delay: Any "F" or "R" to the left of the age line.
- Caution: Place "C" to the right end of any item that the child scores an "F" or "R" where the age line falls between the 75th and 90th percentiles.
- Normal: No delays and a maximum of one caution.
- Abnormal: Two or more delays. Refer for diagnostic evaluation.
- Questionable: One delay or two or more cautions. Suggest to the parent how to stimulate development at home and rescreen within 3 months.

EGO DEVELOPMENT

Ego development should be screened at each well-child visit to determine if the child is progressing appropriately through the expected stages. Erikson's stages of ego development can provide a road map for evaluating and understanding successful transition through the stages of ego growth and development (Table 3–1). There are seven bipolar stages that a child must work through. Each stage has a positive and a negative resolution. For example, in infancy, the bipolar stage is trust (+) versus mistrust (-). If the child's needs are not met, he or she will develop mistrust. If a stage is not successfully completed or a negative resolution occurs, the child may regress to an earlier stage or be fixated and not move on.

COGNITIVE DEVELOPMENT

Cognitive development should also be screened at each well-child visit. Jean Piaget, a Swiss psychologist, thought that the fundamentals of all intellectual development take place during the first 2 years of life. He described the types of intellectual development as perception, learning, cognition, and language. Piaget divided cognitive development into four major stages: sensorimotor, preoperational, concrete operations, and formal operations. He believed that children progress through the stages in a fixed order and that the environment largely influences the rate and pace of development.

There are two processes, organization and adaptation, that actively operate during each of the four stages. Children organize basic sensory information (e.g., images, sounds, experiences) to form more complex ideas and thoughts. Then they adapt through processes of assimilation (i.e., modification of external events to fit already existing schemata) and accommodation (i.e., changes internal structure to fit demands of the environment). The stages of cognitive development are outlined in Table 3–2.

NUTRITION

Nutrition screening is an integral part of pediatric assessment. In-depth assessments of children is not practical in the ambulatory care setting. However, there are several areas that can easily be assessed to determine

TABLE 3–1. ERIKSON'S STAGES OF EGO DEVELOPMENT: BIPOLAR CRISIS

Stage	Positive	Negative	Needs
I. Infancy	Trust	Mistrust	• Meet physical needs • Feeding, diaper changes, adequate
II. Early childhood	Autonomy	Shame or doubt	• Meet needs of toilet training • Development control of body and self-control or willpower • Allow independence • Handle temper tantrums appropriately
III. Play age	Initiative	Guilt	• Separation anxiety • Provide positive reinforcement • Keep your word • Make sure child can trust you • Provide distraction • Provide one-on-one time • Praise • Small tasks that can be accomplished • Allow child to make decisions • Provide some areas of independence • Stop and listen
IV. School age	Industry	Inferiority	• Monitor for disabilities that can lead to feelings of inadequacy • Promote positive self-esteem • Avoid criticism • Praise motivation and the willingness to try
V. Adolescence	Identity	Identity confusion	• Allow child to consider options • Temperament • Meet emotional needs • Provide bonding, comfort, nurturing • Provide protection, love, stimulation • Realize that teens are very idealistic
VI. Young adult	Intimacy	Isolation	• Encourage communication • Encourage responsibility

TABLE 3–2. PIAGET'S STAGES OF COGNITIVE DEVELOPMENT

Stage	Age Group	Description
Sensorimotor	*Birth to 2 years*	
Step 1	First month	• Lack of objective permanence. • Does not realize the bottle being grasped and the object being sucked are related.
Step 2	1 to 4 months	• Motor activities become coordinated. • Looks at object being grasped.
Step 3	4 to 8 months	• Attempts to control and manipulate the environment. • May hear noise and want it repeated, but because child doesn't know what caused the noise, does whatever he or she was doing when noise was heard to try to make it recur.
Step 4	8 to 12 months	• Object permanence. • Displays sense of place and time.
Step 5	12 to 18 months	• If you hide objects under pillow; child will move the pillow to find the objects. • If you hide object under one pillow, then more under second pillow; child will look under second pillow.
Step 6	18 to 24 months	• If you move object in closed fist; child will follow hand and find object.
Preoperational	2 to 7 years	• Ability to represent external world mentally by means of arbitrary symbols that stand for objects. • Transitional period characterized by increased egocentricity. • Makes inappropriate generalizations. • Attributes feelings to inanimate objects (e.g., the clouds "cry" to make rain).
Concrete operations	7 to 11 years	• Conservation: Objects remain the same despite some transformation that changes their appearance. • Compensation: If you stretch a ball of clay into a sausage shape, it becomes longer but is still a ball of clay. • Reversibility: If you roll up the sausage shape into a ball, it reverts to the same ball of clay. • Identity: Nothing has been added or taken away from the ball of clay. • Ability to apply rules of arithmetic becomes easier.
Formal operations	Adolescence	• Complex, abstract, and mature logic develop. • Events can be interpreted in many ways. • There is no final version of the truth.

TABLE 3–3. COMPONENTS OF NUTRITION SCREENING

Age	Medications
Height	Allergies
Weight	Psychological factors
OFC	Family dynamics
Growth history	Socioeconomic status
Diet recall (24 hour)	Religion or cultural beliefs
Feeding pattern and skills	Self-perception
Laboratory findings: Hct or Hgb for	Caretaker
anemia	Child

if a child is receiving proper nutrition (Table 3–3). A thorough nutritional history is critical. Do a 24-hour dietary intake and, if time allows, have the child do a 72-hour dietary intake. There are many physical indications of inadequate nutrition that manifest on the skin; hair; nails; oral cavity; eyes; and musculoskeletal, nervous, cardiovascular, and gastrointestinal systems (Table 3–4). If your initial evaluation indicates a nutritional problem, the child should be sent to a trained nutritionist for complete evaluation.

SCREENING DONE AT SELECTED VISITS

HEMATOCRIT LEVEL

Whenever there is a question of anemia or poor hydration, Hct levels should be obtained. Normal values for each age group are in Table 3–5. In addition, Hct should be checked at least once between ages 1 and 12 months and once between ages 15 months and 5 years. A complete blood count contains the Hct value but also provides more information to assist in the determination of the type of anemia present.

LEAD LEVEL

Lead screening is done to assess for possible lead poisoning. The predominant age of children with lead poisoning is 1 to 5 years. Lead screening should be done at the 12-month and 2-year visits and whenever there is an unexplained change in the child's growth. Children at risk include those living or visiting regularly in houses built before 1950 or before 1978 with ongoing renovation, having a playmate or sibling with lead poisoning, or living in a zip code area with 27% or more of housing built before 1950. Symptoms of lead poisoning are lethargy, myalgia, fatigue, irritability, abdominal discomfort, headache, difficulty concentrating, tremor, vomiting, weight loss, seizures, and coma. If there is no risk, laboratory testing is not performed.

TABLE 3-4. CLINICAL SIGNS OF MALNUTRITION FOUND ON PHYSICAL EXAMINATION

System	Manifestation	Deficiency
General	Edema	Protein
	Pallor	Vitamin E, iron, folic acid, vitamin B12
Nervous	Confusion	Protein, vitamin B1 (thiamine)
Cardiovascular	Enlarged heart	Vitamin B1
	Tachycardia	Iron, folic acid, vitamins B12 and E, copper
Gastrointestinal	Hepatomegaly	Protein, calories
Skin	Xerosis, dry scaling	Fatty acids
	Plaques around hair follicles	Vitamin A
	Ecchymoses, petechiae	Vitamin C
Hair	Lackluster	Protein, calories
	Falls out easily	Protein, calories
Nails	Thin, spoon-shaped	Iron
Mouth	Angular stomatitis	Vitamin B2 (riboflavin)
	Cheilosis	Vitamins B2, B6 (pyridoxine)
	Glossitis	Vitamins B2, B3 (niacin)
	Tongue fissures and edema	Vitamin B3
Eyes	Pale conjunctiva	Iron, folic acid, vitamin B12, copper
	Bitot's spots on whites of eyes (yellow, gray, foamy)	Vitamin A
	Conjunctival or corneal xerosis	Vitamin A
Musculoskeletal	Craniotabes	Vitamin D
	Thickening of wrists and ankle	Vitamin D
	Tenderness of extremities (scurvy)	Vitamin C
	Muscle wasting	Protein, calorie

TABLE 3-5. HEMATOCRIT NORMALS (% OF PACKED RBC VOLUME)

Age	Range (%)
1 day	48–69
2 days	48–75
3 days	44–72
2 months	28–42
6–12 years	35–45
12–18 years	Boys: 37–49
	Girls: 36–46

RBC = red blood cell.

SEXUAL DEVELOPMENT

Tanner staging is used to evaluate children's sexual maturation. Tanner charts are available to help providers explain the normal changes of puberty to older school-age children and adolescents. As with height and weight, pubertal changes occur at various rates of speed but in pattern specific to gender.

The Tanner sexual maturation scale helps providers determine a sexual maturation rating (SMR). Also rate each secondary sex characteristic. For example, a girl might be Tanner I for breast development and Tanner II for hair development. The SMR is calculated by determining where the child falls on each secondary sex characteristic and then averaging the two.

Boys (Fig. 3–1)

In boys, first the testes enlarge and then descend. The scrotum and penis in light-skinned boys change from pale to red and then to dark red; in dark-skinned boys they change from brown to darker brown. Pubic hair appears next. Lastly, the penis elongates and then widens. Ejaculation usually occurs at SMR 3, and semen appears between SMR 3 and 4. Penis and scrotal changes that occur before age 9 years (i.e., precocious puberty) are cause for concern and should be evaluated. Sometimes pubic and axillary hair develop without penis or scrotal changes; this is known as premature pubarche. These children usually experience pubescence at the expected time. However, recent data suggest that children are beginning puberty at earlier ages (Table 3–6).

Girls (Figs. 3–2 and 3–3)

In girls, the breasts start developing first. Pubic hair appears next. Approximately 2 years after public hair appears, axillary hair starts to grow. Menarche occurs approximately 2 years after the beginning of breast development (Table 3–7).

GLASGOW COMA SCALE FOR PEDIATRICS

Whenever a child presents with a head injury of any type, the Glasgow Coma Scale for Pediatrics (Table 3–8) should be used to determine the severity of the injury. The three components of the scale are eye opening, motor response, and verbal response. A score of 15 is excellent, 9 to 12 is worrisome, and less than 8 is critical.

CONCUSSION SCREENING

Whenever a child presents with a head injury of any type, evaluation for concussion should occur. The characteristic features of concussion are confusion and amnesia immediately or several minutes after the injury. Early symptoms include headache, vertigo, decreased awareness of surroundings, nau-

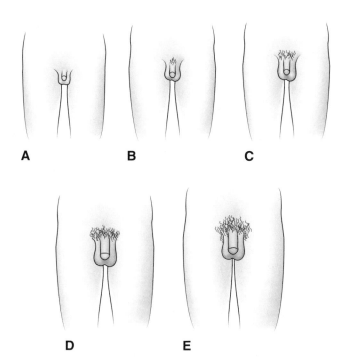

FIG. 3–1. Tanner sexual maturity stages: Male pubic hair and testes. *(A)* Stage I. Prepubertal testes, scrotum, and penis are the same size in proportion as in early childhood. No pubic hair. *(B)* Stage II. Testes and scrotum enlarge. Scrotal skin reddens and coarsens, little change in penis. Sparse growth of slightly pigmented hair at the base of the penis. *(C)* Stage III. Penis enlarges, mainly in length. Growth of the testes and scrotum. Increased pubic hair, becoming coarser, curled, and darker. *(D)* Stage IV. Penis enlarges in width and length. Scrotal skin darkens. Adult pubic hair limited to area. No spread to thighs. *(E)* Stage V. Adult penis and testes. Pubic hair spreads to thighs.

TABLE 3–6. AGES OF SEXUAL MATURITY: NORMS FOR BOYS	
Characteristic	**Age Begins (years)**
Growth of testes	11.5–14.5
Pubic and axillary hair	12–16
Growth of penis	12.5–14.5
Growth spurt	12.5–16

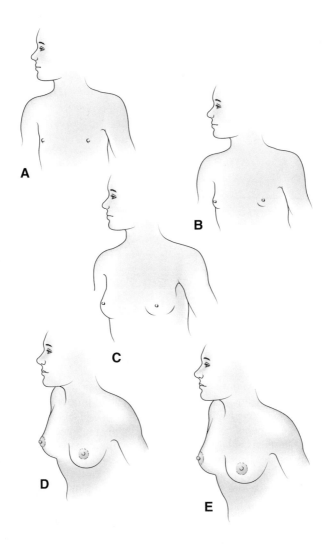

FIG. 3–2. Tanner sexual maturity stages: Female breasts. *(A)* Stage I. Prepubertal. Elevation of papilla (nipple) only. *(B)* Stage II. Breast bud, elevation of breast and nipple enlargement of areola. *(C)* Stage III. Enlargement of breast and areola. No separation of contours. *(D)* Stage IV. Areola projection above the level of the breast mound. *(E)* Stage V. Adult breasts.

sea, and vomiting. Up to 3 months after the injury, the child may continue to experience headaches and dizziness. In addition, the child may exhibit poor attention, poor concentration, memory dysfunction, decreased energy, intolerance of bright lights and noise, sleep disturbances, irritability, and depression. The scale for grading the severity of concussion is seen in Table 3–9.

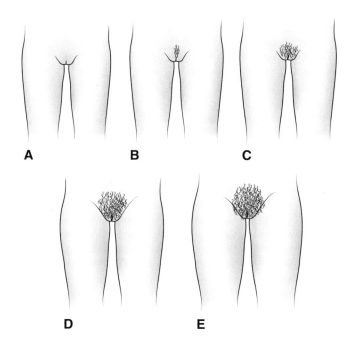

FIG. 3–3. Tanner sexual maturity stages: Female pubic hair. *(A)* Stage I. Prepubertal. No pubic hair. *(B)* Stage II. Sparse growth of slightly pigmented, downy hair, only slightly curled, mainly along labia. *(C)* Stage III. Increased hair becoming coarser, curled, and darker. *(D)* Stage IV. Adult pubic hair limited to the vulva, no spread to thighs. *(E)* Stage V. Adult pubic hair with spread to thighs.

APGAR SCREENING

The Apgar score, which has five parameters, is part of the newborn respiratory assessment measuring successful transition to extrauterine life (Table 3–10). The five parameters are A = appearance (skin, color), P = pulse, G = grimace (irritability), A = activity (muscle tone), and R = respiratory effort. The Apgar score at 1 minute indicates the status of the fetus in utero. It indi-

TABLE 3–7. AGES OF SEXUAL MATURITY: NORMS FOR GIRLS	
Characteristic	**Age Begins (Years)**
Growth of Breasts	11–13.5
Pubic hair	11.5–14
Axillary hair	2 years after pubic hair
Menarche	2 years after beginning breast development
Growth spurt	About 12; range = 11–13.5

TABLE 3–8. GLASGOW COMA SCALE FOR PEDIATRICS: INFANTS

Eye Opening		Motor Response		Verbal Response	
	Score		Score		Score
Spontaneous	4	Spontaneous	6	Coos and babbles	5
To speech	3	Withdraws from touch	5	Irritable cries	4
To pain	2	Withdraws from pain	4	Cries in response to pain	3
No response	1	Abnormal flexion	3	Moans in response to pain	2
		Abnormal extension	2	No response	1
		No response	1		

GLASGOW COMA SCALE FOR PEDIATRICS: CHILDREN

Spontaneous	4	Obeys commands	6	Oriented	5
To speech	3	Localizes	5	Confused	4
To pain	2	Withdraws to pain	4	Inappropriate words	3
No response	1	Abnormal flexion	3	Incomprehensible sounds	2
		Abnormal extension	2	No response	1
		No response	1		

Adapted from Coulter, D. L.: Head trauma. In L. L. Finberg (Ed.), *Saunders' manual of pediatric practice*. Philadelphia: W. B. Saunders, 1998: 883–885

cates cord pH and intrauterine asphyxia. The 5-minute Apgar score indicates how the child is reacting to out-of-utero life. A 10-minute Apgar score should be done if the child had a poor score (<6) at 5 minutes. A score of 8 to 10 is excellent, a score of 4 to 7 is worrisome, and a score of 0 to 3 is critical.

TABLE 3–9. SCALE FOR GRADING THE SEVERITY OF CONCUSSION

Grade 1	Grade 2	Grade 3
Transient confusion	Transient confusion	Any loss of consciousness, either brief (seconds) or prolonged (minutes).
No loss of consciousness	No loss of consciousness	Grade 3 concussion is usually easy to recognize—the person is unconscious for some period of time.
Concussion symptoms or mental status abnormalities on examination resolve in LESS than 15 minutes	Concussion symptoms or mental status abnormalities on examination last MORE than 15 minutes	
Grade 1 concussion is the most common, yet the most difficult form to recognize	Grade 2 symptoms (more than 1 hour) warrant medical observation.	

Adapted from American Academy of Neurology, Quality Standard Subcommittee: Practice parameter. (1997). The management of concussion in sports (summary statement). *Neurology*, 48, 581–585.

TABLE 3–10. APGAR SCORING			
Criterion	**Score**		
	2	1	0
Heart rate	>100	<100	Absent
Respiratory effort	Good crying	Weak crying	Absent
Irritability (response of skin stimulation to feet)	Crying	Some motion	No response
Muscle tone	Well flexed	Some flexion of extremities	Limp
Color	Completely pink	Body pink; extremities blue	Blue, pale

Adapted from Apgar, V., Holoday, D. A. , James, L. S., Weisbrot, I. M., & Berrien, C.: Evaluation of the newborn infant: Second report. *JAMA* 1958:168:1985–1988. Copyright 1958, American Medical Association, with permission.

TEST YOUR KNOWLEDGE OF CHAPTER 3

1. What are the components of screening for the various ages of children?
2. What areas should be assessed to determine nutritional status?
3. What are the clinical signs of malnutrition?
4. What are the components of Erikson's ego development screening for each age group?
5. What are the differences between the stages of cognitive development for each age group?
6. Before performing the Denver Development screening examination, the age of the child should be determined. Explain how this is done.
7. The Denver Development screening examination screens which four areas of development?
8. The Denver Development screening examination can be done until the child is what age?
9. On the Denver Development screening examination, what do the following terms indicate? Caution? Refused? Delay? Normal? Abnormal? Questionable?
10. What questions should be asked to screen for lead exposure?
11. When should diagnostic testing be required for children with possible lead exposure?
12. What is the progression for sexual maturity for boys? Girls?
13. Describe the Glasgow screening examination.
14. Describe how the levels of concussion are determined.

15. What are the five areas tested on the Apgar screening test?
16. What does the Apgar at 1 minute indicate? 5 minutes?

⊛ BIBLIOGRAPHY

Algranati, P. S. (1992). *The pediatric patient: An approach to history and physical examination.* Baltimore: Williams & Wilkins.

Apgar, V., Doloday, D. A., James, L. S., Weisbrot, I. M., & Berrien, C. (1958). Evaluation of the newborn infant: Second report. *Journal of the American Medical Association, 168,* 1985–1988.

American Academy of Neurology, Quality Standards Subcommittee: Practice parameter. (1997). The management of concussion in sports (summary statement). *Neurology, 48,* 581–585.

Coulter, D. L. (1998). Head Trauma. In Findberg, L. L. (Ed.), *Saunders' manual of pediatric practice.* Philadelphia: W. B. Saunders, 1998, pp. 883–885.

Frankenburg, W. K., Dodd, J., Archer, P., Sapiro, H., & Bresnick, B. (1992). Denver II: A major revision and standardization of the Denver Developmental Screening Test. *Pediatrics, 89,* 41–47.

Goldbloom, R. B. (1997). *Pediatric clinical skills.* Philadelphia: Churchill Livingstone.

Jarvis, C. (2000). *Physical examination and health assessment.* Philadelphia: W.B. Saunders.

Siberry, G. K., & Iannone, R. (2000). *The Johns Hopkins Hospital. The Harriet Lane handbook.* St. Louis: Mosby.

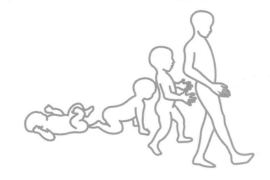

The Medical Interview Process and SOAP Charting

Tracy Call-Schmidt and
Margaret R. Colyar

A thorough medical history is the key to accuracy in diagnosis and treatment. Keen listening skills and a caring attitude lay the framework for a successful interview with children and their family members. Verbal and nonverbal communication help providers determine what is troubling the parent or child, what situation or circumstance caused the problem, and what concerns or fears the parent or child may have about it. Successful interviews incorporate establishing a warm, friendly atmosphere; eliminating distractions; maintaining privacy; keeping eye contact; listening carefully; observing carefully; keeping the discussion focused; and regularly expressing empathy and support.

NEW VERSUS ESTABLISHED CLIENTS

Determine if the child is new to the clinic or an established client. If it is the first time the child is being seen in your setting for a well-child examination or problem visit, a complete history and physical examination are essential.

If the child is an established client, review his or her history thoroughly before entering the examination room. This will prepare you for the encounter and help to establish a therapeutic relationship with the parent.

Parents may have several problems that they wish to discuss related to the child, so be prepared to answer questions in an efficient manner or have referral systems set up to assist them in getting the answers to the questions at hand. Because of time constraints, you may need to focus on only one issue. A statement such as: "You have mentioned several different issues about Sandy. Which one is most important for us to address today?" will help focus the visit.

When approaching the well-child visit, use the age-appropriate guidelines to ensure that issues that need to be discussed are addressed at each visit. Chapters 17 to 23 provide age-specific flow sheets and charts to assist with each visit. Many of these tools are also available on the Websites *www.aanp.org* and *www.napnap.org*. The use of flow sheets may vary from practice to practice, but assessing and addressing important issues are of concern for providers, parents, and children.

If the client is new, do not hesitate to include medical information that the parent or child has brought to the clinic and documents or medical records that were reviewed previously or during the interview. The time it takes for a provider to review the articles should be documented in the history section (i.e., "reviewed Sandy's chart from Dr. Peterson from 1999, 20 minutes").

INTERVIEW AND HISTORY TAKING

History taking is a process you should master. A thorough history helps you to focus the physical examination as well. We will start by discussing the interview techniques and approaches that lead to positive results.

APPROACH

When preparing to have contact with parents and child, keep some things in mind. A professional demeanor is important at all times. When interviewing children, a lab coat, especially a white one, may not be an appropriate choice. Children may be less intimidated by playful scrub attire with badges or stickers, which could help distract them from the medical environment. Be neat and clean but not stuffy. Clean clothes and groomed hair and fingernails are essential when establishing trust and displaying professionalism. Address the parent and child by name. A smile is helpful in establishing a positive relationship.

Infants, Toddlers, and Young Preschoolers

When the provider enters the examination room, many infants and toddlers begin screaming or crying and cling or run to their parents. Suggestions for dealing with this situation are to talk calmly with the parent to gather information and let the child observe. Try putting the stethoscope within the child's reach so that he or she can touch it. Hopefully, when the time comes to do the physical examination, the child will be more comfortable and allow the examination without distress.

Older Preschoolers and School-Age Children

Children in these age groups have usually had many experiences with healthcare providers and are more comfortable with the interview and physical examination process. On entering the room, make eye contact, smile, introduce yourself, and ask the child's name. Ask a few nonthreatening questions before starting the formal interview. For example, say, "Hi, I'm Peggy. What's your name?" and "How old are you?" Be sure to ask children about things they will be able to answer. Direct any questions about medical history, surgical history, family history, immunizations, and medications to the parent.

Adolescents

Adolescents are very sensitive and need to be treated with respect instead of like children. It is best to greet the adolescent before greeting the parent. Gear the conversation to the appropriate level for the teen. Chat about interests and how things are going in general.

The visit flows better if there is an understanding with the parent and the teen about confidentiality at the start of the visit. The adolescent must understand that the interview will be confidential unless there is a problem that needs to be addressed for the health of the client. The parent and adolescent should come to an agreement that the provider will do two interviews, one with the parent and adolescent and one with the adolescent alone.

INTERVIEW POSTURE

Remember that nonverbal communication plays a significant role in the success of the interview. During the interview, try to sit quietly and lean slightly toward the parent and child. This relays interest and respect. Avoid fidgeting positions or moving toward the door until the interview is complete. This makes the client feel unimportant and may block further communication. If the provider's reactions portray disapproval, disgust, anger, shock, embarrassment, or plain boredom, the parent or child may sense this, and the therapeutic relationship could deteriorate. An understanding, caring, and unhurried attitude should be maintained throughout the history taking.

Place your chair at eye level to the parent and child so that it is easy to maintain good eye contact throughout the interview. This also gives parents and children the impression that you are talking to them on their level rather than talking down to them. Place a clock on the wall in each examination room that can be easily viewed to enhance time efficiency. This will also keep you from having to frequently look at your watch, making the parent and child feel hurried or unimportant. Try to avoid interruptions and give the client your full and undivided attention.

INTERVIEW SETTING

The setting of the interview must be comfortable, private, and nonintimidating. Do not place furniture or other items between you and the client. Keep the room well lighted and warm for comfort. Decorative items such as circus animals around the borders of the room, characters on the walls, and colorful examination table paper may place children more at ease. Accessible books or toys could be used to distract or entertain children during the interview or the examination itself if necessary.

Personal space is important in making the parent and child feel comfortable. Try not to invade the child's space during the interview. Personal space is approximately 3 feet in Western cultures. Each individual has a different level of comfort with spacing issues. For example, Eastern cultures, such as Japanese, have a much closer social distance, but they consider direct eye contact to be impolite.

INTERVIEW FORMAT

Start the interview by introducing yourself and stating the purpose of the examination. "Hello, Mrs. Smith, I am Dr. [Mrs.] Jones, [nurse practitioner, physician's assistant] at this clinic. I am here to find out your reason for the visit and to get a history on Johnny." This will put the parent at ease because he or she will know what to expect from the encounter. Wearing a name tag for identification is always a plus.

If you must take notes throughout the interview, be sure the parent and child know you are listening to their information. Stop frequently to reestablish eye contact. Frequent eye contact is especially helpful if you are typing on the computer while collecting information.

COMMUNICATION TECHNIQUES

OPEN VERSUS CLOSED QUESTIONS

Initially, use open-ended questions to determine the parent and child's reason for visiting the clinic. An open-ended question is one that is worded to encourage a descriptive response. For example, "Mrs. Smith, what brings you into the clinic today?" or "Tell me about Johnny." Continue this type of questioning until you think that sufficient general data have been gathered.

TABLE 4–1. COMMUNICATION TECHNIQUES

Communication Technique	Definition	Example
Reflection	Restating the clients' concerns to enhance the communication process	Parent: "Johnny has had a cough for a week now, and I am concerned." Provider: "You are concerned?" Parent: "Yes, when this happened in the past, he had to be hospitalized for 2 weeks" Provider: "Johnny had to be hospitalized?"
Clarification	Repeating the information you have received to present a clearer picture of the event.	Parent: "Johnny has been sick." Provider: "What do you mean when you say Johnny has been sick?"
Confrontation	Directly addressing the issue at hand	Provider "I understand you have been skipping school?"
Silence	Using seconds or minutes of time without speaking to enhance communication	Provider: "What are your financial and health concerns?" Parent: (1 minute with no response) Provider: "Yes?" Parent: "I am afraid of healthcare costs if Johnny is diagnosed with asthma. My friend lost her insurance when this happened to her."

Next, ask closed-ended questions to fill in the information that is missing. For example, "Has Johnny had exposure to anyone who has had a cough?" or "Does he go to daycare?" "Yes" and "no" answers allow completion of the data set so the differential diagnosis can be formulated and the format for the physical examination can be planned.

TYPES OF INTERVIEW QUESTIONS

During the interview, there are several communication techniques you can use as a guide to improve therapeutic relations and enhance communication. These techniques are reflection, clarification, confrontation, and silence (Table 4–1).

Reflection is restating the child or parent's wording to facilitate the communication process. Reflection is used to enable the child or parent to understand that you are aware of their feelings and facts related to the situation. The use of reflection aids your understanding of the problem that needs to be evaluated but also the parent's feelings and fears related to the child.

Clarification is another communication technique that is commonly used to promote effective communication. Use the information the parent or child

41

has given to receive a clearer picture of the event. For example, "Can you describe Johnny's flu symptoms?"

Confrontation may be needed if discrepancies in the story are noted. Confrontation is used to clarify inconsistent statements. Repeat what was said and ask for more detail. For example, "Are you afraid you will be unable to care for Johnny if he becomes ill?"

Silence is a technique that is also used during the interview process. This is extremely helpful when approaching sensitive issues, such as sexuality and abuse. Pause for seconds to minutes to allow the parent or child to process thoughts and express them. Silence can be uncomfortable, but practice and patience promote and improve overall communication and information collection.

SOAP CHARTING

SOAP charting is the accepted format for charting in ambulatory care clinics and practices. SOAP charting includes the subjective (S) information that the parent and child provide; the objective (O) information that the provider observes; the assessment (A) or diagnosis that the provider determines based on the subjective and objective information; and the plan (P) that the provider, parent, and child develop to achieve the desired outcome.

SUBJECTIVE: NEW CLIENT

The subjective portion of the visit includes eight components. They are the chief complaint, history of present illness, medical history, surgical history, family history of disease, psychosocial history, review of systems, and developmental milestones accomplished. Start by collecting the following identifiers: date, time, age, race, and relationship of historian.

Chief Complaint

Determine the parental concerns or chief complaint (CC). This is a statement in the parent's words of why they came to the clinic that day (e.g., "Sandy has had a temperature and was vomiting" or "We're here for a checkup and shots").

History of Present Illness

Another component of the subjective information is the history of present illness (HPI). This is a step-by-step story of the parental concern or chief complaints. This detailed explanation should include specific components in chronological order. One method of obtaining all the correct information is shown in Table 4–2.

An example of an HPI is as follows:

> Sandy, a 2-year-old boy, has had a fever per Mom of 101.3–102.4°F axillary for the past 3 days. He has also been vomiting clear fluid four to six times a day.

TABLE 4–2. COMPONENTS NECESSARY FOR COMPLETE HISTORY OF PRESENT ILLNESS

Component	Comments
Onset	—
Duration of the problem or illness	—
Location	—
Associated symptoms (depends on chief complaint)	For upper respiratory problems, ask about cough, fever, chills, headache, sore throat, runny nose, ear pain, and fever
	For abdominal pain, ask about bowel movements, urination, nausea, vomiting, and fever.
Activity level: Effect of the illness	Determine what effect the illness had on the child' activity level.
	Ask if the child is playing, sleeping, and eating as usual.
	Determine if it was necessary for the child to miss school.
Mood and interaction with the parent	Ask if the child has been fussy, irritable, grouchy, grumpy, and so on
Relieving and alleviating factors	Determine what treatments have been tried and their effectiveness

This started suddenly in the middle of the night and has continued through today. Sandy has been crying a lot. Mom gives him Tylenol every 6 hours, which helps, when he is able to keep it down. Last dose was at 8 AM. Associated symptoms include occasional chills with fever. He is wetting two diapers a day even though Mom has been pushing fluids (formula and Pedialyte). He has been unable to go to daycare, and Mom has missed 2 days of work to take care of him. There are four other children at daycare with similar symptoms. He did have a similar episode 8 months ago, which lasted for 4 days and was diagnosed as viral.

Medical History

The medical history goes beyond the history of present illness to explain the child's overall health status before the present problem began. All medical experiences, including psychiatric disabilities, medications, immunizations, and allergies should be included.

Parents may not remember all medical problems their child has encountered; therefore, specifically ask about common childhood illnesses, such as measles, mumps, chickenpox, whooping cough, ear infections, strep throat, asthma, diabetes, rheumatic fever, and so on. To jog the parent's memory, also ask if there have been any accidents, hospitalizations, or emergency room visits and the problem for which the child was treated.

Medications, including over-the-counter, herbal, and prescription preparations, should be recorded. Determine what immunizations the child has received and when they were administered. Evaluate if the child's immunizations are up to date. If the child is behind schedule, decide what immunizations should be given at the current visit and determine a schedule to provide the remaining vaccinations. Ask about allergies to food, medications, and the environment.

If the child is younger than 2 years old, a detailed evaluation of prenatal care, pregnancy, and labor and delivery should be done. Note any medications (i.e., prescribed, over-the-counter, herbal, recreational) the mother was taking at the time of conception. Determine the mother's nutritional status before conception. Ask about ingestion of alcoholic beverages and tobacco use. Ask about the home environment, including the type of housing, factories or industries close to the home, chemical use in the home, and other teratogen exposure.

Obtain a thorough prenatal and perinatal history. Ask if any prenatal care was obtained and find out about nutritional patterns and weight gain; prenatal tests conducted and their results; accidents and illnesses; unusual medications taken or dental procedures undergone; all potentially harmful environmental exposures (e.g., radiation, chemical fumes); excessive heat (e.g., hot tubs, saunas, fever); and use of tobacco, alcohol, home remedies, and recreational drugs (e.g., marijuana, cocaine, methamphetamine, heroin). Check the mother's previous pregnancy history for previous spontaneous abortions, stillbirths, and problems conceiving.

Ask about the labor and delivery experience of the mother and baby. Note the presentation, difficulties that occurred, length of labor, and whether any asphyxia occurred. Ask about the Apgar score.

Ask if the baby grew consistently throughout the pregnancy or if the growth was too slow or too fast. When did the mother feel the baby move first? Was there any point when movement stopped or became unusually strong? Were the baby's movements always felt in just one part of the abdomen?

Gather data about the child's progress during the first few weeks of life. Note any problems with feedings; weight gain; development; and complications such as infections, jaundice, seizures, floppiness, apnea, fever, or bowel or bladder problems.

If the child is older than 2 years, do a general history of medical problems since birth. Unless there were complications at birth, a general overview of the birth, prenatal care, pregnancy, and labor and delivery is all that is needed.

Surgical History

Ask about any surgical procedures the child had since birth. Ask about common childhood surgeries, such as tonsillectomy, adenoidectomy, myringotomy tubes, and circumcision.

The following is an example of a medical and surgical history:

> Sandy is generally healthy, although he has had two ear infections this year. His mother denies any hospitalizations or surgeries to the current date. She also denies that Sandy has had any major accidents and states that he is placed in an age-appropriate car seat with every car exposure. Sandy's mom states he has never had any emotional problems, and she believes he is active but not overactive. He takes one Flintstones vitamin each day and has no allergies to medications, food, or the environment. He is current on his immunizations for his age.

Review of Systems

A review of systems is a system-by-system evaluation of problems that have occurred since the last visit. You need to be specific and ask directed questions for each system. For example, when screening for the respiratory system, ask: "Has the child had any respiratory problems? RSV? Pneumonia? Asthma? Cough? Shortness of breath? Difficulty breathing?" A list of specific concerns is listed in each of the chapters on assessment of each body system (see Chapters 5 to 15).

Developmental Milestones

Before entering the examination room, review the expected developmental milestones for the age of child you will be assessing. Look at the gross motor, fine motor, language, and social and emotional skills the child should have accomplished. You can use the Denver Development II test as a guide for children up to age 6 years. The Department of Health and Human Services offers a great guide called *Bright Futures* that can be used to focus the developmental assessment. In addition, be cognizant of the stage of ego development (Erikson) and the stage of cognitive development (Piaget) the child should be in for his or her age. Chapter 3 outlines specific developmental stages, and Chapters 17 to 23 discuss assessment by age group.

OBJECTIVE

This section includes all the information gathered through the senses—sight, hearing, smell, and touch, but usually not taste. The findings from the physical examination and any laboratory or diagnostic test results go in this section.

Assessment

Included in this section are the diagnoses that are determined based on the subjective and objective findings. If this is a well-child visit, a diagnosis of "well-child examination" with the specific age of the child should be listed. If other medical problems where assessed, they should also be listed. Examples of diagnoses:

- Well-child visit: No problems
  - Well-child examination: 2 years old
- Well-child visit: Problems
  - Well-child examination: 2 years old
    - ○ Left otitis media (six occurrences in 3 months)
    - ○ Vomiting
    - ○ Baby bottle caries

Plan

If the visit is for a well-child examination, the plan should include five areas of anticipatory guidance and recommended time for the next visit. If it is a well-child visit and problems were addressed, the six components include treatments, medications, referrals, diagnostic tests to be performed, anticipatory guidance, and recommended time for the next visit. An example of the plan for the above well-child visit of a 2-year-old child with otitis media (left ear), vomiting, and baby bottle caries would include:

- BRAT (bananas, rice cereal, applesauce, and toast) diet
- Phenergan suppositories 12.5 mg q 6 hr prn for nausea or vomiting
- Amoxicillin 400 mg/5mL: 1 tsp bid x 7 days
- Auralgan Otic 2 to 3 gtt AS q1–2 hr prn (as needed) ear pain
- Referral to ear, nose, and throat (ENT) specialist for tubes
- Referral to dentist
- Return to clinic in 1 year or prn

Anticipatory Guidance

Anticipatory guidance is essential to address at each well-child examination. Categories that should be addressed for all age groups are growth and development, safety, nutrition, immunization, dental, and discipline. If the client is an adolescent, add sexuality issues and health habits. The *Bright Futures, Guidelines for Health Supervision of Infants, Children and Adolescents Pocket Guide* can be a helpful tool for providers in providing anticipatory guidance.

TEST YOUR KNOWLEDGE OF CHAPTER 4

1. Describe the difference between a new versus an established client visit.
2. What is an appropriate way to focus a client visit?
3. Why is it important to review the medical record before talking with a parent and child?
4. Describe the professional approach to interviewing the children of different ages.
5. Discuss posture and setting issues for interviewing a child and parent.

6. What are common communication techniques? Describe them.
7. What does the acronym SOAP stand for?
8. What are the components of the subjective portion of SOAP charting?
9. What are the components of a thorough history of present illness?
10. How can a provider help a parent focus on the medical and surgical history?
11. How does a provider know which developmental milestones to focus on?
12. What are the components of the objective portion of SOAP charting?
13. What is included in the assessment portion of SOAP charting?
14. What are the five areas of anticipatory guidance?
15. What are the six components to be addressed in well-child visit in which problems are found?

 ## BIBLIOGRAPHY

Boynton, R. W., Dunn, E. S., & Stephens, G. R. (1998). *Manual of ambulatory pediatrics.* 4th Ed. Philadelphia: Lippincott.
Coulehan, J. L., & Block, M. R. (2001). *The medical interview.* Philadelphia: F. A Davis.
Knight, J. R., & Emans, S. J. (2001). *Bright futures.* U.S. Department of Health and Human Services.

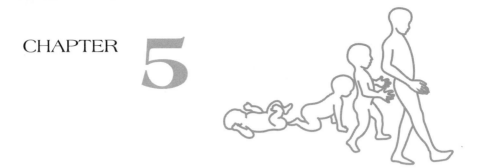

Assessment of the Head and Neck

MARGARET R. COLYAR

OBJECTIVES
- *Establish basic assessment of the head and neck for children.*
- *Develop techniques for using regular and pneumatic otoscopes.*
- *Learn techniques to make the head and neck assessment more acceptable to the child.*

Assessment of the head and neck is stressful for infants and toddlers and usually elicits crying or resistance. This part of the examination should be performed last. Older children are more tolerant. Therefore, the order of the examination depends on the child's comfort level.

HISTORY

Ask about medical history; surgeries; and family history of hearing disorders, sinus problems, cleft palate, and cancer. Include in the history medications, allergies, and immunization status. As part of the review of systems, ask about the occurrence of headaches; head injuries; dizziness; neck pain; limitation of movement; lumps; swelling; and changes in hearing, smell, or taste. For children who are ill, ask if they have been pulling at their ears, putting their hands in their mouths (which sometimes indicates sore throats), or have had feeding difficulties.

TABLE 5–1. HAIR ABNORMALITIES	
Abnormalities	Problem
Kinky	Menkes syndrome
Low-set posterior hairline	Turner's syndrome
Coarse	Mucopolysaccharidoses
Sparse	Ectodermal dysplasias
White streak	Waardenberg's syndrome
Coarse red patches	Kwashiorkor
Dry, gray	Malnutrition
No pigment	Albinism

PHYSICAL EXAMINATION

HEAD

Generally observe the hair, skin, ears, nose, mouth, facial movement, and neck of the child for symmetry, position, and function. Examine the hair for color, consistency, and amount (Table 5–1). In newborns, if the hair is too curly, too long, too much, or if there are more than two whirls, suspect a brain anomaly. Observation of facial features allows you to make a determination of normal versus dysmorphic features. During the examination, watch for smiling, frowning, elevation of the eyebrows, and range of motion of the neck.

Newborns

Measure the head circumference around the most prominent part of the head just above the eyebrows and ears and plot your results on the growth chart (see Chapter 3). Note any decreases or increases in percentile. Palpate the head for lumps, bumps, lesions, or desquamation. Newborns sometimes have overriding sutures caused by the birth process; this is normal. The overriding sutures should even out by 6 months and feel smooth on palpation.

Palpate the fontanels when the child is calm and in the upright position. The anterior fontanel is usually 2 cm by 2 cm in a diamond shape. The anterior fontanel should close between ages 9 and 19 months. The posterior fontanel is usually less than 1 cm. The posterior fontanel may be absent, which is a normal variation. Other palpable fontanels are the sphenoid and mastoid. An unusually large fontanel or delay in closure of the fontanels may indicate a delay in bone growth. Abnormal size or shape may be an indication of hyper- or hypothyroidism. An abnormally large head could indicate hydrocephalus or chromosomal, congenital, or metabolic disorders. Early closure of the fontanels is also of concern because internal structures may not be able to develop properly. Other potential problems are noted in Table 5–2.

Skulls of newborns may indent under pressure and spring back. This is known as craniotabes and is normal. However, if this condition persists after the second month, bone mineralization problems should be considered.

49

TABLE 5–2. FONTANEL EXAMINATION

Normal	Abnormal	Indication
Venous pulsations	Tense, bulging	Intracranial pressure
Flat	Sunken	Dehydration

Older Children

Always evaluate the appearance of the mother, father, and other siblings. In older children, note the condition and amount of hair. Note any areas of alopecia or lesions. Palpate the head for lumps, bumps, and lesions. In infants and older children, check behind the ear margins for lice and nits on the hair shafts.

Ears: External

Placement Examine the placement of the ears from the front, *not* the side or the back. Draw a straight line from the inner canthus of the eye to the outer canthus and then to the ear. The top of the ear should be even to 20% above the line. Low-set ears are seen in children with fetal alcohol syndrome and other chromosomal syndromes.

Size The right ear is usually slightly larger than the left ear. Note any pits, tags, or fistulae around the ear. These occurrences may indicate hearing deficits and should result in evaluation of hearing.

Shape The normal external ear is oval. Darwin's tubercles (or "Spock ears") are a normal variation. A rounded external ear may be a normal deviation but is often associated with Down syndrome.

Earlobe Creases The presence of earlobe creases usually indicates respiratory or cardiac problems.

Ears: Internal

Otoscope Technique Newborns have vernix in the canal; therefore, an otoscopic examination is usually not performed. To safely visualize the ear canal and tympanic membranes (TMs), have the parent or caregiver hold infants and toddlers with head immobile. Hold the otoscope close to the head in the upright or upside-down position (either position is correct). Make sure part of your hand touches the child's head (Fig. 5–1), so that if head movement occurs, your hand will move with the child. This prevents pain and damage to the auditory canal.

Pull the pinna down and back for children younger than age 6 years or up and back if the child is older than age 6 years. Use the largest speculum that will fit in the ear—2.0 for newborns and young infants and 3.0 and 4.0 for older infants and children.

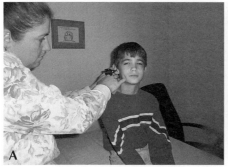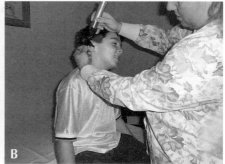

FIG. 5–1. Otoscopic examination of the child. (*A*) Upright position of otoscope. (*B*) Upside-down position of otoscope.

Direct the speculum nasally. Look through the otoscope as you advance the speculum in the ear canal. Do not use the otoscope as a pry bar because this is very painful to the child. Instead, manipulate the pinna to straighten the canal.

Observe the canal. Normal findings include lack of redness, lack of edema, and lack of foreign bodies. The presence of cerumen is normal (Table 5–3). Remove wax only if you must to observe the TM when otitis media is suspected. Also, if the child has tympanostomy tubes in place, they can be seen along the side of the canal just in front of the TM. Abnormalities include redness and edema of the canal, foreign bodies, and purulent drainage. If purulent drainage is present, swab and culture a specimen. Also, smell the drainage because *Pseudomonas* organisms have a sweet odor.

Observe the TM and note the color. Normal variations include pink, gray, and red if the child has been crying or has a fever. The TM should be concave with a light reflex at the 5- or 7-o'clock position. The umbo and long process of the malleus should be visible (Fig. 5–2) Also, if the child has tympanostomy tubes in place, they can be seen. Abnormalities (Fig. 5–3) include a TM that is red, bulging, has a fluid line, or has air bubbles present. Redness of the pars flaccida at the inferior border of the TM may indicate early inflammatory changes. Perforations, scarring, and cholesteastoma may also be present and indicate multiple infections.

Documentation: Ears Document the appearance of external structures and alignment with eyes, canal, and TM. An example is as follows:

TABLE 5–3. CERUMEN TYPES

Yellow, flaky
Brown, sticky
Dark, hard

FIG. 5–2. Normal tympanic membrane.

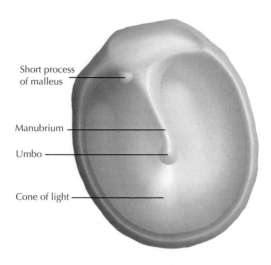

Short process of malleus

Manubrium

Umbo

Cone of light

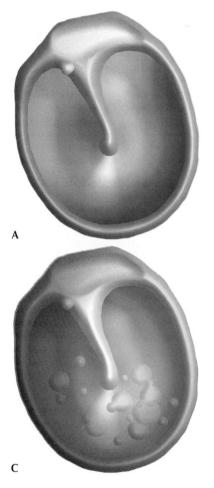

A

B

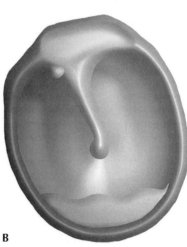

FIG. 5–3. (*A*) Otitis media: red, bulging, with abnormal light reflex. (*B*) Serous otitis: fluid line is visible. (*C*) Eustachian tube dysfunction: air bubbles are visible.

C

Normal ear: Top of ear 10% above eyes, oval without erythema or edema. Canal pink without erythema or edema. Small amount of moist brown cerumen present. Tympanic membrane pearly gray with light reflex at 5 o'clock, no bulging.

Abnormal ear: Low-set ears, round without erythema or edema. Canal erythematous and edematous. Unable to visualize TM because of edema.

Pneumatic Otoscopy Use this procedure only when the diagnosis of otitis media is uncertain. To determine if the TM is bulging from an infectious process, pneumatic otoscopy should be used. Attach the bulb to the head of the otoscope. Use the largest speculum that will fit in the ear canal. A tight fit is necessary to avoid losing air pressure. If a tight fit with the speculum is not made, an alternative is to place a small piece of rubber tubing over the tip of the standard speculum.

When viewing the TM, deflate the bulb and observe for pressure changes. A normal TM moves inward with positive pressure and outward with negative pressure when the bulb is released. An abnormal TM produces no movement with positive pressure. A bulging membrane that does not move with deflation of the bulb indicates middle ear pressure, usually associated with otitis media. A retracted membrane produces minimal or no movement with positive or negative pressure and indicates eustachian tube dysfunction.

Whisper Test Whisper numbers 2 to 4 feet from the ear and have the child repeat them. Cover one ear while testing the other.

Rinne/Weber The Rinne/Weber test (Fig. 5–4) should be performed if hearing problems are suspected to determine if the problem is conductive or sensorineural. The Weber test, which is a test of lateralization, is performed by placing a vibrating tuning fork on the top of the head or upper forehead. Ask the child to tell if the sound can be heard in one or both ears. The Rinne test compares air conduction with bone conduction. Place a vibrating tuning fork on the mastoid process. Ask the child to let you know when he or she can no longer hear the humming or feel the vibrations. Immediately place the tuning fork by the ear. The child should then indicate when he or she can no longer hear the vibrations. Air conduction should be twice as long at bone conduction. When a deficit is found in either of these tests, the child should be referred to an ear specialist.

Tympanometry Tympanometry is an objective technique used to obtain reproducible measurements of TM mobility and determine pressure within the middle ear system. The goal is to evaluate the performance of the middle ear transmission system. It is used to verify middle ear abnormalities, eustachean tube patency, hearing loss, TM perforations, patency of myringotomy tubes, and persistent middle ear effusions. Tympanometry is contraindicated in children younger than 7 months old and when otitis externa or cerumen occlusion is present.

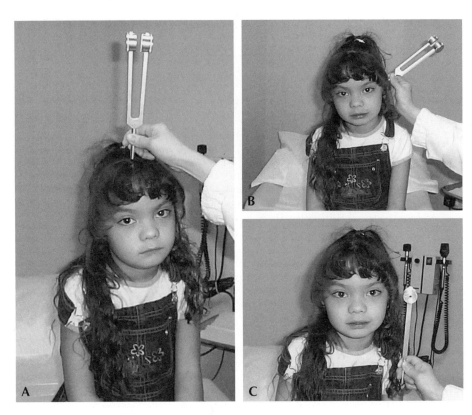

FIG. 5–4. (*A*) Weber test for lateralization. (*B*) Rinne test for bone conduction. (*C*) Rinne test for air conduction.

Audiometry Audiometry is used to quantify the child's ability to hear sound through a range of intensities and frequencies. The goal is to measure the lowest decibel intensity that can be heard for each frequency tested. Audiometry assists in the diagnosis of hearing disorders and degree of hearing impairment. Audiometry is performed when the child has reached an age that allows cooperation with the examination and understanding of his or her responsibilities during the testing. Children must be able to indicate that sounds they are hearing are different. This usually occurs by age 4 years.

Cerumen Removal The two techniques for cerumen removal are cerumen loop and ear irrigation. To use the cerumen loop technique, try to remove soft, moist cerumen using a cerumen loop. Insert the loop approximately 0.25 to 0.5 inches into the ear canal along the superior portion. The superior portion of the ear canal is very sensitive, so do not apply pressure. Sweep down and out gently. Repeat the procedure until enough cerumen is removed to allow visualization of the TM.

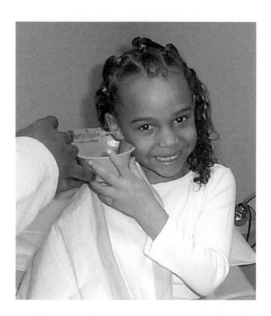

FIG. 5–5. Ear irrigation.

For the ear irrigation technique (Fig. 5–5), aspirate 0.9% saline, warm water, or 1:1 solution of hydrogen peroxide and warm water into a 30- to 60-mL syringe with an 18-gauge intravenous (IV) catheter that has been pared to about 05.–0.5 inch on the end. Drape the child's shoulders and trunk. Have the child tip his or her head toward the collection container, allowing the fluid to run out easily. Insert the catheter into the superior portion of the ear canal approximately 0.5 inch. Gently empty the fluid in the syringe into the canal. Catch the returning fluid in an emesis basin or other container. Repeat the procedure until enough cerumen is removed to allow visualization of the TM.

Nose: External

Observe the nose externally for symmetry and midline placement. When a child has rubbed the end of the nose upward many times (Fig. 5–6), a horizontal crease may form at the end of the nose. This is known as the "allergic salute."

Nose: Internal

Always check for choanal atresia in the newborn. Although there are several procedures to determine the presence of choanal atresia, simply occlude the mouth (a pacifier will work) and occlude one nostril. Because newborns are obligatory nose breathers, this technique causes respiratory difficulty in newborns with choanal atresia. Be sure to check both nares. To inspect the nares internally, tilt the child's head back and place a thumb on the tip by the vestibule (Fig. 5–7). Insert the speculum and observe. Do not touch the septum because doing so is very painful to the child.

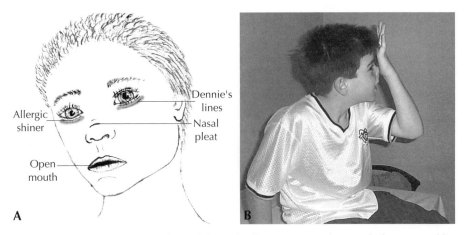

FIG. 5–6. (A) Characteristics of the child with allergies. Note the nasal pleat caused by chronic allergic salute. (B) Child with allergies performing the allergic salute.

There are three turbinates in the nasal passage on the lateral sides, but only the middle and inferior turbinates are visible. Note the floor of the nares. Pale mucosa indicates allergies, and red, swollen mucosa indicates an inflammatory process usually seen with sinusitis. Note any lesions on the septum and lateral structures. Polyps are seen with chronic allergies. They are pale, boggy masses that usually occlude the posterior nasal passage.

Note any exudate. Bilateral nasal discharge is seen with upper respiratory infections. If the nasal discharge is unilateral, the provider should suspect a foreign body.

FIG. 5–7. Nasal examination of the child. Put your thumb at the nasal vestibule. Stabilize the speculum by pressing it against the thumb to prevent injury to the nasal mucosa.

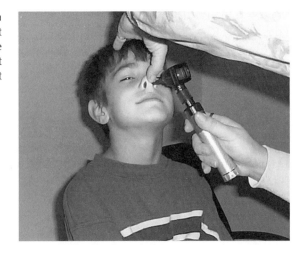

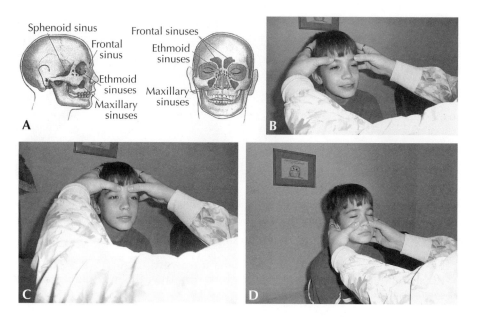

FIG. 5–8. Gently palpate the sinuses. (*A*) Location of the sinuses. (*B*) Maxillary sinuses. (*C*) Ethmoid sinuses. (*D*) Frontal sinuses.

Documentation: Nose Document the external appearance and internal appearance of the nose. An example is as follows:

> Child with allergies: Nose midline, nasal pleat. Nasal mucosa pale, pink, moist, without polyps or purulent discharge.

Paranasal Sinuses

The ethmoid and maxillary sinuses are present at birth but are tiny. The sphenoid sinuses are also present at birth but are small. They cause problems in infancy and toddlerhood. The frontal sinuses develop between age 4 and 7 years. They usually do not cause problems until the child is school age or an adolescent. Periorbital edema and cellulitis may be present with acute sinusitis.

Gently palpate or percuss the sinuses. The maxillary sinuses are located below the eye orbits and above the upper teeth. The ethmoid sinuses are palpated in the medial corner of the eye orbit and against the sides of the nasal bridge. The frontal sinuses can be palpated over and under the eyebrow (Fig. 5–8).

Transillumination Transillumination is another technique used to evaluate the sinus cavities. This procedure should be done in a dark room. To evaluate the frontal sinuses, use a penlight or the light from the otoscope. Place the

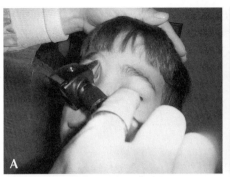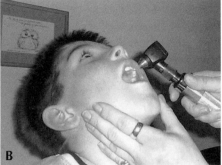

FIG. 5–9. (*A*) Transillumination of the maxillary sinuses. (*B*) Transillumination of the frontal sinuses.

light source under the eyebrow and shine it upward (Figure 5–9A). To evaluate the maxillary sinuses, place the light source over the maxillary area and observe the light inside the mouth (Fig. 5–9B).

Documentation: Sinuses Document which sinuses were tender, if the tenderness occurred on palpation or percussion, and the side on which the tenderness was felt. Also document any edema, heat, or erythema in the area. An example is as follows:

> 10-year-old child with sinus tenderness: Right frontal sinus tenderness on light palpation. No edema, heat, or erythema noted.

Oral Cavity

Examination of the oral cavity is shown in Figure 5–10.

Lips Inspect the outer portion of the mouth. The lips should be moist and symmetrical. Note the color. Cherry red lips are seen with diabetic ketoacidosis and carbon monoxide poisoning. Perioral cyanosis indicates an oxygenation or cardiovascular problem.

Also note any lesions on the lips. Common lesions include hemangiomas, cheliosis (i.e., cracks at the corner of the mouth caused by anemia or yeast infection), impetigo (i.e., crusting lesions), herpes (i.e., vesicles), and cleft lip.

Teeth There are two sets of teeth: temporary (deciduous) and permanent. Development of the temporary teeth begins *in utero*, and eruption begins between age 6 and 24 months. If no tooth eruption has occurred by age 15 months, the child should be evaluated by a dentist. All 20 of the temporary teeth should be present by age 2.5 years (Table 5–4). Between ages 6 and 12 years, the temporary teeth are lost and replaced by permanent teeth (Table 5–5). These permanent teeth appear earlier in girls than in boys and earlier in African-American children than in white children.

58

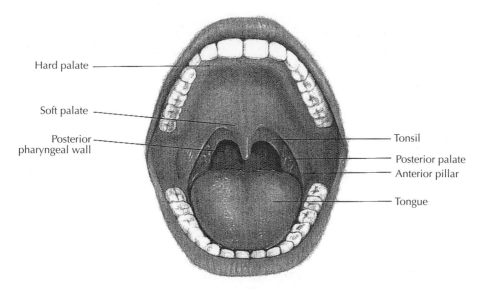

Hard palate

Soft palate

Posterior
pharyngeal wall

Tonsil

Posterior palate

Anterior pillar

Tongue

FIG. 5–10. Parts of the oral cavity.

TABLE 5–4. TEMPORARY TEETH ERUPTION AND LOSS				
Eruption			**Loss**	
Tooth Name	*Upper*	*Lower*	*Upper*	*Lower*
	Months		*Years*	
Central incisor	6–8	5–7	6–7	5–6
Lateral incisor	8–11	7–10	8–9	7–8
Canine incisor	16–20	16–20	9–11	11–12
First molar	10–16	10–16	10–11	10–12
Second molar	20–30	20–30	10–12	11–13

TABLE 5–5. PERMANENT TEETH ERUPTION AND LOSS		
	Eruption	**Loss**
Tooth Name	*Upper (years)*	*Lower (years)*
Central incisor	7–8	6–7
Lateral incisor	8–9	7–8
Canine incisor	11–12	9–11
First premolar	10–11	6–7
Second premolar	10–12	11–13
First molar	6–7	6–7
Second molar	12–13	12–13
Third molar	17–25	17–25

TABLE 5–6. COMMON TONGUE PROBLEMS SEEN IN CHILDREN

Problem	Description
White patches	Thrush
Beefy red, smooth	Anemia
Big	Retardation, hypothyroidism, acromegaly, Down syndrome
Dry	Dehydration
Small	Malnutrition
Increased saliva	Neurological dysfunction
Ulcers > 2 weeks	Aphthous ulcers, herpes
Strawberry tongue	Group A beta-hemolytic Streptococcus

Infants and toddlers who have been bottle fed must be checked for baby bottle caries, which occur when the child's teeth constantly come in contact with carbohydrates. This occurs when the child is given a bottle with milk or sugar containing fluid while in bed or is allowed to carry a bottle around. Note any caries or brown spots. Check for malocclusion, including underbite (i.e., mandibular protrusion) or overbite (i.e., maxillary protrusion).

Gingival and Buccal Mucosa The gingival or buccal mucosa should be pink without overgrowth between the teeth. Black lines at the gingival margins indicate heavy metal (e.g., lead, mercury, arsenic) exposure and should be evaluated. Overgrowth of gums is usually seen when the child is taking anticonvulsant agents.

Tongue Note the movement of the tongue. It should be freely moveable without constant fasciculations. It should move in all directions and lack sustained quivering or trembling. The tongue should be pink, even, and moist. Check the size of the tongue. Macroglossia is a sign of congenital hypothyroidism (i.e., cretinism), Down syndrome, and other disorders. Normally, the surface is roughened because of papillae. The geographic tongue is a normal variation. Ask the child to touch the roof of the mouth with the tongue. The ventral surface should look smooth and glossy with veins easily visible. Common tongue problems seen in children are noted in Table 5–6. Note the frenulum under the tongue. If the frenulum is too tight (i.e., the child cannot stick the tongue out), feeding and speech difficulties may occur.

Hard and Soft Palate Palpate the hard and soft palate for closure. Check for congenital defects of cleft palate, which can be found both on the hard and the soft palate.

Tonsils: Grading There should be no exudate on the tonsils. Some children have small craters that collect whitish cellular debris, which is normal. Tonsil size is graded as 1+ (visible), 2+ (halfway between the tonsillar pillars and the uvula), 3+ (touching the uvula), and 4+ (touching each other). Large, nonerythematous tonsils are common in toddlers, preschoolers, and school-age children (Fig. 5–11).

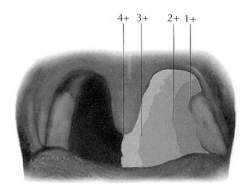

4+ 3+ 2+ 1+

FIG. 5–11. Grading of tonsils.

Documentation: Oral Cavity Document the appearance of all structures in the oral cavity and note abnormalities with appropriate description. An example is as follows:

> A 2-year-old has not been eating well recently: Lips pink and moist without lesion. Teeth: 10 upper and 12 lower. Gums pink/moist without lesion. Oral mucosa and tongue with white patches. Uvula, anterior and posterior pillars erythematous without edema. Tonsils: 2+ on right, 4+ on left with patches of purulent exudates. Gag reflex present.

Anterior and Posterior Pillars The anterior pillars are located anterior and lateral to the tonsils, and the posterior pillars are located posterior and lateral to the tonsils. They should not be red or swollen.

Pharynx The posterior pharynx is the back of the throat. Observe for color, exudates, and swelling. The posterior pharynx is usually dark pink without exudate or edema. Exudate can be seen as white patches (viral or bacterial etiology), gray film (diphtheria), or yellow-green color high up in the posterior pharynx from sinus drainage. Swelling is most notable as cobblestoning, seen with allergic rhinitis. With streptococcal infection, the entire pharynx is beefy red with or without white patches and sometimes petechiae on the soft palate.

Uvula The uvula is usually unified, but a bifid uvula is a normal variation. A bifid uvula looks partially severed and is common in Native Americans. The length of the uvula is approximately 1 to 2 cm, but it may be larger in children. If the uvula is long but does not appear sore, red, or with exudate, consider it normal. Have the child say "ahh," growl, or inhale. The uvula should deviate upward. If the uvula deviates sideways, suspect a neurological deficit.

Epiglottis The epiglottis is easily visible in younger children. It can be seen at the base of the posterior tongue and posterior pharynx. It should be pink and moist without redness or edema. If the epiglottis is red and edematous, stop the oral examination, suspect epiglottitis, and transfer the child to the emergency department of the nearest hospital.

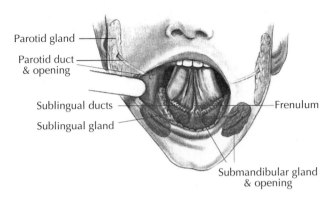

Parotid gland

Parotid duct & opening

Sublingual ducts

Sublingual gland

Frenulum

Submandibular gland & opening

FIG. 5–12. Note the placement of the parotid and submandibular glands with their duct system.

Parotid and Submandibular Salivary Glands The parotid gland is located just below the anterior ear and down the lateral mandible (Fig. 5–12). The ducts of the parotids (Stenson's ducts) are located inside the oral cavity just below the second upper molar. They are dimpled in appearance. If a duct is red or swollen with drainage, suspect parotitis.

The submandibular gland is located just below the mandible laterally (see Fig. 5–12). The ducts of the submandibular gland (Wharton's ducts) are located under the tongue on each side of the frenulum. They appear as raised dimples and should be pink and moist without edema.

Frenulum There are two frenula in the mouth. One is between the upper lip and gingivae in the maxillary area, and the other is under the tongue. Check for frenula that decrease the mobility of the lips and tongue because they could cause feeding and speech problems.

NECK

Observe the neckline to determine that the trachea is midline. Note any webbing, which is associated with Turner's syndrome and Noonan's syndrome. Note any unusual masses. Note torticollis, which is present with sternocleidomastoid muscle damage and prochlorperazine (Compazine) ingestion.

Lymph Nodes

Place both of your hands on the child's neck and palpate. Many children have shotty nodes, which are pea-sized nodes up to 1 cm in size, nontender, and easily moveable. These are normal in toddlers and preschool-age children. Enlarged nodes that are bigger than 1 cm should be measured and documented. After they are enlarged, a node usually does not return to flat and can be palpated as small lumps in the neck. Nodes are at their peak size between ages 6 and 9 years. The lymph nodes are shown in Figure 5–13.

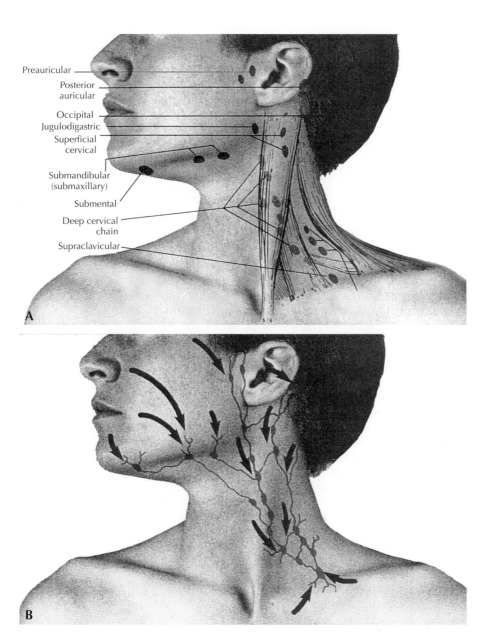

Preauricular

Posterior
auricular

Occipital
Jugulodigastric
Superficial
cervical

Submandibular
(submaxillary)

Submental

Deep cervical
chain

Supraclavicular

A

B

FIG. 5–13. (*A*) Lymph node placement in the neck. (*B*) Drainage pattern of lymph
nodes.

Observe the movement of the child's neck. Younger children will usually
follow a light or toy, and older children will do range of motion on verbal
directions. The neck should be able to move freely back and forth, side
to side, and rotate right and left. If nuchal rigidity is suspected, have the

63

child attempt to touch the chin to the chest. This will not be possible when nuchal rigidity is present. Also perform the Brudzinski's and Kernig's tests (see Chapter 11) if nuchal rigidity is suspected. The most common problems that present as pain in the neck are meningitis (nuchal rigidity), swollen lymph nodes, and tense neck muscles.

Documentation: Lymph Nodes Document lymph nodes that are palpable by location, size, and mobility. An example is as follows:

> 4-year-old child with sore throat: Bilateral tonsillar nodes 2 cm, moveable.

Thyroid Gland

Because many children are ticklish, touching the neck may elicit squirming, scrunching up the neck, and giggling. Therefore, sit the child on a chair or examination table and ask him or her to take a sip of water. Observe the area just above the sternal notch and observe the thyroid gland movement while swallowing. Next observe for thyroid enlargement by having the child hyperextend the neck. The examination of the thyroid gland is shown in Figure 5–14.

In newborns, the thyroid cannot usually be palpated. If you can palpate it, then it is enlarged. Place your hand under the newborn's scapula and raise the baby's shoulders. Allow the newborn's head to fall back gently, and observe the thyroid gland for enlargement. Palpate with one finger on either side of the gland.

To palpate the thyroids of infants, toddlers, and preschool children, place your fingers on the front of the trachea by the cricoid and palpate for lumps.

For school-age children and adolescents, place your fingers on both sides of the trachea from the back by the cricoid and ask the child to swallow. Note any lumps in the thyroid as it rises. Then have the child tilt the head to one side. Displace the trachea in the opposite direction and palpate the thyroid gland. Repeat with displacement to the other direction.

TABLE 5–7. PALPATION OF THE THYROID	
Consistency of Thyroid Gland	**Disorder**
Soft	Normal
Soft to firm, nontender	Graves' disease
Firm	Hashimoto's disease
Hard	Carcinoma
Goiter	
Soft to firm, nontender	Graves' disease
Diffusely swollen, tender	Subacute thyroiditis
One or more nodules that are smooth, firm, round, or oval	Toxic nodular goiter
Central, rounded midline mass between thyroid and chin; moves upward when child sticks tongue out; not fixed	Thyroglossal duct cyst

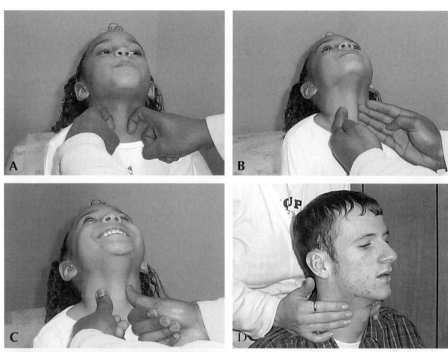

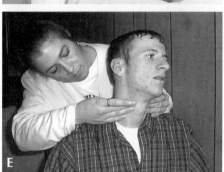

FIG. 5–14. (A) Palpation of thyroid in the young child, anteriorly. (B) Palpation of thyroid in the young child, anteriorly. (C) Palpation of thyroid in the young child, anteriorly. (D) Palpation of the thyroid of the older child, posteriorly. (E) Have the child bend to one side, displace the trachea gently to the opposite side, and palpate the thyroid.

Table 5–7 shows the difference in consistency of the thyroid gland. A thyroglossal duct cyst may also be found as a midline mass between the thyroid and the chin. This cyst moves upward when the child sticks out the tongue. If distinct lumps are palpated on the thyroid, the child has a goiter.

Documentation: Thyroid Gland Document consistency, size, any nodules felt, and placement. Examples are as follows:

15-year-old with thyroid nodule: 1 cm hard nodule left midthyroid gland.

15-year-old with normal thyroid: Soft, without nodules, no thyromegaly.

TEST YOUR KNOWLEDGE OF CHAPTER 5

1. What questions should be included in the review of systems?
2. Why is comparison of the child's features with the parents' so important?
3. Which fontanels are usually palpable in the newborn? Describe their placement and size.
4. Discuss overriding sutures and closure of fontanels.
5. How does assessment of the head in a newborn or infant differ from assessment in an older child?
6. What are the characteristics of external ears of a normal child?
7. What findings on external ear examination would alert you to potential problems?
8. Discuss the technique for doing an internal ear examination.
9. What are the characteristics of a normal ear canal and TM?
10. How and why is pneumatic otoscopy useful?
11. What are the differences between tympanometry and audiometry?
12. How is cerumen removed safely and effectively in a child?
13. What external and internal nasal characteristics alert you to chronic allergies?
14. When can the paranasal sinuses be evaluated in children?
15. What external and internal oral characteristics would alert you to a problem?
16. What is the progression of tooth eruption and loss (temporary and permanent)?
17. Discuss the grading of enlarged tonsils.
18. What are the lymph nodes in the neck area, and what areas do they drain?
19. How do you palpate the thyroid in children?

BIBLIOGRAPHY

Algranati, P. S. (1992). *The pediatric patient: An approach to history and physical examination*. Baltimore: Williams & Wilkins.

Goldbloom, R. B. (1997). *Pediatric clinical skills*. Philadelphia: Churchill Livingstone.

Jarvis, C. (2000). *Physical examination and health assessment*. Philadelphia: W. B. Saunders.

Seidel, H. M., Ball, J. W., Dains, J. E, & Benedict, G. W. (2001). *Mosby's guide to physical examination*. St. Louis: Mosby.

6

Assessment of the Visual System

MARGARET R. COLYAR

OBJECTIVES
- Develop basic assessment of the visual system of children.
- Determine age-related visual system assessment.
- Ascertain problem areas and when to refer clients to specialists.

An intact visual system is important for normal intellectual growth and development. Vision accounts for 80% of a child's sensory input. Many ocular and systemic diseases can cause changes with the visual system, so conducting a reliable visual examination is very important.

🏐 HISTORY

Ask about the child's medical history, surgeries, and family history of visual disorders. Include in the history medications, allergies, and immunization status. As part of the review of systems, ask about the occurrence of visual difficulties, strabismus, diplopia, redness, swelling, itching, watering, discharge, glaucoma, cataracts, and if the child wears glasses or contacts. Also note whether the child is squinting, cross-eyed, stumbling, or walking into things.

DIFFERENCES IN THE VISUAL SYSTEM BY AGE

NEWBORNS

The sclera of newborns is blue/white because the sclera overlying the choroids is thin. The color of the iris is usually blue at birth because of poorly defined pigmentation. The iris usually changes color between ages 3 and 6 months. The internal structures may be visualized with an ophthalmoscope. The retina is pale, and the macula is barely visible because the fundus is so pale.

Because of the trauma of the birth process, scleral and retinal hemorrhages may occur. These are usually harmless and disappear within 2 weeks. Parents many need reassurance if these occur.

Newborns' eyes can fix and follow. Their eyes should move together, and the red reflex should be round and present bilaterally. However, the red reflex is not always red; it may be tan or brown and usually corresponds with the child's skin pigmentation. Newborns' pupils should be equal, round, and reactive to light (PERRL), but newborns are not able to accommodate well. Newborns can focus best at arm's length but are unable to focus on distant objects. They can see black and white well and fix their eyes on contrasting patterns (Fig. 6–1). Eye movements sometimes appear irregular or disconjugate in newborns.

Additionally, the nasolacrimal duct may be blocked at birth. This blockage usually resolves spontaneously. In 10% of the cases, it remains blocked until age 1 year. If it does not resolve by age 1 year, refer the child for possible surgical correction.

EYE CHANGES IN INFANTS, TODDLERS, AND SCHOOL-AGE CHILDREN

Infants start developing tears at age 2 months. The ability to focus on colored objects improves next. By age 3 months, the child should be able to differentiate between red, green, and yellow. Eye movements become symmetrical, and focus improves. Children between ages 1 and 2 years have vision about 50% of adult vision. Between ages 3 and 5 years, visual acuity improves to 20/40, and color vision is apparent. By age 5 years, the visual acuity is 20/30, accommodation is well defined, and the development of amblyopia is unlikely. Vision of 6-year-old children is well developed, and visual acuity is 20/20. Eye changes in infants, toddlers, and school-age children can be found in Table 6–1.

EXAMINATION TECHNIQUES

Different eye examinations are done for children in the different age groups based on their ocular and general development (Table 6–2).

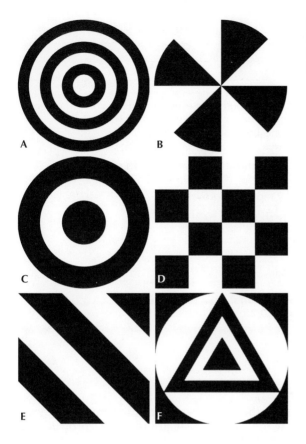

FIG. 6–1. (*A* through *F*) Newborns and infants up to 3 months can focus well on black and white shapes.

TOOLS NEEDED FOR WELL-CHILD EYE EXAMINATIONS

Tools needed for well-child eye examinations include:

- Ophthalmoscope
- Illiterate E, pictoral Snellen, or regular Snellen charts (Fig. 6–2)
- Black-and-white pictures (for newborns)
- Ishihara color chart (for children ages 4 years and older)

PHYSICAL EXAMINATION

INSPECTION AND OBSERVATION

Head Position

If the child has light vision, the head should be held straight up and down. Tilting will occur if the child has blindness, ptosis, photophobia, or diplopia (Table 6–3).

TABLE 6–1. EYE CHANGES FOR INFANTS AND SCHOOL-AGE CHILDREN	
Age	**Change**
Infant	
Age 2 months	Child starts developing tears
3 months	Child focuses on mouth and eyes and simple colored objects
	Can differentiate between red, green, and yellow
	Eye movements become regular or conjugate
	Focus improves
Toddler	Vision is 50% of the adult vision of 20/40 to 20/50
Preschool	Visual acuity rapidly improves
3 years	Visual acuity should be 20/30
4 years	Color vision
School Age	
5 years	Accommodates well
	Visual acuity 20/30
	Development of amblyopia is unlikely
5 years	Visual acuity 20/20

Eye Structures (Fig. 6-3)

Compare one side of the face with the other. Facial features are either symmetrical or dysmorphic. Note if the eyes appear jittery or are protruding. Slight horizontal nystagmus can be normal, but vertical nystagmus and continuous horizontal nystagmus are not normal and should be examined by a neurologist.

TABLE 6–2. EYE EXAMINATION FOR CHILDREN						
Age	Red Reflex	Corneal Light Reflex	EOMs	Cover/ Uncover Test	Visual Acuity Examination	Fundoscopic Examination
Newborn	X	X				
Infant	X	X	Try			
Toddler	X	X	X	Try	Picture	Try
Preschool	X	X	X	X	HOTV Illiterate E Picture	X
School age	X	X	X	X	Letter	X
Adolescent	X	X	X	X	Letter	X

EOM = extraocular movement

TABLE 6–3. REASONS FOR HEAD TILTING

Tilt Pattern	Cause
Tilted any way	Blindness
Back	Ptosis
Down and away from light source	Photophobia
Sideways	To prevent diplopia
	To stabilize nystagmus

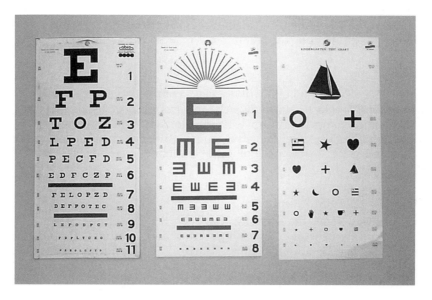

FIG. 6–2. Eye charts: Snellen, Illiterate E, and Pictorial Snellen.

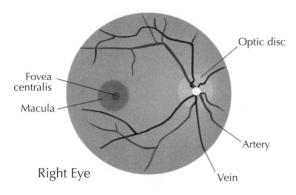

FIG. 6–3. Structures within the eye.

Optic disc

Fovea centralis

Macula

Right Eye

Artery

Vein

Colobomas

Colobomas are missing sections of any of the eye structures. They are commonly seen on the iris and eyelids.

Pupils

The pupils should be equal, round, and reactive to light. Note whether they appear wide set (i.e., hypertelorism) or set close together (i.e., hypotelorism).

Globes

The globes should be the same size. If one appears larger or smaller, check for eyelid lag, ptosis, or exophthalmos.

Eyelids

Observe for eyelid lag (eyelid will not close completely), ptosis (droopy eyelid), entropion (eyelashes curl inward), or ectropion (eyelashes curl outward and lower eyelid appears droopy). Angioedema (swelling of the eyelid) can occur with allergies. Swelling also occurs with crying and lacrimal duct inflammation. While you are looking at the child's eyelids, check the eyelashes for nits or lice.

Palpebral Fissures

Palpebral fissures are the openings between the upper and lower eyelids. The palpebral fissures should be symmetrical and of equal width bilaterally. They should also be straight across. Narrow or slanted palpebral fissures may be a normal variation but are often seen in individuals with many chromosomal syndromes, including Down syndrome. However, most Asian children also have slanted palpebral fissures.

Epicanthal Folds

Epicanthal folds are the vertical folds of skin that cover the inner canthus. They are normal in Asian children. Twenty percent of white children also have epicanthal folds, but they usually disappear by age 10 years. They are also seen in several chromosomal syndromes.

Sclera

The sclera is blue/white in newborns; otherwise, white is normal. A red sclera indicates several problems (Table 6–4).

Lacrimal Gland

The lacrimal gland (Fig. 6–4) is located above the eye and under the eyebrow laterally. If it is edematous, suspect infection or inflammation and ask if the child has been crying recently.

TABLE 6–4. INDICATIONS FOR COLOR OF THE SCLERA

Color	Indication
White	Normal
Blue/white	Normal in newborns only
Red	
Patch	Subconjunctival hemorrhage
Lower margins red, injected	Bacterial conjunctivitis: Usually staphylococcal infection
Overall redness	Viral conjunctivitis
Around cornea	Corneal ulcerations, acute uveitis
Overall bright red and pupils will not dilate	Iritis

Lacrimal Sac

This is located from the inner canthus of the eye down the side of the nose bilaterally. Note whether this area is red or edematous. If so, suspect dacrocystitis.

TESTING: EXTRAOCULAR MOVEMENTS

All of the following tests will check for weakness in the extraocular muscle groups.

Corneal Light Reflexes

This is a simple test to perform and can be done just with observation (Fig. 6–5). Look at the child's eyes. Using a light source or just the overhead light in the room, determine where the light falls on each of the child's eyes. If the extraocular movements (EOMs) are intact, the light should be in the exact same location on the eyes whichever way the child looks.

Documentation An example is as follows:

Normal: Corneal light reflex equal position bilaterally.

Abnormal: Corneal light reflex unequal position bilaterally.

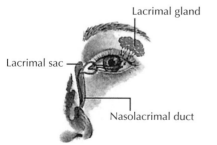

Lacrimal gland

Lacrimal sac

Nasolacrimal duct

FIG. 6–4. Lacrimal gland, sac, and duct.

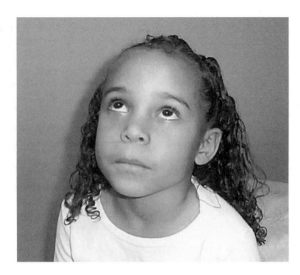

FIG. 6–5. Corneal light reflex, normal.

Extraocular Movements

For toddlers and older children, use an object of interest to the child, a light source, or your finger. The child must hold his or her head still and follow your finger with the eyes as you move the object. If the child is unable to hold the head still, stabilize it with your nondominant hand. Slight horizontal nystagmus (i.e., vibration) in the lateral fields is normal. Vertical nystagmus is never normal and warrants a consultation with a neurologist.

For infants, two tests can be done: try spinning first and twisting as a last resort.

- Spinning: Surprise prompts the eyes to open (Fig. 6–6).
  - Hold the child up in the air, facing you, at a 30-degree incline.
  - Then turn around in place two to three times. The child's eyes should deviate in the direction of the turn. Next turn the opposite way and observe.
- Twisting: Twist the child in all six fields and watch the eye movements (Fig. 6–7).

Documentation Examples are as follows:

Normal: EOMs equal in six cardinal fields of gaze.

Abnormal: EOMs with nystagmus. EOMs unequal in lateral fields.

Cover/Uncover Test

The cover/uncover test checks for weakness and deviation in alignment of the eyes (Fig. 6–8). The test should begin as early as possible to detect strabismus and prevent amblyopia. Remember that disconjugate gaze is normal in newborns. Unfortunately, it is difficult to get younger children to cooper-

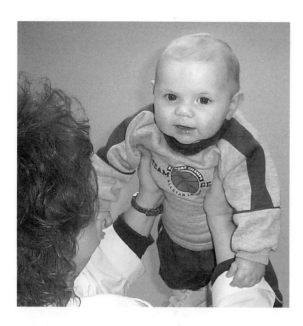

FIG. 6–6. Spinning.

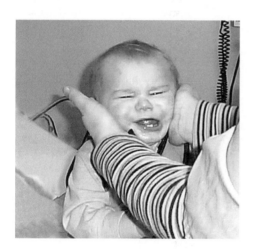

FIG. 6–7. Twisting.

ate fully. To perform this test, cover one of the child's eyes with your hand or a card. Have the child look directly at your nose. Uncover the eye and look at the previously covered eye. Check for fixation. The covered eye should have a fixed, steady gaze. It is out of alignment if it moves to fixate.

Documentation Examples are as follows:

Normal: Cover/uncover negative.

Normal: No movement with cover/uncover.

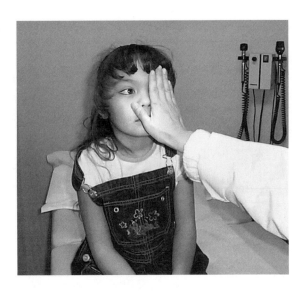

FIG. 6–8. Child performing the cover/uncover test.

Normal: No strabismus with cover/uncover.

Abnormal—Esophoria: Right eye (eye is medial when eye is uncovered).

Abnormal—Exophoria: Right eye (eye is lateral when eye is uncovered).

Testing: Accommodation

While testing the EOMs, bring your finger toward the nose in front of the child's eyes. The eyes should converge (i.e., move closer together) and constrict. Now move your finger away from the child's nose. The eyes should move apart and dilate.

TESTING: VISUAL ACUITY
Newborn/Infant: Fix and Follow

Place a black-and-white chart at arm's length from the child's eyes and move the chart. If the child can see, he or she should be able to fixate on the black and white chart and follow the images (see Fig. 6–1).

Younger Children

Use the HOTV, Illiterate E, or pictoral Snellen charts for the younger child.

Older Children

When the child knows the English alphabet, the letter Snellen chart can be used.

Technique

Have the child stand 20 feet from the chart. First cover one eye and have the child read the lowest line possible. Then test the other eye. Lastly, the child should read the lowest line possible with both eyes uncovered. The lowest line of which the child can read at least half is the score line.

Interpretation

The first number is the number of feet the child is standing from the chart. The second number is the number of feet at which a normal-sighted child can read the letters or pictures. Therefore, 20/40 indicates that while standing at 20 feet, the child can read what the normal-sighted child can read at 40 feet. The higher the second number, the worse the client's visual acuity. If there is a two-line difference between eyes, the child should be referred for further eye testing.

Documentation Examples are as follows:

Normal: 20/20 right eye (OD), left eye (OS), both eyes (OU).

Abnormal: 20/30 OD, 20/60 OS, 20/40 OU.

TESTING: RED REFLEX

Check the red reflex on children of all ages. Using the ophthalmoscope, point the light source toward the pupil. Starting at a 15- to 20-degree lateral angle about 2 feet away from the eye, look through the ophthalmoscope and observe the red circle that appears. The red circle is the light reflected off the retina. If the reflex is irregular or has black areas, suspect opacified cornea, cataract, or retinoblastoma and refer the child to an ophthalmologist.

FUNDOSCOPIC EXAMINATION

OPHTHALMOSCOPE

The ophthalmoscope has five apertures (Table 6–5). In the ambulatory care setting, the small and large apertures are used most frequently. Use the small aperture for constricted pupils and the large aperture for dilated pupils. In addition to the five apertures, the ophthalmoscope has a switch that allows you to filter light to see different parts of the inner eye (Table 6–6). Lastly, there is a wheel on the side of the ophthalmoscope head that allows for changes in diopter. The diopters are + (green) or − (red).

TECHNIQUE

To begin the examination, set the diopters to match your vision by looking through the lens at the palm of your hand approximately 3 to 6 inches away. Move the diopter wheel until you can see the lines of your palm crisply. Next turn off the room light.

TABLE 6–5. APERTURES OF THE OPHTHALMOSCOPE	
Aperture	Use
Small	To view the fundus with the undilated pupil
Large	To view the fundus with the dilated pupil and general exam of the eye
Fixation	To observe and measure lesions of the retina without masking the macula
Slit	To determine various levels of lesions and edema of the disc
Cobalt filter	To visualize corneal abrasions with fluorescein dye and herpes simplex dendrites

Newborns and Infants

Lay the newborn and infant on the examination table, have someone stabilize the head if the child tries to twist away, and then proceed to visualize the inner eye. Make a repetitive sound such as clicking to hold the child's attention, decrease anxiety, and gain cooperation.

Toddlers

With the child sitting upright or lying on the examination table, stabilize the child's head with your hand on the child's forehead and proceed to visualize the inner eye. Encourage the child to hold the eyes still. You may have to remind the child several times. If the child is uncooperative, try making repetitive sounds or talking as you do the examination to distract the child.

Preschoolers, School-age Children, and Adolescents

Direct the child to look at a spot on the wall. This allows the pupil to dilate for better visualization. To keep from bumping heads with the client, place your nondominant hand on the child's forehead to stabilize him or her. To prevent bumping noses, view the child's right eye with your right eye and the child's left eye with your left eye. Then, starting at a 15- to 20-degree angle laterally, look through the ophthalmoscope and move toward the child's eye.

FUNDOSCOPIC EXAMINATION
Red Reflex

As you start your observation, note the red reflex as you move toward the eye.

Vessels

There are both veins and arteries in the fundus of the eye. The veins are darker and thicker than arteries. The ratio width of arteries to veins is 2:3. The vessels get smaller as you move away from the optic disc. Start at the

TABLE 6–6. FILTER SWITCHES* OF THE OPHTHALMOSCOPE

Switch	Use
Left: Red-free light exudates, and (under green dot)	Used to observe vessels, small hemorrhages, and macular changes Background appears gray The optic disc appears white The macula appears yellow The fundus reflex is intense The vessels appear darker (vein: blue; arteries: black)
Middle: No filter	Normal visualization
Right: Crossed linear polarizing	Used to eliminate annoying glare from the cornea

* Each filter can be used over all the apertures.

distal end of the vessels in one quadrant and move your ophthalmoscope toward the center region of the disc. Do this in all four quadrants, observing for nicking, twisting, or hemorrhages of the vessels. Nicking and twisting are seen in individuals with hypertension and diabetes.

Optic Disc

The optic disc is in a medial position or nasal side of the retina. It is a creamy yellow-pink color; however, the color can be darker because it tends to vary with race. The optic disc appears approximately 1.0 to 1.5 cm in size. The edges should be crisp, round, and even. If the edges of the disc appear to bulge or are fuzzy, suspect papilledema caused by intracranial pressure. This is a medical emergency, and you should immediately send the child to an ophthalmologist or emergency department. Note the size of the disc. The location of all abnormalities is measured in disc diameters from the optic disc.

Macula

The macula is responsible for central vision. It is hard to visualize. The macula is located two disc diameters (DDs) from the optic disk temporally. Check this structure last because light penetration of the fovea (i.e., the central structure of the macula) tends to cause pain and tearing.

Documentation An example is as follows:

> Normal: Red reflex round and present bilaterally. Fundus red, A:V 3:2, optic disc round and smooth without edema, macula 2 DD temporally.

Abnormalities

Describe where the abnormalities are located and the number of DDs from the optic disc using clock placement.

Documentation An example is as follows:

> Abnormal: Red reflex irregular left eye. Fundus red, A/V nicking, optic disc edematous, macula not seen.

CORNEAL STAINING

Any unexplained red eye warrants corneal staining to determine the cause (see Chapter 29). If you suspect a foreign body imbedded in the child's eye or a corneal abrasion, then corneal staining should be done. In neonates and infants with unexplained crying, photosensitivity, unilateral tearing, and conjunctival inflammation, corneal staining should be performed. Do not stain with chemical acid or alkali exposure, history of high-velocity injury, deeply embedded foreign object, or eyelid lacerations.

Refer the child to an ophthalmologist if the abrasion is close to the central line of vision, corneal opacities or "rust ring" occurs, there is increasing pain or loss of vision, abrasion does not resolve, or preseptal cellulitis with periorbital cellulitis occurs.

TEST YOUR KNOWLEDGE OF CHAPTER 6

1. What are the components of the visual history and review of systems?
2. Describe the differences in vision between the different age groups.
3. What are the normal and abnormal findings in the external eye structures?
4. What tests are done to examine EOMs?
5. How are EOMs tested in infants?
6. Why should a cover/uncover test be performed, and what is the technique?
7. How is visual acuity tested in the different age groups?
8. What can the red reflex tell us about the vision of a child?
9. What are the different components of an ophthalmoscope?
10. What can be seen on the funduscopic examination?
11. When is corneal staining indicated or contraindicated?

BIBLIOGRAPHY

Algranati, P. S. (1992). *The pediatric patient: An approach to history and physical examination.* Baltimore: Williams & Wilkins.

Goldbloom, R. B. (1997). *Pediatric clinical skills.* Philadelphia: Churchill Livingstone.

Jarvis, C. (2000). *Physical examination and health assessment.* Philadelphia: W. B. Saunders.

Seidel, H. M., Ball, J. W., Dains, J. E, & Benedict, G. W. (2001). *Mosby's guide to physical examination.* St. Louis: Mosby.

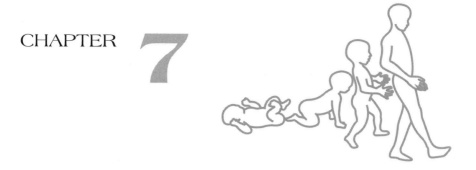

CHAPTER 7

Assessment of the Respiratory System

MARGARET R. COLYAR

OBJECTIVES
- Understand basic techniques used for the respiratory assessment of children.
- Develop age-related respiratory assessment techniques.
- Differentiate between normal respiratory assessment and abnormal findings.

The thoracic cavity is a body structure that is narrower at the top. It consists of a sternum, 12 pairs of ribs, and 12 thoracic vertebrae and is separated from the abdomen by the diaphragm. Ribs 1 to 7 are attached directly to the sternum, ribs 8 to 10 are attached to cartilage, and ribs 11 and 12 are floating. The thorax grows as the child grows. In newborns, the thorax is round and soft to elliptical shape. By age 6 years, a child's thorax is shaped like an adult's (Table 7–1). The bifurcation of the trachea is at the third vertebra in infancy and at the fourth vertebra as the child ages. Infants are nose breathers, and abdominal or diaphragmatic breathing usually does not occur until age 6 to 7 years. The most common chief complaints heard for respiratory problems are cough, wheeze, noisy breathing, recurrent colds, rhinorrhea, chest pain, dyspnea, and hyperventilation.

HISTORY

Ask about the child's medical history; history of surgeries that involve the respiratory system; and family history of chronic respiratory illnesses such

81

TABLE 7–1. CHANGES IN CHEST DIAMETER WITH AGE	
Age	Transverse:Anteroposterior Diameter
Newborn	1:1
1 year	1:25
6 years	1:35

asthma, allergies, and cystic fibrosis. As part of the review of systems, ask about the occurrence of cough, shortness of breath, chest pain with breathing, wheezing, trouble breathing, fever, history of respiratory infections, cigarette smoking, or exposure to secondary smoke. Determine the medications the child is currently taking and exposure to environmental factors such as smoking, inhalants, molds, dust, sprays, perfumes, grass, trees, pollens, and pets. Prenatal and birth history should include the details of the mother's pregnancy and birth (Table 7–2).

APGAR

The Apgar score is part of the respiratory assessment of newborns. It measures successful transition to extrauterine life (Table 7–3). The five parameters of the Apgar score are heart rate, respiratory effort, muscle tone, reflex irritation, and color.

PHYSICAL EXAMINATION

INSPECTION AND OBSERVATION

Newborns and Infants

The chest wall of newborns and young infants is thin with little musculature. The ribs are soft and pliant, and the distal tip of the xyphoid process protrudes. Normally, newborns and infants are diaphragmatic breathers with a paradoxical breathing pattern in which the abdomen goes out when the lungs go in. If a newborn or infant exhibits an increased abdominal breathing pattern, it is abnormal, and pulmonary disease should be suspected. The

TABLE 7–2. HISTORY FOR RESPIRATORY SYSTEM		
Mother's Pregnancy History	Birth History	Medical History
Maternal infections	Gestational age	Difficulty feeding
Drug use	Birth weight	Apnea
Cigarette smoking	Apgar score	Cyanotic episodes
Problems during labor and delivery	Need for resuscitation, oxygen, or ventilation	Allergies, asthma, or other respiratory problems

TABLE 7–3. APGAR SCORING		
Score At 1 Minute	Condition	Needs
7–10	Good	None
3–6	Moderately depressed	Resuscitation and close observation
0–2	Severely depressed	Full resuscitation Ventilatory assistance Intensive care

chest circumference of a newborn is 30 to 36 cm and is usually 2 cm smaller than the head circumference until age 6 months to 2 years.

The thorax is rounded in newborns and infants. The anteroposterior diameter is equal to the transverse diameter. The ratio of transverse to anteroposterior diameter changes with age (see Table 7–1). Other variations seen in the child include pectus excavatum (i.e., funnel chest) and pectus carinatum (i.e., pigeon chest), which are normal (Fig. 7–1). Harrison's groove, which is a flaring of the lower ribs, is considered normal but is also seen in those with rickets. The presence of scoliosis may compromise the respiratory system (see Chapter 12).

Respiratory Effort

Children should have an ease of respiration without nasal flaring or substernal or intercostal retractions. Abnormal indications of acute respiratory effort are shown in Table 7–4.

Rate

Count respirations for 1 full minute. Count when the newborn or infant is sleeping if possible to get a more accurate rate. Increased rate during sleep may suggest cardiac disease. See Chapter 2 for normal values by age.

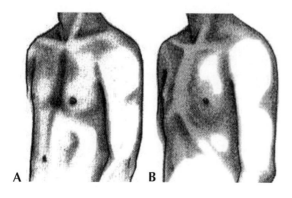

FIG. 7–1. (A) Funnel chest (pectus excavatum). (B) Pigeon chest (pectus carinatum).

A   B

TABLE 7–4. ABNORMAL INDICATIONS OF ACUTE RESPIRATORY EFFORT

Respiratory Problem	Description
Nasal flaring	Lateral margins or nares flares
Intercostal retractions	Space between ribs pulls inward with inspiration
Tachypnea	Faster than normal for age
Apnea	Periods of nonbreathing (periods > 15 seconds in newborns)
Dyspnea	Difficulty breathing
Orthopnea	Must sit up to breathe
Tripoding	Sits in tripod position with chin forward
Stridor	High-pitched crowing sound with inspiration
Wheezing	High-pitched musical sound caused by narrowed airways Heard on inspiration and expiration

Depth

Deep breathing is known as hyperpnea, and shallow breathing is known as hypopnea. A child will demonstrate both normally. However, an increase of either should be further evaluated.

Rhythm

The child's respiratory rhythm should be regular. Newborns have irregular breathing patterns with periods of apnea up to 10 to 15 seconds, which is considered normal if no other cardiovascular symptoms are present.

Documentation: Inspection of the Chest Document chest diameter, respiratory rate, depth, rhythm, and effort. Examples are as follows:

Normal: Chest diameter 1:2, rate 32 breaths/minute, regular rate and rhythm.

Abnormal: Barrel chest, rate 60 breaths/minute, irregular, with substernal retractions.

Finger Clubbing

Early finger clubbing (i.e., straightening of the angle between the nail and nail bed; see Chapter 8) is seen with children with cystic fibrosis and other chronic respiratory problems but can also occur with cardiovascular and gastrointestinal disorders.

Noisy Breathing

The type of sounds made can help to indicate the disease process (Table 7–5). To determine whether the breathing problems are upper or lower respiratory in origin, place a stethoscope by the nose and over the lung area. If the lungs sound just like the nasal sounds, then it is nasal in origin.

TABLE 7–5. NOISY BREATHING: COUGH

Characteristic	Disease
Dry, loose, rattling	Bronchitis; viral syndrome
Dry, tight, wheezy	Asthma; viral syndrome; respiratory syncytial virus
Bark (stridor)	Croup
Spasmodic, repetitive	Pertussis
Paroxysmal, dry, staccato	Pneumonia caused by *Chlamydia pneumoniae* infection
Brassy or vibratory	Tracheomalacia
Honk	Psychogenic

Tracheal Position

Tracheal position should be midline. If deviated to right or left, then suspect a space-occupying lesion or pneumothorax.

Skin and Nailbeds

Skin should be warm and dry and always be free of cyanosis and pallor. Capillary refill should be less than 3 seconds.

AUSCULTATION

Listen to the lungs both anteriorly and posteriorly in the intercostal spaces. Compare one side with the other side (Fig. 7–2). Use an age-appropriate stethoscope to better localize sounds. Auscultate with both the diaphragm and bell. Breath sounds are louder and harsher in infants and young children because of their thin chest walls. Newborns have crackles normally. Infants and toddlers are usually uncooperative with deep breathing; many of them bat at the stethoscope and cry. Try distraction with a toy, book, song, or clicking sound. By preschool age, children are usually cooperative and try to deep-breathe as instructed. Demonstrate to children how you want them to breathe and have them mimic it. If they are unable to deep-breathe easily, have them pretend your finger is a candle and have them blow it out.

Sounds

Bronchial, bronchovesicular, and vesicular breath sounds are normal (Table 7–6). Adventitious or abnormal breath sounds are described in Table 7–7.

Differentiating Between Upper and Lower Airway Problems

Upper airway problems are extrathoracic, that is, above the lungs. Examples of upper airway problems include colds, sinus problems, rhinitis, strep throat, tonsillitis, laryngitis, epiglottis, croup, and tracheomalacia. Lower

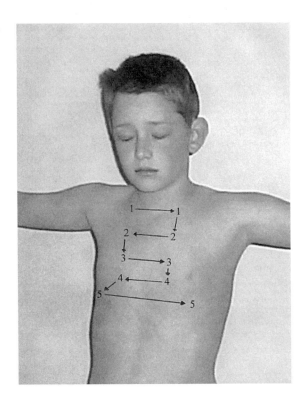

FIG. 7–2. Auscultate, comparing one side with the other.

airway problems are intrathoracic, or inside the lungs. Examples of lower airway problems include asthma, bronchitis, foreign body inhalation, pneumonia, and tuberculosis.

Techniques that use auscultation should also be used when lower respiratory tract problems are suspected. They include egophony, bronchophony, and whispered pectoriloquy (Table 7–8). Pathology that increases lung density also enhances transmission of voice sounds. Normal voice transmission is muffled, soft, and indistinct.

TABLE 7–6. NORMAL BREATH SOUNDS			
Sound	Characteristic	Duration	Where
Tracheal (bronchial)	Loud, tubular, high pitched	Inspiration < expiration	Over trachea
Bronchovescular	Higher pitched	Inspiration = expiration	Over major bronchi
Vesicular	Soft, lower pitched	Inspiration > expiration	Axillary area and lung bases

86

TABLE 7–7. ADVENTITIOUS BREATH SOUNDS

Sound	Description	Where and When	Indication
Crackles	Popping	Upper lung fields Lower lung fields Late inspiration (one field) Over entire chest: Persistent, fine, scattered	Cystic fibrosis Heart failure Pneumonia Bronchiolitis
Gurgles	Bubbling, loud, low pitched	Early inspiration	Pulmonary edema Pneumonia, fibrosis
Wheezes	Squeaking, high-pitched musical	Entire chest: Expiratory	Asthma
	Moaning, low pitched	Entire chest: Expiratory Only in one area	Bronchitis Pneumonia
Rubs	Harsh grating sound	Only in one area	Pneumothorax

Documentation: Lung Sounds Document normal and abnormal lung sounds indicating placement. Examples are as follows:

Normal: Lungs clear bilaterally to auscultation, anterior and posterior.

Abnormal: Coarse crackles right lower lobe posterior; otherwise clear.

PALPATION AND PERCUSSION

Use palpation and percussion when a lower respiratory problem is suspected. Percussion assists in determining if the underlying tissues are filled with air, fluid, or solid. Because percussion penetrates only about 5 to 7 cm, deep lesions cannot be detected. Use the following techniques when lung consolidation or obstructions are suspected.

TABLE 7–8. AUSCULTATION TECHNIQUES FOR ABNORMAL BREATH SOUNDS

Technique	Abnormal Finding	Indication
Egophony: Child says "ee-ee" while chest is auscultated	"Ee-ee" changes to "aa-aa"	Consolidation or compression
Bronchophony: Child says "99" while chest is auscultated	Clear "99	Consolidation
Whispered pectoriloquy: Child whispers "1-2-3" while chest is auscultated	Clear "1-2-3"	Consolidation

FIG. 7–3. Palm placement for tactile fremitus testing.

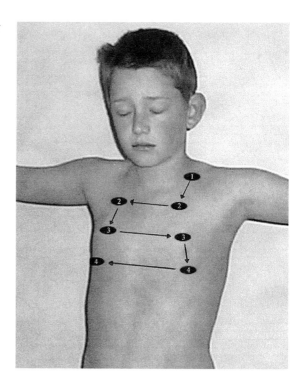

Palpation Techniques

Palpate for local tenderness, crepitus, and supraclavicular nodes. The following techniques may be performed to further substantiate a respiratory problem.

Respiratory Excursion Place the palms of your hands on the child's lower ribs with your thumbs close together and your fingers around the client's lateral rib cage. As the child breathes, watch the movement of your thumbs laterally for symmetry. Lag or impaired thoracic movement on one side indicates lung or pleura problems.

Tactile Fremitus Using the palm of your hand at the base of your fingers, palpate the anterior and posterior chest for vibrations transmitted through the chest wall when the child speaks (Fig. 7–3). Ask the child to say "99" or "1-1-1." Vibration is increased over areas of lung consolidation and decreased or absent when the bronchus is obstructed or occupied by fluid or solid tissue.

Percussion

The lungs are percussed by tapping between each intercostal space (Fig. 7–4). Resonance should be heard. If dullness is heard, suspect consolidation caused by pneumonia, pleural effusion, atelectasis, or tumor.

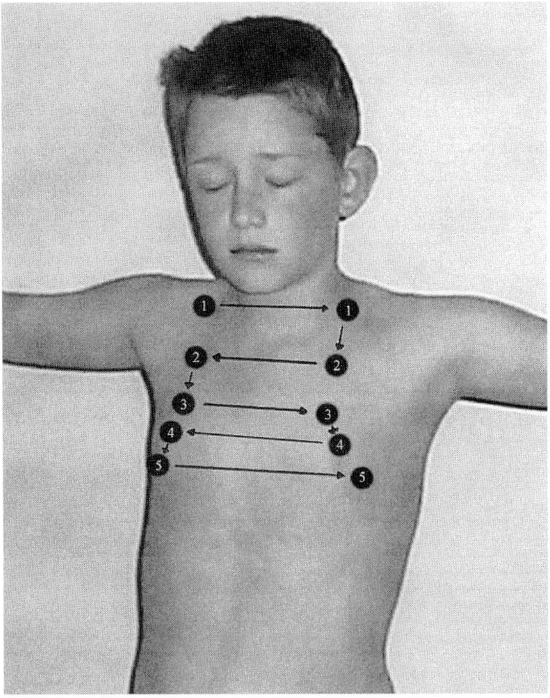

FIG. 7–4. Percuss between intercostals.

Diaphragmatic Excursion Diaphragmatic excursion is used to determine abnormalities of pleural effusion, diaphragm paralysis, or atelectasis. This can be done in older children, but younger children may not be able to cooperate. Have the child inspire and hold his or her breath. Percuss the posterior lung field until the sound changes, and place a mark on the chest. Then percuss the same area when the child expires and holds his or her breath. Measure the area between the marks.

TEST YOUR KNOWLEDGE OF CHAPTER 7

1. What are the differences in a child's thorax by age group?
2. What history and review of systems should be focused on in the respiratory system assessment?
3. What are the indicators of normal and abnormal respiratory functioning?
4. How can one determine if an adventitious sound is coming from the upper or lower respiratory system in a child?
5. What are some techniques used to gain cooperation of the child while performing a respiratory examination?
6. If a lower respiratory tract problem is suspected, what techniques can be performed to further differentiate the problem? Describe the techniques.

7. What are the indicators of abnormal acute respiratory effort?
8. What are the characteristics of normal breath sounds, noisy breathing, and adventitious breath sounds? What do they indicate?

 BIBLIOGRAPHY

Algranati, P. S. (1992). *The pediatric patient: An approach to history and physical examination*. Baltimore: Williams & Wilkins.

Goldbloom, R. B. (1997). *Pediatric clinical skills*. Philadelphia: Churchill Livingstone.

Jarvis, C. (2000). *Physical examination and health assessment*. Philadelphia: W. B. Saunders.

Seidel, H. M., Ball, J. W., Dains, J. E, & Benedict, G. W. (2001). *Mosby's guide to physical examination*. St. Louis: Mosby.

CHAPTER 8

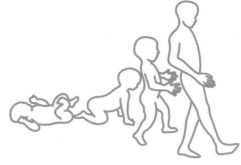

Assessment of the Cardiovascular System

MARGARET R. COLYAR

OBJECTIVES
- *Use basic cardiovascular assessment in children.*
- *Determine when to refer a child with cardiovascular signs and symptoms.*
- *Differentiate between innocent and organic heart murmurs in children.*

A congenital cardiovascular anomaly occurs in approximately 1% of live births (or 13 of every 1000). There are three types: obstructive lesions, left-to-right shunts, and cyanotic lesions (Table 8–1). Symptoms that accompany these three types of cardiovascular problems include respiratory distress, fatigue, excessive perspiration, poor weight gain, squatting, central cyanosis, hypoxic spells, angina, peripheral edema, and orthopnea (Table 8–2). The three most common manifestations seen in the ambulatory care setting are murmurs, cyanosis, and respiratory difficulty.

A thorough clinical assessment can spare many children with cardio-vascular complaints from unnecessary or inappropriate procedures. Recognition of characteristic manifestations peculiar to congestive heart fail-ure in early infancy is of paramount importance. It is also important to deter-mine the presence or absence of central cyanosis. Of all cardiovascular prob-lems encountered in children beyond early infancy, by far the most common is the need to assess the clinical significance of a systolic murmur, which is

91

TABLE 8–1. CARDIOVASCULAR ANOMALIES	
Type of Lesion	**Problem**
Obstructive	Aortic stenosis
	Coarctation of the aorta
	Pulmonary stenosis
Left-to-right shunts	Ventricular septal defect
	Atrial septal defect
	Patent ductus arteriosus
Cyanotic (central)	Tetralogy of Fallot
	Transposition of the great arteries
	Tricuspid atresia

present in up to 40% of preschool children. The overwhelming majority of such murmurs are innocent.

 HISTORY

Ask about the medical history of congenital heart defects and other cardiovascular problems. Ask if the child has had any cardiovascular surgical procedures. When determining the family history, include questions about myocardial infarction (especially in those younger than age 52 years), transient ischemic attack, cerebrovascular accident, syncope, congestive heart failure, bypass surgery, shortness of breath, and apnea. Determine if the child is taking any medications that would affect the cardiovascular system. Include in the review of systems questions about palpitations, syncopal episodes, chest pain, dyspnea, orthopnea, cough, fatigue, cyanosis, pallor, edema, nocturia, feeding, activity or exercise intolerance, poor weight gain, and delayed development.

TABLE 8–2. CARDIOVASCULAR SYMPTOMS ASSOCIATED WIH ANOMALIES	
Type of Lesion	**Symptom**
Obstructive	Angina
Left-to-right shunts	Fatigue
	Excessive perspiration
	Poor weight gain
	Peripheral edema
	Orthopnea
Cyanotic	Tachypnea
	Squatting (tires easily): Tetralogy of Fallot
	Hypoxic spells: Tetralogy of Fallot
	Central cyanosis

PHYSICAL EXAMINATION

INSPECTION AND OBSERVATION

For each age group, it is important to observe the child thoroughly. First look over the child, observing for color of skin and nail beds, creases in the ear-lobes, activity, respiratory effort, clubbing of the digits, and edema. There are two types of cyanosis: peripheral and central.

Peripheral Cyanosis

Peripheral cyanosis is seen commonly in newborns and is known as acro-cyanosis. That is, the hands and feet are bluish in color. This is a normal occurrence that resolves within the first 3 days of life. Harlequin sign is another instance of nonproblematic cyanosis in newborns. The newborn is literally blue on one side of the body and pale on the other. This is also nor-mal; it lasts only a few seconds and indicates transient vascular instability. Peripheral cyanosis in older children is seen as pale or bluish nail beds. This is related to cardiovascular or respiratory problems and is a precursor of cen-tral cyanosis.

Central Cyanosis

Central cyanosis has a worse etiology and usually indicates some type of cardiovascular problem. Central cyanosis includes cyanosis of the lips, ear-lobes, nose, and trunk.

Earlobe Creases

Although creases in the lower third of the earlobes can be seen in newborns with severe cardiovascular problems, they are usually noted in older chil-dren with chronic cardiovascular and respiratory disorders.

Activity

Squatting may be seen with children with cyanotic heart defects such as tetralogy of Fallot. These children tire easily and squat, which assists in increasing systemic oxygen saturation by decreased right-to-left shunting.

Because metabolism demands increase during feeding, infants with car-diovascular problems tire easily and do not feed well. In addition, these chil-dren may become diaphoretic during feeding and respirations may increase. If this occurs, suspect shunt problems and congestive heart failure.

Tachypnea or bradycardia may reflect a problem with the respiratory, car-diovascular, or central nervous system. Dyspnea and orthopnea are not obvious in infants and are usually seen with pulmonary edema.

Nasal flaring and intercostal retractions may indicate hypoxia, which occur more often in children with acute respiratory problems.

Clubbing of the fingers is seen in clients with chronic respiratory and cardiovascular problems. With early clubbing, the angle between the nail and the nail base straightens out. With late clubbing, the angle between the nail and the nail base exceeds 180 degrees.

Edema in infants and young children first manifests as periorbital edema and is preceded by tachycardia, dyspnea, and enlargement of the liver. Pretibial and presacral edema are late symptoms in children.

PALPATION

Nail Beds

Check for capillary refill. Press the nail beds in the fingers or toes. In dark-skinned children, press the fat pads of the fingers and toes. The tissue should turn white with pressure and return to pink in less than 3 seconds. If the process of blood return takes longer than 3 seconds, an oxygenation or cardiovascular problem should be suspected.

Pulses

Palpate all the peripheral pulses (Fig. 8–1). The pulses should be equal bilaterally. Use the fat pads of your index and middle fingers to palpate the pulses. Be sure not to apply too much pressure and obliterate the pulses.

Pulses may be described in several ways. They may be described as bounding, normal, diminished, or absent. Also, a numerical classification of 0 to 4 may be used (Table 8–3). For newborns and infants, simultaneously palpate the right brachial and right femoral arteries. These two pulses should be the same in volume and timing. If the right femoral pulse feels weaker, is absent, or lags behind the right brachial pulse, coarctation of the aorta should be suspected.

Heart

Press gently on the precordium to the left of the xyphoid process at the fourth or fifth intercostal space. A faint impulse is normal. Lift is a prominent pulsation felt at the point of maximal impulse (PMI) or apical impulse. If lift is felt, suspect respiratory or cardiac problems and volume overload.

A thrill is a vibratory feeling that is abnormal. Palpate for thrills in five different areas on the anterior chest: PMI (right ventricle), left sternum fourth or fifth intercostal space, second left intercostal space at sternal border (pulmonary artery), substernal notch (aortic arch), and apical area (apical portion of heart).

Liver

Also palpate the liver to determine its size (see Chapter 9). Enlargement of the liver is usually seen in clients with pulmonary edema.

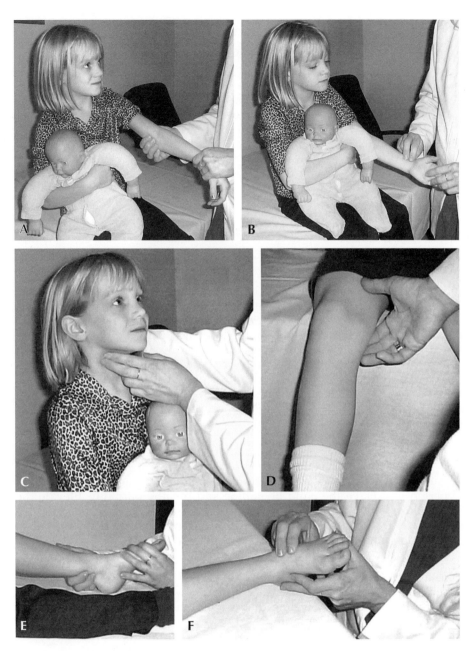

FIG. 8–1. Palpate all the pulses. (*A*) Brachial. (*B*) Radial. (*C*) Carotid. (*D*) Popliteal. (*E*) Posterior tibial. (*F*) Dorsalis pedis. Femoral not shown.

TABLE 8–3. CLASSIFICATION OF PULSES

Numerical Classification	Description
0	Completely absent
1	Weak
2	Normal
3	Increased
4	Bounding

OTHER TESTS

If cardiovascular problems are suspected, the following tests may be done.

Pulsus Paradoxus

Pulsus paradoxus is an indication of cardiac tamponade. Have the child lie supine and breathe normally. Elevate the child's arm. Apply the blood pressure cuff and inflate. While observing the child's respiration, gradually decrease the cuff pressure and note the level at which Korotkoff sounds are heard (point A). Gradually increase the cuff pressure until no Korotkoff sounds are heard (point B). The difference between point A and point B represents the difference in inspiratory and expiratory systolic blood pressure. Excesses over 8 mm Hg indicate the level of "paradox." Children with asthma normally have an increased difference, so it is difficult to interpret this procedure in these children.

Pulsus Alternans

Pulsus alternans is associated with myocardial failure and left ventricular hypertension. Have the child lie supine and breathe normally. Elevate the child's arm. Apply the blood pressure cuff and inflate. Lower the cuff pressure slowly toward the systolic level. Note alternating loud and soft sounds or a sudden doubling of the heart rate as the cuff deflates.

PERCUSSION

For the cardiovascular assessment, percuss the heart and liver.

Heart

To determine the size of the heart, do the scratch test (Fig. 8–2). This test is performed by placing the stethoscope on the child's chest over the heart. As you auscultate, gently scratch the chest, starting at the left midaxillary line. Scratch toward the heart. When the sound changes, mark the chest. Do the same procedure, scratching toward the heart area from the right midclavicular line, the left clavicle, and the left bottom rib. The area inside the four

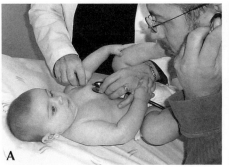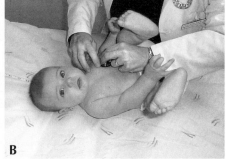

FIG. 8–2. Scratch test.

marks indicates the size of the heart. A child's heart should be approximately the size of his or her fist.

Liver

See Chapter 9 for the liver percussion technique. If enlargement is suspected, as seen with congestive heart failure, percussion of the liver is needed.

AUSCULTATION

Blood Pressure

Blood pressure (BP) must be taken at every well-child visit with a properly sized cuff. When the cuff size is too small, the BP measurement will be elevated. When the cuff size is too large, the BP measurement will be lower than the actual value. The stethoscope should have the pediatric diaphragm, tubing approximately 18 inches in length, with no sharp edges. Place the earpieces angled toward the tympanic membrane to get better sound. The cuff bladder should be 40% of the length of the upper arm and encircle 80% to 100% of the arm.

Heart Rate and Rhythm

Always auscultate the apical rate in newborns and infants. Bradycardia and tachycardia vary according to the age of the child (see Chapter 2). Bradycardia is a heart rate less than the lower end of the range for the age of the child, and tachycardia is a heart rate greater than the higher end of the range for the age of the child. Determine if the heart rate is in the normal range for the child's age group. Assess the heart rate for 1 full minute because newborns and infants may have irregular heart rhythms. Also, older children often have a sinus arrhythmia with irregular heartbeats. Evaluate for other indicators of cardiovascular problems if any irregularities in rate or rhythm occur.

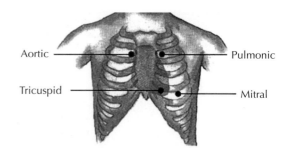

FIG. 8–3. Auscultation of the four heart areas: aortic, pulmonic, tricuspid, and mitral.

Aortic — Pulmonic

Tricuspid — Mitral

Heart Sounds

Auscultate the heart with the child standing, sitting, and supine. Listening in at least two positions is very important because some murmurs are heard better or only heard in certain positions. Auscultate in four areas (Fig. 8–3) using the appropriate size of stethoscope. Listen first with the diaphragm and then with the bell. When listening with the bell, place it on the chest and hold it lightly. Pressing firmly alters the sounds. S_3 (third heart sound) and S_4 (fourth heart sound) can be heard only with the bell.

Listen for S_1 (first heart sound) and S_2 (second heart sound). S_1 is the "lubb" sound that indicates ventricular depolarization and systole. It is heard best at the apex. Next, listen to S_2, or "dup" ("dub"). S_2 is ventricular repolarization, or diastole, and is best heard at the base. You should be able to hear S_1 and S_2 in all four areas of auscultation.

Also listen for S_3 and S_4 with the bell of the stethoscope. S_3 is heard immediately after diastole and sounds like S_1, S_2, S_3. S_4 is heard immediately before systole and sounds like S_4, S_1, S_2. The third and fourth heart sounds are heart muscle sounds. The third heart sound is caused by high blood flow. Third heart sounds are usually heard in children with thin chest walls. The fourth heart sound indicates poorly compliant ventricles; fourth heart sounds are always abnormal.

Documentation: Normal Heart Sounds Document the normal heart sounds and presence or absence of abnormal heart sounds. An example is as follows:

S_1, S_2 without murmurs, clicks, rubs, lifts, or thrills (Fig. 8–4).

Murmurs

Murmurs are caused by turbulence in blood or tissue vibration. They can be organic and innocent (benign) and occur separately or simultaneously. Murmurs are classified as systolic and diastolic (Table 8–4). Systolic murmurs occur on S_1 and sound like "swish dup." Systolic murmurs may be innocent or organic in nature. Diastolic murmurs occur on S_2 and sound like "lub swish." Diastolic murmurs are always organic in nature. Some murmurs, such as Still's murmur and pulmonary ejection flow murmur, are best heard while the patient is in the supine position. Some murmurs, such as

TABLE 8–4. TYPES OF MURMURS		
Area	Type	Disorder
Systolic	Regurgitation (sounds like breath sound)	Ventricular septal defect Mitral insufficiency Tricuspid insufficiency
	Obstructive (organic)	Aortic and pulmonic stenosis (coarse and loud)
	Vibratory (innocent; musical, mid-pitch and hum)	Still's murmur
	Flow (sounds like vibratory murmur; in pulmonary area but has FIXED split S_2 and does NOT change with respiration)	Atrial or septal defect
Diastolic (all are organic)	Regurgitation	Aortic or pulmonic insufficiency
	Obstructive	Mitral or tricuspid stenosis
	Flow	Ventricular septal defect Atrial septal defect
	Continuous	Venus hum Patent ductus arteriosus

venous hum, disappear when the patient supine. If the murmur disappears when the patient is supine, the murmur is an innocent one (Table 8–5). An innocent murmur is never heard in diastole and is never associated with clicks or rubs or other signs of cardiac disease such as cyanosis, syncope, absent pulses, and shortness of breath. Some murmurs, such as pulmonic flow murmurs that first occur in school-age children, disappear with sitting.

Grading of Murmurs When a murmur is auscultated, you must give it a grade based on its intensity (Table 8–6).

Documentation of Murmurs Indicate the grade; whether the murmur is systolic, diastolic, or holosystolic (both systolic and diastolic); where it is best heard; and if it radiates. An example is as follows:

Grade 2/6, systolic, mitral, radiates to the neck.

Abnormal Heart Sounds

Abnormal heart sounds indicate a problem with the heart or vessels. They include snaps, clicks, and bruits. Snaps are heard when the mitral and tricuspid valves open, and they signal the beginning of diastolic flow of the blood into ventricles. Ejection clicks are heard with the opening of the pulmonary and aortic valves, and they signal the beginning of blood flow to the

TABLE 8–5. INNOCENT MURMURS BY AGE GROUP

Age Group	Murmur	Description
Infants	Peripheral pulmonic stenosis	Short, midsystolic blowing
		Grade 2/6
		Heard along the distribution of the pulmonary arteries; equally heard in the anterior chest, back, and axilla
		Disappears by age 3 months
Toddlers and school-age children	Still's murmur	Low-pitched systolic ejection murmur
		Musical or vibratory quality
3 to 6 years		Heard halfway between the lower left sternal border and apex
		Increases in intensity when supine; increases or disappears with change in position (turn to side) or Valsalva maneuver
		Louder with exercise and fever
		Grade 1–3/6
	Venous hum	Continuous blowing systolic and diastolic murmur
		Heard on the right side of chest at the level of clavicles
		May be obliterated by turning the head away from the side of the murmur or compressing internal jugular vein on side of murmur
		Disappears in the supine position
	Carotid bruit	Harsh systolic ejection murmur
		Heard best over the right supraclavicular area and over the carotid arteries
		Approaches aortic or pulmonic areas
		Disappears in the supine position
		Increases with light pressure over the carotid arteries
		Grade 1–3/6
8 to 14 years	Pulmonary murmur	High pitched systolic ejection murmur
	Ejection flow murmur	Heard best at upper left sternal border in the supine position
		Disappears when sitting and standing
		Grade 1–3/6
Any age	Hemic murmur	High-pitched systolic ejection murmur
		Associated with anemia, fever, or increased cardiac output
		Best heard over the aortic and pulmonic areas
		Disappears with stabilization of anemia, fever, or cardiac output
		Common in pregnant women

TABLE 8–6. GRADING OF MURMURS	
Grade	Intensity
I	Very faint; heard with concentration
II	Faint; heard immediately
III	Moderate
IV	Loud; associated with a thrill
V	Loud; heard with the stethoscope on the chest
VI	Very loud; heard with the stethoscope off the chest

body. Bruits sound like swishing when blood flow is interrupted such as when there is occlusion of a vessel present (i.e., thrombus, atherosclerosis) or outpouching of a vessel (i.e., aneurysm). Place the bell of the stethoscope gently over the vessel to be auscultated. Have the child hold his or her breath and auscultate for swishing sounds, which indicates a problem with blood flow.

TEST YOUR KNOWLEDGE OF CHAPTER 8

1. What are common manifestations of cardiac problems in children?
2. What are the components of a cardiac history and review of systems in children?
3. Which pulses should be palpated in children, and where are they located?
4. Discuss the differences between a lift, thrill, bruit, and murmur.
5. What is an effective way to percuss the heart to determine size?
6. What are organic and innocent murmurs?
7. What are common innocent murmurs in children?
8. How do you document a murmur?

BIBLIOGRAPHY

Algranati, P. S. (1992). *The pediatric patient: An approach to history and physical examination*. Baltimore: Williams & Wilkins.
Goldbloom, R. B. (1997). *Pediatric clinical skills*. Philadelphia: Churchill Livingstone.
Jarvis, C. (2000). *Physical examination and health assessment*. Philadelphia: W. B. Saunders.
Seidel, H. M., Ball, J. W., Dains, J. E, & Benedict, G. W. (2001). *Mosby's guide to physical examination*. St. Louis: Mosby.

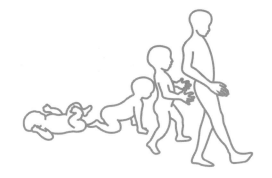

Assessment of the Gastrointestinal System

Margaret R. Colyar

Abdominal assessment involves the assessment of many of the gastrointestinal and genitourinary organs, which are the source of many common complaints of children, ranging from presenting symptoms (e.g., vomiting and diarrhea) to illness (e.g., urinary tract infections) to associated symptoms (e.g., abdominal pain with pneumonia). Assessment of the abdomen is slightly different in children than in adults because the placement of organs changes as the child grows. For example, the urinary bladder lies between the symphysis pubis and the umbilicus in children. The liver and spleen enlarge as the child grows. Additionally, children's abdominal walls are less muscular, which makes their internal organs easier to palpate.

HISTORY

Ask about the medical history of gastrointestinal problems, abdominal surgeries, and family history of abdominal problems or cancer. Determine what medications the child is taking, if he or she has any allergies, and what the immunization status is. Include in the review of systems appetite, dysphagia, feeding difficulties, food intolerances, abdominal pain, fever, nausea,

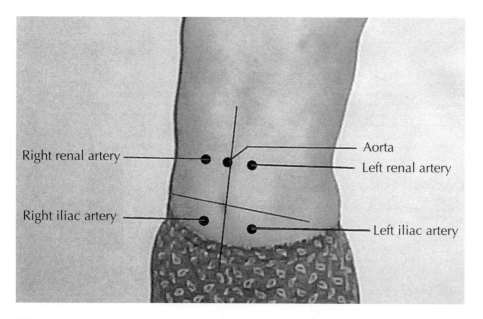

FIG. 9–1. Auscultating bruits on the abdomen. (a) Aorta, (b) Renal artery, (c) Iliac artery, and (d) Femoral artery.

vomiting, diarrhea, constipation, normal bowel habits, rectal conditions (specifically encoporesis), rectal bleeding, and nutrition. For adolescent girls, determine the date of the last menstrual period and if it was normal.

OVERVIEW

Visualize the organs in each of the four quadrants of the abdomen (Fig. 9–1) as you inspect, auscultate, palpate, and percuss. The internal anatomy is listed in Table 9–1. It is important to help the child relax during the examination. Talking to the child about school, family, and friends may take his or her mind off what you are doing. Ask the child to point to any areas of discomfort and to report tenderness or pain during the examination. With younger children, watch the child's face for facial grimaces. Examine the area of discomfort last to avoid guarding. Make sure that a good light source is available to assist in observation.

PHYSICAL EXAMINATION

INSPECTION AND OBSERVATION

Observe the abdomen while the child is standing and supine. Stand above the child and observe the abdomen, and then stoop down to view the abdomen tangentially. Visually observe the abdomen for contour, peristalsis, pulsations, scarring, symmetry, and masses.

TABLE 9–1. INTERNAL ABDOMINAL ORGAN PLACEMENT

Quadrant	Organ
RUQ	Liver and gallbladder
	Duodenum and part of the ascending and transverse colon
	Head of the pancreas
	Right kidney
LUQ	Stomach
	Spleen
	Left lobe of the liver
	Body of the pancreas
	Left kidney
	Part of transverse and descending colon
RLQ	Right ureter
	Right ovary and tube
	Right spermatic cord
	Appendix
LLQ	Left ureter
	Left ovary and tube
	Left spermatic cord
	Part of the descending colon
	Sigmoid colon
Midline	Aorta, uterus, bladder, umbilicus

LLQ= left lower quadrant; LUQ = left upper quadrant; RLQ= right lower quadrant; RUQ = right upper quadrant.

Contour

The abdomen should be flat, scaphoid, or slightly convex (rounded). A prominent abdomen is normal for toddlers and until puberty occurs. The abdomen should be symmetrical without masses or deformities. A fine, superficial venous pattern may be seen in thin children. Assess for protuberance or any bulges (Table 9–2). If the abdomen is protuberant, suspect peritoneal problems, tumors, or organomegaly.

Peristalsis

If the child is thin, peristalsis is easily seen. Increased peristaltic waves may indicate an intestinal obstruction and, in young infants, pyloric stenosis.

Pulsations

The normal aortic pulsation is visible in the epigastric area. If the pulsation is increased, suspect an aortic aneurysm or increased pulse pressure.

Scarring

Document any scarring and inquire as to the cause.

TABLE 9–2. COMMON ABDOMINAL BULGES IN CHILDREN		
Bulge	Description	Treatment
Umbilical hernia	Umbilicus protrudes, laxity around the umbilicus may be palpated	None unless hernia does not resolve by age 5 years
Diastasis recti	Separation of the two rectus abdominis muscles from under breast to pubic area When the child sits up, a ridgelike bulge appears	Disappears gradually
Epigastric hernia	Small, fatty nodule midline Felt through linea alba from the xyphoid to the umbilicus Caused by herniated fat	Surgical correction may be needed if painful
Pyloric tumor	Olivelike muscle tumor in the RUQ beneath the right rectus muscle	Surgical correction

RUQ = right upper quadrant.

Umbilicus

Note any bulging of the umbilicus (i.e., umbilical hernia), poor healing, erythema, or purulent discharge. Umbilical hernias are common in children of African-American descent and usually resolve by age 5 years. Erythema or purulent discharge (i.e., omphalitis) may be seen in children with poor hygiene, and proper hygienic procedures must be instituted. The umbilicus of newborns may not heal properly. This is a common occurrence that can easily be taken care of with application of silver nitrate to the area.

AUSCULTATION

Auscultation is the next technique to be used on the abdomen. With other body systems, palpation and percussion come first. If these techniques are used first on the gastrointestinal system, the bowel sounds may be altered. When a child is ticklish, have the child hold the head of the stethoscope and place it over the appropriate areas of the abdomen. Auscultate the abdomen in all four quadrants, noting bowel sounds (Table 9–3), using the diaphragm of the stethoscope. Listen for 1 minute and up to 5 minutes when bowel sounds appear to be absent. Bowel sounds should be of the same frequency and character throughout the abdomen. Hyperactive bowel sounds heard in one area and then absent in another area may indicate an obstruction between the two areas. Hyperactive bowel sounds should also be auscultated throughout the abdomen when diarrhea is present and in the epigastric area when vomiting is present.

Auscultation of bruits in seven areas using the bell should be performed whenever a child is hypertensive or arterial insufficiency in the legs is suspected. Bruits sound like heart murmurs and may indicate vascular prob-

TABLE 9–3. ASSESSMENT OF BOWEL SOUNDS*	
Description	**Frequency per Minute**
Normoactive	5–20 sounds
Hypoactive	< 5 sounds
Hyperactive	> 20 sounds

* Note: Hyperactive bowel sounds in one area with hypoactive or absent bowel sounds below the area usually indicate an obstruction.

lems in the abdominal area (Table 9–4). Listen over the aorta, renal artery, iliac artery, and femoral artery (see Fig. 9–1).

PERCUSSION

Percussion is useful for measuring the liver, spleen, ascitic fluid, and masses. Although not usually performed during well-child examinations, percussion should be performed if abdominal problems are suspected. The normal sounds percussed in the abdomen are dullness over organs, feces, and a full bladder. Tympany is heard over the intestines.

Liver

The liver is dull on percussion. To determine the size of the liver, you must palpate both its length and width. To percuss the width of the liver, start midway in the right upper quadrant. Then percuss upward toward the rib cage until the percussion sound changes from tympany to dullness. Mark this change in sound. Then percuss downward from the anterior chest below the nipple line until a change in sound is heard. Mark where the sound changed and measure.

To percuss the length of the liver, start percussing at the right midaxillary line toward the abdomen just above the right costal margin. Mark the change in sound. Then percuss from the middle of the abdomen at the level of the right costal margin toward the midaxillary line. Mark the change in sound (Fig. 9–2). The normal liver size for boys is 2.4 cm at age 6 months and

TABLE 9–4. ABNORMAL VASCULAR SOUNDS IN THE ABDOMINAL AREA	
Problem	**Sound**
Aortic aneurysm	Harsh murmur, systolic or continuous
Renal artery stenosis	Soft, low- to medium-pitched murmur
	Midline and toward flank
Partial obstruction of the femoral arteries	Venous hum: Periumbilical
	Medium pitch, continuous
	Heard with cirrhosis and portal hypertension

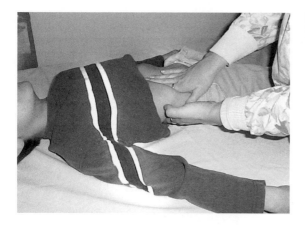

FIG. 9–2. Percussion of the liver.

7.4 cm at age 18 years. The normal liver size for girls is 2.7 cm at age 6 months and 6.1 cm at age 18 years.

Spleen

The spleen is normally dull and approximately the same size as or slightly smaller than the liver. Use the same technique in the left upper quadrant to percuss the spleen as used to percuss the liver.

Stomach

The stomach has a hollow or tympanic sound to percussion. It is located in the midepigastric and left upper quadrant area.

Kidney

Place your left palm flat over the client's back at the costovertebral angle and gently strike it with the ulnar surface of your right fist (Fig. 9–3). This should elicit a jar or thud but not pain unless kidney infection is present.

PALPATION

Palpation is done to identify areas of inflammation, infection, and masses. Light palpation is helpful to identify muscular resistance, abdominal tenderness, and superficial masses. Deep palpation is required to feel the abdominal organs and deep masses. Palpate all four quadrants systematically. Palpation in the left lower quadrant may reveal a fecal mass in children with constipation. If a rigid abdomen is felt, do an assessment for the surgical abdomen (see Chapter 10).

Flat palpation and hooking are two techniques that can be used to palpate the liver and spleen easily. The first technique is to place your dominant hand flat just below the child's rib cage and push up from the back with your

FIG. 9–3. Percussion of the kidneys.

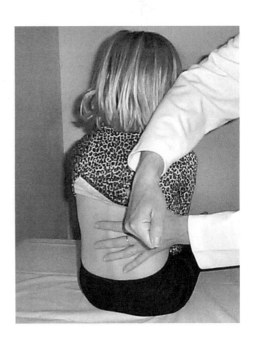

opposite hand. When the child takes a deep breath, push the hand on the abdomen up under the rib cage and palpate the lower edge of the liver or spleen. Another technique is to hook your fingers up under the client's rib cage and palpate the lower edge of the liver or spleen (Fig. 9–4).

Sometimes a child is ticklish or resists the examination by tensing the abdominal muscles. To decrease resistance, several techniques can be used. For children who tense the abdominal muscles, have them bend their knees and place their feet flat on the table (Fig. 9–5). For children who are ticklish, have them place their hands over yours and assist with the palpation (Fig. 9–6).

FIG. 9–4. Palpation: Hooking technique.

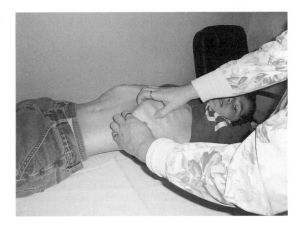

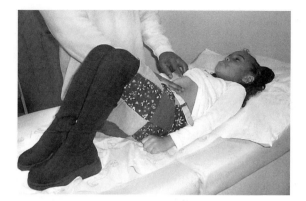

FIG. 9–5. Flat palpation. Have the child bend the knees during the examination if abdominal muscles are tense.

Liver

The liver is smooth and firm and is located in the right upper quadrant. The liver may normally be palpated 1 to 2 cm below the right costal margin on newborns and infants, especially during inspiration.

Spleen

The spleen is located in the left upper quadrant under the left anterior ribs. It is not normally palpable. However, in newborns and young infants, the tail of the spleen (1 to 2 cm) may be palpated during inspiration. The spleen is enlarged in children with mononucleosis, sickle cell anemia, or trauma. It may be friable and can rupture easily, so care should be taken when palpating the spleen.

Kidneys

The kidneys are smooth and rounded. They are prominent in newborns and frequently palpable in young infants. You may feel the lower pole of the right kidney in older children; otherwise, the kidneys are not palpable unless there is a large mass present.

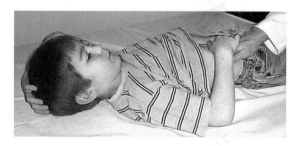

FIG. 9–6. To decrease the tickling sensation, place the child's hand over yours.

Inguinal Nodes

Palpate the inguinal nodes bilaterally. In young children, shotty (pea-sized) nodes are commonly found. If the nodes are larger than 1 cm, note their size and location. Larger nodes indicate infection or inflammation in the groin or lower extremities.

TEST YOUR KNOWLEDGE OF CHAPTER 9

1. What are the components of a thorough abdominal history and review of systems?
2. When observing the abdomen, what components should be checked?
3. Why should the abdomen be auscultated before it is palpated or percussed?
4. What do hypoactive and hyperactive bowel sounds indicate?
5. When auscultating abdominal bruits, which areas should be auscultated, and which part of the stethoscope should be used?
6. Describe the percussion of the liver, spleen, and kidneys.
7. What two techniques can be used with abdominal palpation of the liver and spleen?
8. Which internal abdominal organs are assessed in each quadrant?
9. What are common abdominal bulges in children?

 # BIBLIOGRAPHY

Algranati, P. S. (1992). *The pediatric patient: An approach to history and physical examination*. Baltimore: Williams & Wilkins.

Goldbloom, R. B. (1997). *Pediatric clinical skills*. Philadelphia: Churchill Livingstone.

Jarvis, C. (2000). *Physical examination and health assessment*. Philadelphia: W. B. Saunders.

Seidel, H. M., Ball, J. W., Dains, J. E, & Benedict, G. W. (2001). *Mosby's guide to physical examination*. St. Louis: Mosby.

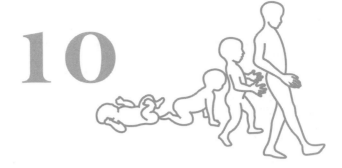

Assessment of the Surgical Abdomen

Margaret R. Colyar

Although not included in the well-child examination, the assessment of the surgical abdomen is a necessity whenever a child presents with abdominal pain in any area, bloating, nausea, vomiting, constipation, or diarrhea. When acute inflammatory disease is suspected, identification of peritoneal irritation is necessary, which may be caused by leaking fluid (i.e., blood, gastric fluid, pancreatic or intestinal contents, or pus. Common surgical problems include pyloric stenosis, bowel obstruction, cholecystitis, appendicitis, hernia, gastrointestinal (GI) hemorrhage, and ectopic pregnancy. Other problems that should be considered are listed is Table 10–1.

 HISTORY

Ask about past medical problems, abdominal surgeries, and family history of abdominal problems and GI and genitourinary cancer. Determine any current and past medications the child is taking (including homeopathics and herbals), allergies, and immunization status. In the review of systems,

TABLE 10–1. DIFFERENTIAL DIAGNOSIS FOR ABDOMINAL PAIN: NONSURGICAL

Anxiety: Family dysfunction, psychogenic causes, school phobia	Megacolon
	Mittelschmerz
Crohn's disease	Mononucleosis
Constipation	Pancreatitis
Disk space disease	Pelvic inflammatory disease
Duodenal ulcer disease	Peptic ulcer disease
Helicobacter pylori disease	Pregnancy
Inflammatory bowel disease	Pyleonephritis
Gastroesophageal reflux disease	Synovitis of the hip joint (referred pain)
Hepatitis	Urinary tract infections
Lower lobe pneumonia	Vaginal infections

include appetite, dysphagia, food intolerances, abdominal pain, nausea, vomiting, constipation, diarrhea, normal bowel habits (consistency and frequency), rectal conditions, blood in stool, and recent exposure to infectious disease. Do a 24-hour nutritional intake to determine if the problem has a food origin.

HISTORY OF PRESENT ILLNESS

Explore the basic chronological sequence of events related to the chief complaint. Use the anatomy of a symptom questioning technique to determine all the nuances of the current abdominal problem with a child (Table 10–2).

TABLE 10–2. ANATOMY OF ABDOMINAL SYMPTOMS

Item	What to Ask
Onset	When did it begin?
Timing	How often does it occur?
Duration	How long does it last?
Character	What does it feel (look) like?
Severity	How severe is it? Have the child use the 0 to 10 pain rating scale if able. For younger children, use the faces pain scale and have them point at it.
Location	Where is it, and to where does it radiate? Have the child point to where it hurts.
Associated symptoms	Are you experiencing any other problems such as fever, vomiting, diarrhea, cough, urinary tract infection symptoms, or pain? Find out when the last bowel movement occurred. Ask the parent or caregiver to tell you what the child ate the day before and before the office visit.
Alleviating or aggravating factors	What makes it better? What makes it worse?

PHYSICAL EXAMINATION

INSPECTION AND OBSERVATION

Gait and Stance

Children with peritoneal irritation walk cautiously and sometimes bent over.

Contour

Assess for any bulges or pulsations (see Chapter 9). Note distention that occurs with obstruction.

Color

Assess for Cullen's sign, which is faint, irregularly formed hemorrhagic patches around the umbilicus that occur with acute pancreatitis, massive upper GI hemorrhage, and ruptured ectopic pregnancy. Also note any petechiae or striae.

AUSCULTATION

Bowel Sounds

Check all four quadrants for presence or absence of bowel sounds. If the bowel sounds are hypoactive (< 5 per minute), listen for a full 2 minutes to determine if they are absent. An absence of bowel sounds in one quadrant with hyperactive bowel sounds in the previous quadrant indicates an obstruction between the quadrants.

PERCUSSION

Percuss to determine the size and location of masses. The scratch test is useful in determining size (see Chapter 8).

PALPATION

Soft or Hard

Note if the abdomen is soft or hard. Be aware of muscle tensing by the child. To decrease tension, have the child interlock his or her hands together and pull or have the child bend the knees and put the feet flat on the table.

Tenderness

To determine where the problem lies, try eliciting rebound tenderness. To do this test, push in one area, let up quickly, and note where the pain is elicited.

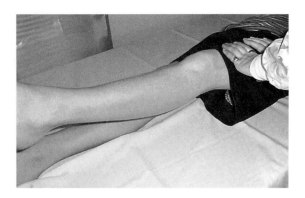

FIG. 10–1. Iliopsoas testing. Have child do a straight leg lift while you press downward on the lower portion of the thigh.

Masses

Note the position of any masses. Clients with pyloric stenosis present with a hard nodule just below the sternum. Hernias can commonly be found at the umbilicus, inguinal, and femoral areas.

OTHER TESTING

There are several tests that must be done when a surgical abdomen is in your differential diagnosis. They include iliopsoas, obturator, Rosving's sign, and Murphy's sign. These tests assist in localizing the pain.

Inflamed Appendix

The iliopsoas, obturator, and Rosving's tests should always be performed if an inflamed appendix is suspected. In older children, another test includes having the child jump from the step of the examination table. If this causes severe abdominal pain, suspect peritoneal irritation. It is not feasible for infants or toddlers to jump off the examination table step. With this age group, just tap the bottom of the client's foot, and the pain will be elicited, as evidenced by an increase in crying.

Iliopsoas

Have the child raise his or her leg while you push down on the lower part of the child's thigh (Fig. 10–1). If peritoneal irritation is present, pain will usually be elicited over the appendix.

Obturator

With the child in the supine position, pick up the ankle in one hand and hold the knee with the opposite hand. Flex the hip and knee 90 degrees and then rotate the leg internally and externally, holding the ankle stable (Fig. 10–2). If the child is reluctant to cooperate, try pretending that you are "exercising" the legs. If peritoneal irritation is present, pain will usually be elicited over the appendix.

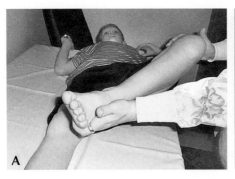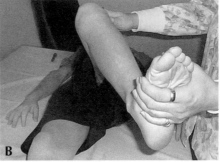

FIG. 10–2. Obturator testing. (A) With the child supine, pick up the ankle in one hand and hold the knee with the opposite hand. (B) Flex the hip and knee 90 degrees, then rotate the leg internally.

Rosving's Sign

Press deeply and evenly in the left lower quadrant. Quickly withdraw pressure. The test result is positive if pain is elicited in the right lower quadrant during left-sided pressure *or* if right lower quadrant pain is elicited on quick withdrawal of pressure.

Inflamed Gallbladder

If an inflamed gallbladder is suspected, check for Murphy's sign.

Murphy's Sign

Palpate the liver area. When a child has an inflamed gallbladder, he or she usually feels sharp pain with deep palpation and abruptly stops inspiration midway.

TEST YOUR KNOWLEDGE OF CHAPTER 10

1. What are the components of a surgical abdomen history and review of systems?
2. What should be included in the differential diagnosis of abdominal pain?
3. What questions should be asked of a child with abdominal pain?
4. What are the common surgical abdominal problems in children?
5. What do examination techniques such as Rosving's, iliopsoas, and obturator test for?
6. Describe the techniques for performing the Rosving's, iliopsoas, and obturator tests.
7. Describe the examination techniques that test clients with gallbladder inflammation.

⊛ BIBLIOGRAPHY

Algranati, P. S. (1992). *The pediatric patient: An approach to history and physical examination*. Baltimore: Williams & Wilkins.

Goldbloom, R. B. (1997). *Pediatric clinical skills*. Philadelphia: Churchill Livingstone.

Jarvis, C. (2000). *Physical examination and health assessment*. Philadelphia: W. B. Saunders.

Seidel, H. M., Ball, J. W., Dains, J. E., & Benedict, G. W. (2001). *Mosby's guide to physical examination*. St. Louis: Mosby.

CHAPTER 11

Assessment of the Neurological System

MARGARET R. COLYAR

OBJECTIVES
- *Develop basic neurological examination in children.*
- *Determine ways to elicit cooperation of the child during a neurological examination.*
- *Ascertain what neurological tests indicate.*

Neurological examinations can be made fun for children through the use of simple toys and instruments. Avoid overlooking important neurological findings. Keep the following categories in mind: (1) higher cortical function, (2) cranial nerves (CNs), and (3) trunk and extremities. Cortical function includes the parietal, frontal, and temporal lobes. Table 11–1 shows the problems that may occur in each lobe.

HISTORY

Check the birth and prenatal history for neurological problems, whether new or ongoing, and surgeries that would affect the neurological system. Check on medications the child is taking, allergies, and immunization status. Ask about family history of neurological problems such as seizures, migraines, and endocrine disorders. In the review of systems, include headache, head injury, dizziness (vertigo or syncope), seizures, tremors,

TABLE 11-1. CORTICAL FUNCTION PROBLEMS

Lobes	Indication
Parietal	Sensory perception abnormalities
	Impaired two-point discrimination
	Impaired graphesthesia
	Apraxia (inability to perform a series of tasks)
Frontal	Upper motor neuron dysfunction
	Personality changes, irritability, lethargy
	Lack of spontaneity
	Sphincter incontinence
	Re-emergence of primitive reflexes
Temporal	Aphasia
	Impaired comprehension of word elements
	Altered ability to read, write, and understand speech
	Distorted spatial relationships
	Decreased learning
	Psychotic aggressive behavior
	Memory deficits
	Visual problems

weakness, incoordination, numbness, tingling, difficulty swallowing, and difficulty speaking.

APPROACH

Do a systematic examination with the three categories (higher cortical function, CNs, and trunk/extremities) in mind. When a problem is noted, determine if it is upper motor neuron lesion (UMNL) or a lower motor neuron lesion (LMNL) (Table 11-2). UMNLs are associated with central nervous system (CNS) dysfunction, which involves the intracranial region, brainstem, or spinal column. LMNLs are associated with peripheral neurologic system dysfunction, which involves intracranial horn cells, nerves, the neuromuscular junction, and the muscles.

TODDLERS AND PRESCHOOL CHILDREN

Involve the child in the assessment by making a game of the examination.

SCHOOL-AGE CHILDREN AND ADOLESCENTS

School-age children and adolescents will usually assist with the examination. First establish rapport by asking open-ended questions about non-threatening subjects such as school, friends, TV, and sports.

TABLE 11–2. SIGNS OF LOWER AND UPPER MOTOR NEURON LESIONS

Lower Motor Neuron Lesion		Upper Motor Neuron Lesion
Parameters	Peripheral Nervous System	Central Nervous System
Coordination	Weakness hinders	Impaired: Cerebellum problems
CNs	Impaired	Abnormalities: Brainstem problems
Fasciculations	Presence: Anterior horn cell problem	None
Intellect	Normal	Impaired: Cortical problems
Power	Markedly reduced: Neuromuscular Junction problem	Slightly decreased
Reflexes	Difficult to elicit	Hyperactive: Pyramidal problems
Sensation	Impaired	Intact
Tone	Reduced	Spastic: Pyramidal problems

PHYSICAL EXAMINATION

INSPECTION AND OBSERVATION

Watch the child as he or she walks into the room and plays. Note the shape and size of the head, shape and position of the eyes and ears, presence of any skin lesions, symmetry of the facial features, and speech patterns.

STRENGTH, POWER, AND TONE

Watch the child walk. Note any weakness or wasting of muscles (i.e., neuropathy). A waddling gait is seen in children with muscular dystrophy. Usually proximal muscle weakness is associated with myopathy and distal muscle weakness with neuropathy.

Coordination and Gait

Note any spasticity or limb held in an unusual position. Spasticity (i.e., difficulty relaxing muscles) is commonly seen in children with myotonic dystrophy. Observe for choreiform movements (Table 11–3).

Cranial Nerves

Cranial nerves II through VII can easily be checked in well-child examinations. The olfactory nerve (CN I) is usually not tested. Table 11–4 shows easy-to-perform tests for each CN.

Spinal Nerves

There are 31 pairs of spinal nerves that supply the body (Table 11–5). They contain both sensory and motor fibers. The sensory afferent fibers enter and exit through the dorsal roots of the spinal cord. The motor efferent fibers

119

TABLE 11–3. ABNORMAL MOVEMENTS AND SENSATION: CHOREIFORM MOVEMENTS

Reflexes	Description
Involuntary posturing in unusual position	Dystonia
Quick, nonrhythmic muscle contractions	Myoclonus
Repetitive movements without purpose or vocalizations	Tics
Writhing movements	Athetosis (seen in individuals with cerebral palsy)

enter and exit through the ventral roots of the spinal cord. Each nerve innervates a particular portion of the body. Dermatomes are skin areas that are supplied from one spinal cord segment through a particular spinal nerve (Fig. 11–1). Because dermatomes overlap, the sensations can be transmitted by the dermatome above or below when one nerve is severed.

TABLE 11–4. CRANIAL NERVE ASSESSMENT

Cranial Nerve	Test
I Olfactory	Start testing at preschool age; have the child blow his or her nose to clear mucus, which may alter the test results; with the child's eyes closed, ask the child to identify bubble gum, peppermint, coffee, or chocolate; never use an irritant such as ammonia
II Optic	Test each eye separately; there are four parts to testing the optic nerve: visual fields, visual acuity, fundoscopy, and pupillary response
III Oculomotor	EOMs, corneal light reflex, eyelid elevation, "doll's eyes"
IV Trochlear	Clench teeth
V Trigeminal	Whisper numbers 2 to 4 feet from the child's ear and have the child repeat the numbers; cover one ear while testing the other
VI Abducens	Close eyes tight, wrinkle forehead, show teeth; cotton wisp or blow on cornea (blink occurs).
VII Facial	Rinne and Weber tests: Do these tests if problems are suspected
VIII Acoustic	Check palatal movement, gag, uvula deviation upward
IX Glossopharyngeal	Have child say "b," "d," and "k" sounds
X Vagus	Have child push against your hand with mandible
XI Spinal accessory	Have younger child lie supine, push head laterally; the child will resist
XII Hypoglossal	Have child move the tongue side to side; fasciculations indicate anterior horn cell disease

EOM = extraocular movement.

120

TABLE 11–5. SPINAL NERVES*		
Number of pairs	Name	Area Innervated
8	Cervical	Head, neck, shoulders, arms, upper chest, cervical vertebrae
12	Thoracic	Chest, abdomen, thoracic vertebrae
5	Lumbar	Groin, thighs, legs, lumbar area
5	Sacral	Genitals, perineum, and sacrum
1	Coccygeal	Coccyx

* There are 31 pairs.

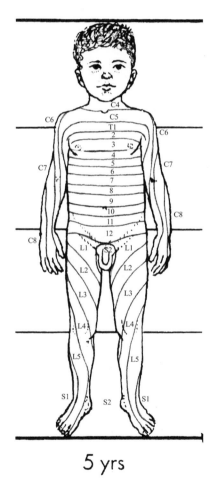

5 yrs

FIG. 11–1. Dermatomes.

121

TABLE 11–6. PRIMITIVE REFLEXES BY AGE

Reflex	Appears	Disappears	Abnormal Indicates
Rooting: Stroke cheek; face will turn toward stroked cheek and begin suck	Birth	3 to 4 months	Absence: Serious CNS disease
Sucking	Birth	10 to 12 months	Weak or absent: Neurological disorder, prematurity, CNS depression, or medications used during pregnancy
Palmar grasp: Place finger at base of metacarpals; fingers will curl downward	Birth	3 to 4 months	Diminished response: Prematurity No response: Neurological deficit Asymmetric: Fracture of humerus or peripheral nerve damage Lasts past age 4 months: Cerebral dysfunction
Plantar grasp: Place finger at base of metatarsals; toes will curl downward	Birth	8 to 10 months	Diminished response: Prematurity
Tonic neck: Supine with head turned to one side, infant will flex arm and leg on opposite side of body; arm and leg are extended on side head is facing (also known as fencing)	2 months	4 to 6 months	No response: Neurological deficit
Moro (startle): With loud noise or sudden movement, infant will extend limbs and spread fingers, then retract limbs	Birth	3 to 4 months	Persists after age 6 months: Brain damage Asymmetric response: Injury to slower part Absent response: CNS injury If present at birth but disappears shortly after: Cerebral edema, intracranial hemorrhage
Babinski: Stroke lateral edge of bottom of foot; toes fan outward	Birth	Within 2 years	If positive response (i.e., toes fan out) after 2 years: Pyramidal tract disease (white matter of spinal cord regulates motor and reflex activities of muscles)
Stepping: Hold infant upright with feet touching table; infant will move legs and feet as if stepping	Birth	2 to 3 months	Asymmetric response: Leg or hip injury, CNS damage, or peripheral nerve injury

Reflexes

Newborns Motor activity in newborns is under control of the spinal cord and medulla. There is very little cortical control, and the neurons are not yet myelinated. Primitive reflexes (Table 11–6) should be assessed in children who are younger than age 1 year. Each reflex occurs and resolves at certain ages. Document all primitive reflexes that are present and all that are absent.

Infant During the first year of life, cerebral cortex development and primitive reflexes are inhibited. CNS dysfunction should be suspected if primitive reflexes persist. The process of myelinization occurs cephalocaudad and proximodistally, so it is in this order (i.e., head, neck, trunk, extremities) that infants gain control.

PERCUSSION
Deep Tendon Reflexes

When you tap a tendon with a reflex hammer, the muscle stretches and impulses are sent to the spinal cord. The impulse is sent back to the muscle fibers and the muscle contracts. Thus, the deep tendon reflexes (DTRs) reflect problems with the spinal cord and peripheral nervous system. However, the cerebral cortex also exerts an inhibitory effect. So cortical lesions result in hyperactive reflexes, as seen with cerebrovascular accidents (CVAs). Each deep tendon is innervated at a certain position in the spinal cord (Table 11–7).

Deep tendon reflexes are rated using a reflex response scale from 0 to 4+ (Table 11–8). Abnormal variations can give you clues to neurological problems (Table 11–9). There are five reflexes that should be tested when a complete well-child assessment is performed: biceps, triceps, brachioradialis, patella, and Achilles. Assess each DTR bilaterally and compare responses. The numbers in parentheses below refer to the sites in Table 11–7.

Biceps Deep Tendon Reflex (C6) Lay the arm with the thumb up resting on the child's leg. Place your thumb on the biceps tendon at the antecubital space on the ulnar side. Tap your thumb with the reflex hammer. The client's arm should contract, and the hand should deviate medially (Fig. 11–2A).

TABLE 11–7. DEEP TENDON REFLEX INNERVATION SITES

Reflex	Portion of the Spinal Cord Tested
Biceps	C6
Triceps	C7
Brachioradialis	C6
Patella	L3
Ankle	S1

TABLE 11–8. DEEP TENDON REFLEX RESPONSE SCORING SYSTEM

Score	Response	Indication
0	No response	Blocked somewhere in reflex arc
1+	Slight muscle contractions with little or no movement of the arm or leg	Normal depending on other findings
2+	Visible muscle twitch and movement of arm or leg	Normal reflex
3+	Brisk, slightly exaggerated muscle twitch and movement of the arm or leg	Normal depending on other findings
4+	Exaggerated jerk of the muscle and arm or leg with repetitions (clonus)	Abnormal; lack of cortical inhibition

Triceps Deep Tendon Reflex (C7) Hold the child's arm up at shoulder height, bent at the elbow with the forearm hanging. Locate the triceps tendon just above the olecranon process. Place your thumb on top of the tendon and tap with the reflex hammer. The arm should swing outward (Fig. 11–2B).

Brachioradialis Deep Tendon Reflex (C6) With the child's arm resting on the leg, locate the brachioradialis tendon approximately 1 inch above the wrist on the radial side. Place your thumb on top of the tendon and tap with the reflex hammer. The arm and thumb should flex. This is often difficult to see because tapping with the reflex hammer often jars the hand. Another technique is to hold both of the child's thumbs together in one hand while tapping the brachioradialis tendon lightly with the reflex hammer (not illustrated).

Patellar (Knee Jerk) Deep Tendon Reflex (L3) Have the child (i.e., toddler,

TABLE 11–9. ABNORMAL DEEP TENDON REFLEX PATTERN VARIATIONS

Deep Tendon Reflex	Indication	Cause
Reflexes on same side of body different	Problem with reflex arc	Herniated disk Spinal abnormality
Reflexes different from one side of body to the other	Cortical damage	CVA
Reflexes different above and below waist	Spinal cord	Spinal
	Peripheral	Neuropathies
Slow relaxation phase	Hormonal	Hypothyroidism

CVA = cerebrovascular accident.

124

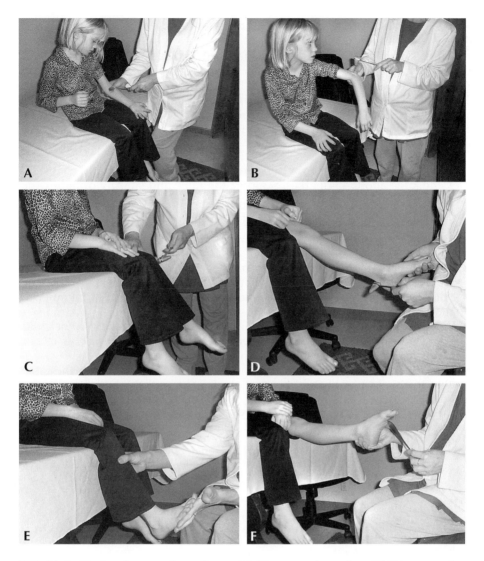

FIG. 11–2. Testing deep tendon reflexes. (*A*) Biceps tendon reflex. (*B*) Triceps tendon reflex. (*C*) Patellar tendon reflex. (*D*) Achilles tendon reflex. (*E*) Ankle clonus. (*F*) Babinski's reflex.

preschooler, school-age child, adolescent) sit on the examination table with legs dangling over the side. Locate the tendon just below the patella. Tap the tendon with the reflex hammer. The lower leg should extend (Fig. 11–2C). To test the patellar DTR in an infant, drape the leg over your arm with the knee slightly bent and gently tap the tendon.

Achilles Deep Tendon Reflex (S1) Have the child (i.e., toddler, preschooler, school-age child, adolescent) sit on the examination table with legs dangling over the side. Grasp the foot with your nondominant hand and dorsiflex gently. Tap the Achilles tendon slightly medially. The foot should plantarflex (Fig. 11–2D). Use the same procedure to test the Achilles DTR in infants; however, the infant may be lying on the examination table or in the caregiver's lap.

Ankle Clonus If the DTRs are hyperreactive, ankle clonus should be tested. Flex the knee about 45 degrees. Support the knee and sharply dorsiflex the foot, maintaining the foot in dorsiflexion. Sustained rhythmic oscillations between plantarflexion and dorsiflexion may indicate upper motor neuron disease (Fig. 11–2E).
Hints to elicit DTRs include:

- An easy way to find the tendon is to place your thumb over the appropriate area and flex the joint while you palpate. You should be able to feel the pull of the tendon. This is the location you tap with the reflex hammer to elicit the reflex.
- If the child is having a hard time relaxing the legs and feet, have the child focus on something in the room, clench his or her teeth, or put his or her hands together and pull. Tap the tendon as the child relaxes.
- For the Achilles tendon examination, have the child kneel on the table with the heels over the edge.

Documentation: Deep Tendon Reflexes Document the name of the tendon, the response, and the side of the body. Examples are as follows:

> Normal DTRs: Bicep and tricep DTRs 2+ bilaterally.

> Abnormal DTRs: Bicep and tricep DTRs 2+ on the right and 4+ on left.

Other Reflexes

Document all reflexes that are tested and the child's response to the examination.

- **Cremasteric (L1, L2):** Stroke the inner thigh. The testes should rise.
- **Anal wink (S3, S4, S5):** Scratch the skin around the anus and observe for contraction of the anal ring.
- **Abdominal (T8–T12):** While the child is in the supine position, gently stroke the abdomen from lateral to medial toward the umbilicus. The muscle should contract.
- **Plantar (Babinski) (L4, L5, S1, S2):** Stroke the lateral aspect of the sole of the foot from the heel to the ball of the foot, curving medially across the ball with a pointed (not sharp) object. For infants up to age 18 months, the toes should flare. After 18 months, the toes should plantarflex. Dorsiflexion of the great toe with fanning after 18 months indicates an upper motor neuron disease (Fig. 11–2F).

TABLE 11–10. MUSCLE STRENGTH SCALE	
Grade*	**Description**
5	Active movement against full resistance without fatigue
4	Active movement against gravity and some resistance
3	Active movement against gravity
2	Active movement of the body part with gravity eliminated
1	A barely detectable trace of contraction
0	No muscular contraction

* Document as 1/5 or 3/5.

Strength, Tone, and Power

Muscle strength may be graded on a scale of 0 to 5 (Table 11–10). Observe the extremities and compare. Note any leg or arm weakness and muscle wasting.

Upper Extremities Have the child simultaneously grip two of your fingers with his or her hands. Have the child push and pull. Make it fun—push in and pull out. Then place your hands on the child's elbows and have the child push you away (i.e., abduct). Then place your hands on her or his inner forearms and have the child push in (i.e., adduct).

Lower Extremities Place your hands on the child's knees and have the child raise the knees. Then place your hands on the front of the lower legs and have the child kick or push out. Then, with your hands on the back of the lower legs, have the child pull back. Ask the child to raise the toes up (toes to nose, or "smiley toes") and down ("frowny toes").

Coordination

Gait Have the child hop on one foot, do deep knee bends, and duck walk to test to proximal strength. Have the child heel/toe walk or do three pirouettes while walking to test for cerebellar functioning. Also have the child kick an object.

Point-to-Point Testing Ask the child to touch your index finger and then his or her own nose alternately several times. Move your finger to different locations so the child has to alter directions. Observe the child's accuracy and if the child crosses midline. Have the child switch hands and repeat. Another fun test is to have the child touch his or her nose with the index finger and then perform the test with the eyes closed. Repeat with each hand. For the lower extremities, have the child place the heel on the opposite knee and run it down the shin to the big toe. Awkwardness, tremor, or inaccurate movements may indicate cerebellar disease.

127

Rapid Alternating Movements There are two tests you can have children perform. Both are fun for children. First have the child place the hands on the knees and tap as fast as he or she can, turn the hand over and back as rapidly as possible. Then have the child touch each of his or her fingers with thumb in rapid sequence. Test cognition by having the child count forward and backward when touching the fingers and thumb together. Next ask the child to tap your hand as quickly as possible with the ball of each foot in turn. Slow, jerky, and awkward breaks in rhythm indicate cerebellar disease.

Sensation

Tickle the child on various parts of the body. If you are concerned about sensation, check for discriminative sensations, light touch, pain, position, temperature, and vibration. Be sure to demonstrate what you are planning to do to the child. Then have the child close his or her eyes for each test.

Discriminative Sensations There are five tests for discriminative sensations. Damage to the sensory cortex is indicated if pain, temperature, or touch senses are impaired. The posterior column is impaired if two-point discrimination and the ability to identify objects in the hand are diminished. The five tests are:

1. **Stereognosis:** Place a familiar object such as a key in the palm of the hand and ask the child to identify it.
2. **Number identification:** Using the end of a pen, draw a large number in the palm of the child's hand and ask the child to identify it.
3. **Two-point discrimination:** Using two ends of an opened paper clip, touch a fingerpad in two places simultaneously or in only one place and ask the child to tell you if his or her hand was touched in two places or only one.
4. **Point localization:** Have the child close his or her eyes. Touch a place on the child's skin. Then have the child open his or her eyes and touch the same area.
5. **Extinction:** Simultaneously touch both sides of the child's body. Ask the child to point where you touched.

Light Touch Using a cotton ball, ask the child to indicate when you touch his or her body.

Pain Using something pointed (not a needle) and something dull, touch different parts of the body (e.g., arms, hands, legs, feet). Make sure the child closes the eyes. Ask if the touch is sharp or dull.

Position Grasp the big toe by its sides and move it up and down. Ask the child to point in the direction where the toe is moved. Also check the upper

TABLE 11–11. ABNORMAL REFLEXES (SIGNS OF MENINGEAL IRRITATION)

Sign	Method	Abnormal Response
Brudzinski's	Flex chin on chest	Resistance and pain
Kernig's	Raise leg straight or flex thigh on abdomen and extend knee	Resistance to straightening; pain in lower posterior thigh

extremities starting with the thumbs. If position sense is impaired, move to the next proximal joint.

Temperature Use two test tubes, one filled with hot water and the other filled with cold water. Touch the skin in alternating areas and ask the child to determine if the object is hot or cold.

Vibration Vibration sense is often the first sensation to be lost. Therefore, you would not need to check pain if vibration is lost. Use a tuning fork; touch the vibrating tuning fork to bony prominences distal to proximal and ask the child what he or she feels.

Proprioception: Romberg's Test

Have the child close his or her eyes. This deprives the child of visual input for maintaining balance, forcing the child to rely on proprioception. With the eyes closed and the feet together, have the child extend the arms in front, laterally at shoulder height, or just keep the arms at the sides. Have the child maintain each position for about 5 to 10 seconds. You may want to tap the child's shoulder and try to make him or her lose balance. Make sure you warn the child first. A negative test result is normal (i.e., the child did not lose balance), and a positive test result is abnormal (i.e., the child lost balance with his or her eyes closed).

Meningeal Irritation

When nuchal rigidity is found or meningeal irritation is suspected, check for Brudzinski's and Kernig's signs (Table 11–11).

TEST YOUR KNOWLEDGE OF CHAPTER 11

1. What are the components of a neurological history and review of systems?
2. Differentiate between upper motor neuron and lower motor neuron lesions.
3. How are cranial nerves tested in children?
4. Why is it necessary to be aware of the dermatomes?

5. Describe the common primitive reflexes, including when they occur and when they resolve.
6. Describe where to elicit all five deep tendon reflexes and which spinal nerves are being tested.
7. Describe how to easily locate deep tendon reflexes.
8. When should ankle clonus be performed?
9. What is the pattern of reflex development in newborns and infants?
10. How is muscle strength examined and graded?
11. Describe the tests for evaluating coordination.
12. Describe the tests for evaluation sensation.
13. How do you test proprioception in children?
14. What are the signs of meningeal irritation?

BIBLIOGRAPHY

Algranati, P. S. (1992). *The pediatric patient: An approach to history and physical examination*. Baltimore: Williams & Wilkins.

Goldbloom, R. B. (1997). *Pediatric clinical skills*. Philadelphia: Churchill Livingstone.

Jarvis, C. (2000). *Physical examination and health assessment*. Philadelphia: W. B. Saunders.

McHugh, J. & McHugh, W. (1999). How to assess deep tendon reflexes. *Nursing 99* (August).

Seidel, H. M., Ball, J. W., Dains, J. E., & Benedict, G. W. (2001). *Mosby's guide to physical examination*. St. Louis: Mosby.

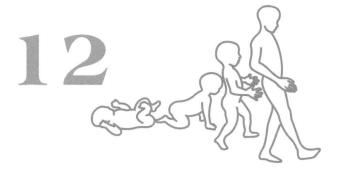

12

Assessment of the Musculoskeletal System

Margaret R. Colyar

> **OBJECTIVES**
> * *Develop musculoskeletal examination techniques for children*
> * *Ascertain common musculoskeletal problems that occur in different age groups*

The musculoskeletal system consists of bones, joints, muscles, tendons, ligaments, and cartilage. Understanding normal variants helps you avoid performing unnecessary and expensive tests. Learning when to expect changes with children's musculoskeletal development helps you determine when intervention is needed. Become familiar with skeletal movements so that your documentation will be understandable to all other providers. This will assist all healthcare personnel involved when abnormal findings occur.

HISTORY

Ask about medical history and surgeries (i.e., muscle, tendon, ligament, joint, bone) that affect the musculoskeletal system. Ask about family history of bone-related abnormalities, spontaneous fractures, cancer, and surgeries. Determine medications the child is taking, allergies, and immunization status. The review of systems should include joint pain, stiffness, swelling, heat, and limitation of motion. Determine if the child has had muscle pain, cramping, or weakness. Also ask about bone pain, deformity, and trauma

131

TABLE 12–1. GRADING MUSCLE STRENGTH		
% of Function	Activity Level	Grade
0	No evidence of muscle contractility	None
15	Evidence of slight contractility; no effective joint motion	Trace
25	Full ROM without gravity	Poor
50	Full ROM against gravity	Fair
75	Complete ROM against gravity; some resistance	Good
100	Complete ROM against gravity; full resistance	Normal

ROM = range of motion.

Source: Adapted from Jarvis, C. (1992). *Physical examination and health assessment.* Philadelphia: W. B. Saunders.

(i.e., fractures, sprains, and dislocations), including falls and injuries during play or sports.

PHYSICAL EXAMINATION

MUSCLES

Bilaterally inspect the muscles for symmetry, redness, swelling, nodules, atrophy, and skin changes. Palpate the muscles for tenderness, heat, crepitation, deformities, nodules, and strength. If you combine this procedure with palpation of the joints, it can be done quickly and easily. The scale for grading muscle strength is noted in Table 12–1.

UPPER EXTREMITIES

Have the child shrug the shoulders against resistance (Fig. 12–1). Test the grips by having the child push and pull. Place your hands on the child's lateral forearms and have the child push outward. Then place your hands on the child's medial forearms and have the child push inward.

LOWER EXTREMITIES

Have the child raise the knees against resistance. Then place your hands on the child's outer thighs and have the child push outward. Next place your hands on the medial knees and have the child push inward. Place your hands on the front of the ankles and have the child push toward you. Place your hand on the back of the ankles and have the child pull back toward the examination table. Ask the child to point the toes toward the ceiling and then toward the floor.

Check for pelvic girdle muscle weakness (i.e., Gowers's sign), which is seen in children with muscular dystrophy. With Gowers's sign, when children squat, they are unable to stand up without holding onto something or pushing themselves up using their hands on their legs (Fig. 12–2).

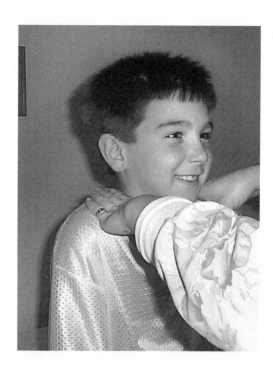

FIG. 12–1. Shoulder shrugs against resistance.

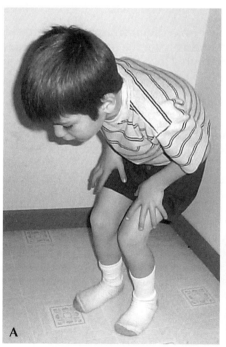

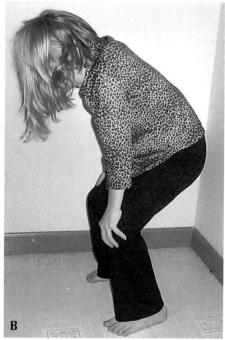

A   B

FIG. 12–2. (*A*) and (*B*) Gowers's sign.

133

TABLE 12–2. BONE AND JOINT CHANGES THROUGHT CHILDHOOD

Age Group	Expected Changes
Newborns	Tibial bowing, pes planus
Infants	Genu varum, pes planus, intoeing or out-toeing, wide-based stance
Toddlers	Genu varum or valgum, pes planus, lordosis, in-toeing or out-toeing, wide-based stance
Preschoolers	Genu valgum
School-age children	Scoliosis
Adolescents	Osgood-Schlatter, scoliosis

JOINTS

Bone and joint changes occur throughout childhood (Table 12–2).

Temporomandibular

Place finger on either side of the jaw in front of the ears. Have the child open and close the mouth several times. Check for audible and palpable clicks. Have the child open the mouth as wide as possible. Normal width is 3 to 6 cm.

Next, ask the child to protrude the jaw (mandible) and move it from side to side. Have the child clench the teeth and palpate the temporalis and masseter muscles for size, firmness, and strength. Have the child open his or her mouth against resistance.

Neck (Cervical Spine)

Watch the child throughout the examination (Fig. 12–3). Usually the child will perform complete range of motion (ROM) just by curiously watching you move around. If you are unsure, have the child move his or her neck back and forth (touching the chin to the chest), rotate side to side, and lay the ear on the shoulder. Nuchal rigidity, which is associated with meningitis, is the inability to move the neck back and forth. Side-to-side neck movement is usually intact.

Torticollis occurs many times during the birth process but is also related to medication use (e.g., prochlorperazine), abuse, and sports injuries. Torticollis is caused by damage to the sternocleidomastoid muscle. The child presents with head tilted to one side and inability to tilt to the opposite side.

Back

Observe the back. Palpate the scapula for symmetry. Palpate each vertebra for pain, subluxation, deviation, and curvature. The normal curvature of a younger child's spine is lordotic. Note the level of the shoulders and hips,

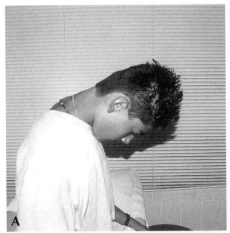

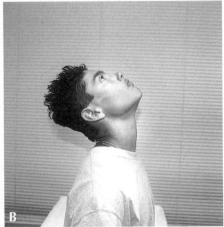

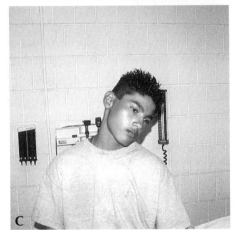

FIG. 12–3. Range of motion. (*A*) Forward flexion. (*B*) Backward flexion. (*C*) Lateral flexion. Note: Rotation not shown.

which should be even. Have the child stand and flex to each side. Normally, children can touch the head of the femur with their fingertips without difficulty. Next, have the child straddle a chair (stabilizes hips), cross arms (stabilizes shoulders), and rotate at the waist while sitting (tests spinal rotation).

Scoliosis Start checking for scoliosis (Fig. 12–4) in the early school-age years. There are three areas to be inspected for scoliosis: the shoulders, scapula, and hips. First, when the child is sitting on the examination table, note whether the shoulders are straight or uneven. Have the child stand and turn his or her back to you. Again, check the level of the shoulders. Next check that the iliac crests are level. Last, have the child bend over as if to touch the floor. The arms and head must be hanging down. Now look at the level of the scapula. With scoliosis, the shoulders, iliac crest, and scapula are uneven. If the deviation is subtle, back muscle exercises can be instituted. If it is caused by wearing a backpack, maybe just wearing the backpack on the

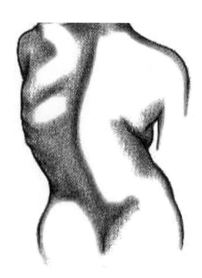

FIG. 12–4. Scoliosis. Note lateral curvature of the spine, one scapula and one shoulder higher.

opposite shoulder will do the trick. If the deviation is great, refer the child to an orthopedist for evaluation and treatment.

UPPER EXTREMITIES

Note any asymmetry, deformity, swelling, or redness. Compare one extremity with the other. Palpate, flex, and extend each major joint, noting heat, crepitation, and tenderness. Do ROM of all joints (Table 12–3). Make a game of it; this can be fun for the child. Common single and multiple joint problems are listed in Table 12–4.

Hands

Note small pinpoint dark spots on the nail bed, which represent small vasculitic infarcts seen in individuals with connective tissue disease. Palpate each finger for joint pain, crepitus, and effusion. Have the child spread and close his or her fingers and then make a fist. Note any swelling of the interphalangeal joints with flexion contractures, which is seen in children with juvenile arthritis.

Wrists and Elbows

Have the child flex and extend the wrist. Normal flexion and extension is 80 to 90 degrees. Also have the child bend the elbows to 90 degrees. Ask the child to pronate (palms down) and supinate (palms up) the forearm to assess the distal and proximal radial and ulnar joints (Fig. 12–5). Inspect and palpate the wrist for swelling along the joint line (effusion). Note any swelling seen on the dorsum of the wrist. Have the child open and close his or her fist. If the swelling moves, suspect tenosynovitis of the extensor tendon sheaths. Flex and extend the elbow while palpating for heat, edema, and nodules.

136

TABLE 12–3. NORMAL RANGE OF MOTION OF ALL JOINTS

Joint	Extension (degrees)	Flexion (degrees)	Right/Left (degrees)
TMJ	3–6 cm		
Neck: Forward	55	45	
Neck: Lateral bending			40
Neck: Rotation			70
Back	30	90	
Trunk: Lateral bending			35
Trunk: Rotation	30		
Hips: Flexion with knee straight	0	90	
Hips: Flexion with knee flexed	0	120	
Supine: Internal rotation	40		
Supine: External rotation	45		
Abduction	45		
Adduction	30		
Prone: Hyperextension		15	
Prone: Extension	0		
Knees	130	0	
Ankle Dorsiflexion		20	
Ankle Plantarflexion		45	
Ankle Eversion	20		
Ankle Inversion	30		
Shoulder: Forward/back	50	180	
Shoulder: Internal rotation			90
Shoulder: External rotation			90
Shoulder: Abduction	180		
Shoulder: Adduction	50		
Elbow	0	160	
Elbow: Pronation	90		
Elbow: Supination	90		
Wrist	70	90	
Wrist: Ulnar deviation	55		
Wrist: Radial deviation	20		
MCP	30	90	
PIP	0	120	
DIP	0–10	90	

DIP = distal interphalangeal; MCP = metacarpophalangeal; PIP = proximal interphalangeal; TMJ = temporomandibular.

Shoulders

Note the normal rounded curve of the shoulder. Uneven curvature may indicate dislocation or rheumatoid arthritis. Test mobility of the shoulder joints by having the child reach as high as possible and then put the hands behind the neck (external rotation). Then have the child lower the arms and put them behind the small of the back (internal rotation). Limited external rotation is often the first sign of juvenile rheumatoid arthritis shoulder joint disease. Also have the child forward flex, abduct, adduct, and reach forward and backward with the arms at shoulder height.

137

TABLE 12–4. ETIOLOGY OF SINGLE AND MULTIPLE SWOLLEN JOINTS

Single swollen joint
Trauma
Infection
Malignancy
Rheumatic
Hematological
Mechanical
Multiple swollen joints
Hepatitis B
Epstein-Barr virus
Adenovirus
Rubella
Mycoplasma

Lyme disease
Salmonella infection
Shigella infection
Yersinia infection
Acute onset
Kawasaki disease
Serum sickness
Lupus
Endocarditis
Chronic onset
Juvenile rheumatoid arthritis
Scleroderma
Polyarteritis nodosa

If tendonitis is suspected, have the child raise the arm laterally to shoulder height. Put your hand on the child's arm and ask the child to raise it. If this causes pain in the shoulder area, suspect tendonitis. If rotator cuff problems are suspected, do the drop arm test. Have the child abduct the shoulder and lower the arm slowly. If the arm drops suddenly, suspect a rotator cuff tear.

Newborns and Infants Check symmetry and spontaneous movement of the upper extremities. Birth trauma can cause three types of paralysis: Erb's palsy, Klumpke's paralysis, and entire brachial plexus.

Erb's Palsy Erb's palsy is paralysis of shoulder girdle and upper arm muscle. This problem is caused by C5 and C6 nerve root damage. Eighty percent of children with Erb's palsy recover. With this type of paralysis, the child is unable to move the upper arm but still has palmar grasp.

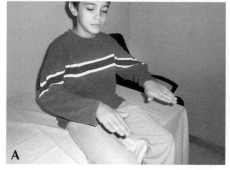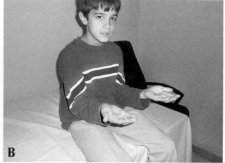

FIG. 12–5. Checking forearms. (*A*) Ulnar pronation. (*B*) Ulnar supination.

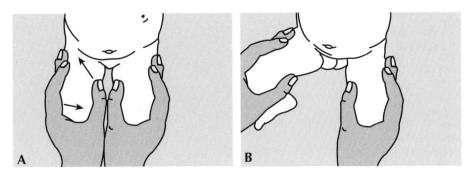

FIG. 12–6. Checking for hip displasia. (A) Ortolani maneuver. (B) Barlow maneuver.

Klumpke's Paralysis Klumpke's paralysis is paralysis of the forearm, wrist, and hand movements, caused by C7, C8, and T1 damage. Fewer than 50% of children recover. With this type of paralysis, the child has a flaccid hand, but the arm works.

Entire Brachial Plexus With entire brachial plexus paralysis, there is no movement in the entire arm and hand. This problem has a poor prognosis and is usually permanent.

LOWER EXTREMITIES

Hips: Newborns and Infants

Until an infant is walking, the provider should check for hip dysplasia. There are three areas that should be assessed to determine hip dysplasia (Fig. 12–6). Perform the Ortolani and Barlow maneuvers to check for hip joint instability. Also check leg length and posterior thigh creases. In infants, also check hip flexion and external rotation in the supine position. Place one hand on the thigh and gently roll the hip internally and externally while feeling for any resistance that will occur with muscle spasm secondary to hip joint irritability.

Ortolani Maneuver Place your hands over the child's thighs with your fingers extended from knee to tip of femur. The thumb is on the medial lesser trochanter (thigh). Abduct the hips 90 degrees. With the index finger, palpate the hip joint for clicks, clunks, or dislocation.

Barlow Maneuver Hand placement is the same position as for the Ortolani maneuver. However, with this test, the thumb presses the thigh backward and outward. Note any lateral movement of head of the femur.

Leg Length Flex the knees and place the feet flat on the examination table. Note any discrepancy in the size of the leg from the foot to knee. With hip dysplasia, one leg will be shorter.

139

FIG. 12–7. Measure leg length from the anterior superior iliac spine to the medial malleolus.

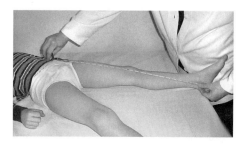

Thigh Creases Observe both legs both anteriorly and posteriorly. With hip dysplasia, there are more thigh creases on one leg than the other.

Hips: Older Children

Hip problems in older children include Legg-Calvé-Perthes disease, slipped capital femoral epiphysis, flexion deformity, hip girdle weakness, transient synovitis, and tendonitis. With the child in the supine position, measure the leg length from the anterior superior iliac spine to the medial malleolus (Fig. 12–7). Watch the child's gait. If the child will cooperate, have him or her walk on the tiptoes, then on the heels, and then duck-walk (Fig. 12–8). These maneuvers give valuable information about the child's neurological status; muscle strength; and the flexibility of the hip, knee, and ankle joints.

Slipped Capital Femoral Epiphysis Slipped capital femoral epiphysis usually occurs in adolescents, but short, obese children with delayed puberty and children during a growth spurt are also prone to this problem. With the child in the supine position, move the child's leg laterally (abduction) and medially (adduction) (Fig. 12–9). Have the child turn over onto the abdomen (prone). Flex the knee 90 degrees and externally rotate, then internally rotate. Decreased abduction and internal rotation are early signs of Legg-Calvé-Perthes disease and slipped capital femoral epiphysis problems.

Avascular Necrosis of the Femoral Head (Legg-Calvé-Perthes Disease) This usually occurs in children between the ages of 2 and 10 years. It may have an acute or insidious onset. Symptoms include limping, decreased ROM of the hip, and hip pain.

Flexion Deformity Check for a flexion deformity by using the Thomas test. With the child supine, flex the knees to the chest. Check to ensure that the lumbar spine is flat on the examination table. Place one hand under the lumbar area to note changes in positioning. Extend each leg separately to the table. If the child is unable to extend the leg to the table without moving the lumbar spine into lordosis, suspect a fixed flexion deformity.

Hip Girdle Weakness To check for hip girdle weakness, perform the Trendelenburg test. Have the child stand on one leg. The normal pelvis will rise on the opposite side. If the hip abductor muscles are weak, the pelvis will drop on the opposite side.

140

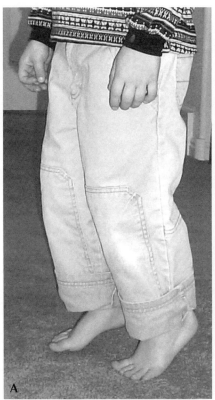

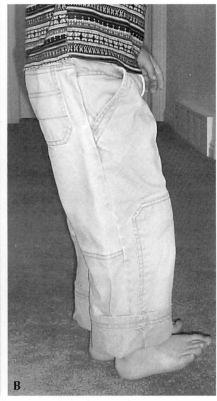

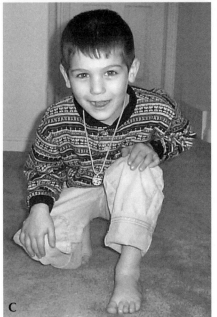

FIG. 12–8. Checking gait. (*A*) Tiptoe. (*B*) Heel walk. (*C*) Duck walk.

FIG. 12–9. Have the child lie supine and move the leg laterally and medially.

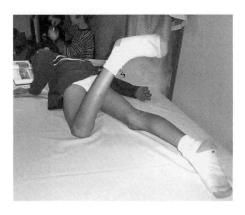

Knees and Legs

Inspect for edema, erythema, or bruising. Growing children have many problems with their knee joints. Draw a line from the inguinal ligament to the midpoint of the ankle. The line should cross the patella. Note any genu varum (bowleg) or genu valgum (knock knee). Mild bowing of the tibia is normal in newborns, infants, and young children. An infant may have varum, appear normal at 18 months, and again develop valgum between 2 and 4 years of age. The valgum should resolve by age 7 to 8 years. If the varum or valgum is greater than 15 degrees or asymmetrical, refer the child to an orthopedist for further evaluation.

Knee Joint Effusion If edema is noted above the patella, elicit the "bulge sign." Milk upward on the medial aspect of the knee and then tap the lateral side of the patella. Observe the medial aspect for a bulge that indicates returning fluid.

Baker's Cyst Palpate the popliteal area for a soft tissue swelling.

Synovitis and Tendonitis With the knee flexed 90 degrees, palpate the knee joint line for tenderness, which is seen in individuals with synovitis. If there is point tenderness, suspect tendonitis. The most common type of tendonitis in children (usually older school-age children and teens) is Osgood-Schlatter disease, which includes swelling over the tibial tuberosity.

Meniscal Tear To check for a meniscal tear, perform the McMurray test. Hold the child's heel in one hand and the knee in the other. Rotate the tibia externally and internally while slowly extending the knee, palpating for a click or clunk with possible pain associated.

Ankle and Foot

Check for edema, erythema, and asymmetry. Palpate for tenderness. Note gait and the occurrence of limping. Dorsiflex and plantarflex, invert, and

142

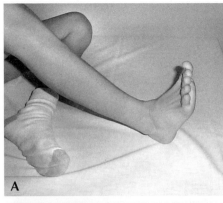

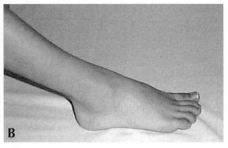

FIG. 12–10. Checking ankles. (A) Ankle dorsiflexion. (B) Ankle plantarflexion. (C) Ankle inversion. Note: Ankle eversion not shown.

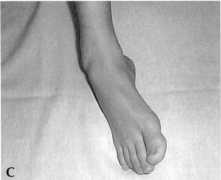

evert each ankle (Fig. 12–10). Palpate the metatarsals individually. Compress the distal metatarsals to check for tenderness.

Note the alignment of the toes, metatarsals, and forefoot. Hold feet in your hand and observe. Look at resting position and spontaneous movement. Note the curvature of the ankles. If spontaneous movement corrects curvature, then there is no problem. If spontaneous movement accentuates curvature, surgical correction is needed. Two common problems found in the newborns and infants are metatarsus adductus and clubfoot (talipes equinovarus) (Fig. 12–11).

Metatarsus Adductus With metatarsus adductus, passive ROM can be performed. This problem usually resolves within 2 months.

Clubfoot (Talipes Equinovarus) With clubfoot, passive ROM cannot be performed. This problem needs surgical correction.

Flat Feet (Pes Planus) Flat feet are normal if the child is younger than age 3 years. If an older child appears to be flat-footed, check the longitudinal arch on the bottom of the foot with the child sitting on the examination table. The arch should appear.

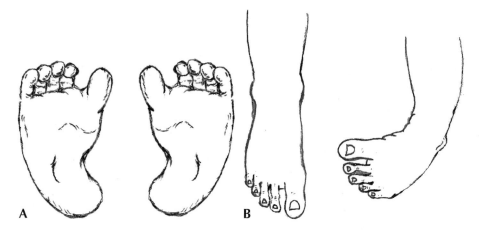

FIG. 12–11. Foot problems. (*A*) Metatarsus abductus. (*B*) Talipes equinovarus (club-foot).

Toe Walking Toe walking is usually caused by Achilles tendon tightening and gastrocnemius spasm. Intermittent toe walking is normal. If the toe walking is persistent, suspect cerebral palsy or muscular dystrophy. With cerebral palsy, note tight heel cords, increased muscle tone, and hyperreflexia. Children with cerebral palsy also circumduct their legs (scissorlike) when walking. Children with muscular dystrophy have proximal muscle weakness (Gowers's sign).

Wide-Based Stance A wide-based stance is expected as a child begins to walk. As the child improves in skill, the wide-based stance should decrease.

In-toeing and Out-Toeing In-toeing or out-toeing are also expected as a child begins to walk. As the child improves in skill, the in-toeing or out-toeing usually resolves. If in-toeing or out-toeing is greater than 30 degrees (Fig. 12–12), refer the child to an orthopedist. The three common problems causing exaggerated in-toeing or out-toeing are internal femoral torsion, external tibial torsion, and external rotation of the hips:

● Internal femoral torsion (femoral anteversion) is intoeing with patellar strabismus (i.e., one knee is rotated more than the other as in Fig. 12–13). To test for this problem, gently rotate the knees so that both patella face forward. If the feet point straight forward, then internal femoral torsion is the problem. Another test for this problem is to have the child lie prone and flex the knees 90 degrees. Allow the leg to fall outward by gravity (internal rotation). Then allow the leg to fall inward (external rotation). Measure the degree of rotation. Normally, external rotation is greater than internal rotation. With internal femoral torsion, the degree of internal rotation is greater than 70 degrees.

144

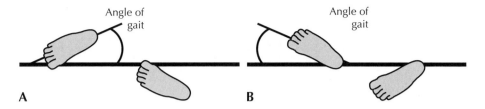

FIG. 12–12. In-toeing and out-toeing. (*A*) In-toeing. (*B*) Out-toeing.

- Internal tibial torsion is in-toeing with the patella pointing forward and the feet normal. This appears between age 6 to 18 months and disappears by age 2 years.
- External rotation of the hips is out-toeing, which may be caused by external rotation of the hips or external tibial torsion. To test for this problem, rotate the hips to a normal position, and it will correct. This does not interfere with walking and spontaneously corrects in 6 to 12 months after first occurrence.

Toes Palpate each metatarsophalangeal joint and each phalange individually. Examine the toes for swelling or deformity.

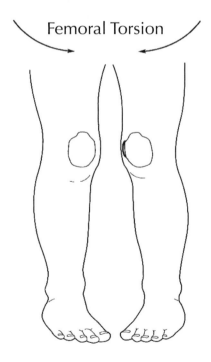

FIG. 12–13. Internal femoral torsion with patellar strabismus.

TEST YOUR KNOWLEDGE OF CHAPTER 12

1. What are the components of the history and review of systems for the musculoskeletal system?
2. Describe how muscles are tested in children.
3. How is muscle strength graded?
4. What are common bone and joint changes seen throughout childhood?
5. For each joint, describe examination techniques in children.
6. What are three areas of examination used to rule out scoliosis?
7. For newborns, what three upper extremity problems may occur during birth? Describe them.
8. How is hip dysplasia determined in newborns and infants?
9. Describe three hip problems seen in older children.
10. Describe three knee problems seen in older children.
11. Differentiate between metatarsus adductus and talipes equinovarus.
12. Differentiate between genu varum and genu valgum.
13. Describe in-toeing and out-toeing. When should the child be referred to an orthopedist?
14. Describe two problems with the legs that are caused by intoeing and out-toeing.

 BIBLIOGRAPHY

Algranati, P. S. (1992). *The pediatric patient: An approach to history and physical examination*. Baltimore: Williams & Wilkins.

Cassidy, J. T., & Petty, R. E. (1995). *Textbook of pediatric rheumatology*. Philadelphia: W. B. Saunders.

Goldbloom, R. B. (1997). *Pediatric clinical skills*. Philadelphia: Churchill Livingstone.

Jarvis, C. (2000). *Physical examination and health assessment*. Philadelphia: W. B. Saunders.

Seidel, H. M., Ball, J. W., Dains, J. E, & Benedict, G. W. (2001). *Mosby's guide to physical examination*. St. Louis: Mosby.

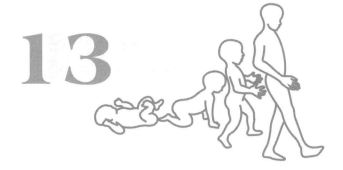

Assessment of the Endocrine System

MARGARET R. COLYAR

OBJECTIVES
- *Determine how the hormone feedback system works.*
- *Ascertain common endocrine indicators.*
- *Develop an endocrine-focused physical examination.*

Many endocrine diseases are life threatening, so it is vital for healthcare providers to recognize their presence. Common concerns are that a child is too small, too heavy, too thin, too tall, or developing sexually in a premature fashion. First you must understand the feedback system relationship of gland to hormones, hormonal relationship to the body systems, and disorders caused by hormonal imbalance. A thorough examination of the child will assist you in determining if a hormonal imbalance is occurring.

⑤ OVERVIEW OF THE FEEDBACK SYSTEM

Hormones are produced and regulated by a negative feedback system. The feedback system works in the following manner: The hypothalamus secretes releasing hormones to the anterior and posterior pituitary, which causes the pituitary to release stimulating hormones into the bloodstream. The bloodstream transports hormones to glands and targets cells, where they exert their effects. The target cells respond only to those hormones for which they have receptors. When glands and cells have responded appropriately, feedback is provided to the hypothalamus to release inhibiting hormones to the pituitary, which slows or stops the secretion of the hormones into the bloodstream.

 # HISTORY

Ask about the client's medical history of hormonal problems. Ask if the child has had any hormone-related surgical procedures. In the family history questions, ask about hypothalamus, pituitary, thyroid, parathyroid, thymus, adrenal, and pancreatic problems. Determine if the child is taking any medications that may affect the endocrine system. In the review of systems, include questions about polyuria, polydypsia, polyphagia, hair loss, unusual hair growth, intolerance to heat or cold, fatigue, irritability, constipation, or feeding problems.

 # PHYSICAL EXAMINATION

A thorough head-to-toe examination should be completed. Table 13–1 outlines the specific areas to focus on and indicators of possible endocrine dysfunction that can occur. The table discusses every gland and outlines common disorders.

COMMON DISORDERS OF THE PITUITARY IN CHILDREN

Pituitary Deficit: Growth Hormone Deficiency

Growth hormone deficiency (GHD) is usually a result of idiopathic hypothalamic-pituitary failure of growth hormone secretion. Midline defects often associated with GHD are cleft palate, choanal atresia, optic nerve hypoplasia, and single upper central incisor. Growth hormone is a major counter-regulatory hormone to insulin, so children with GHD are susceptible to hypoglycemia during fasting periods or when they are ill. Symptoms include limping, glassy eyes, stupor, and possible unresponsiveness to verbal commands.

Monitor height and weight percentiles of all children. Children with GHD present with an increased weight-to-height ratio. These children appear younger than their chronological age and have a rounded face; chubby limbs; delayed tooth eruption; fine, wispy hair; and poorly developed musculature. Always investigate growth of less than 5 cm per year in children from the age of 5 years until puberty. In older children, GHD is usually caused by a destructive lesion (i.e., tumor) and manifests as new onset growth failure (Table 13–2).

TABLE 13–1. GUIDELINES FOR PHYSICAL ASSESSMENT OF ENDOCRINE SYSTEM FUNCTION

Area of Assessment	Abnormal Finding	Possible Endocrine Problem
Vital Signs	Low core temperature	GHD
	Systolic hypertension with wide pulse pressure; tachycardia	Hyperthyroidism
	Bradycardia; weak arterial pulse; distant heart sounds	Hypothyroidism
	Hypertension	Conn's disease
Weight	Weight loss	Hypoinsulinism, androgen deficit, adrenal deficit
	Poor weight gain	Adrenal excess
Height	Poor statural growth	Adrenal excess
	Increased weight-to-height ratio	GHD
	Increased weight-to-height ratio	GH excess
General	Lethargy	Hypercalcemia
	Listlessness	Androgen insufficiency, Hypercalcemia
	Nervousness, irritability	Hypercalcemia, excess or decreased insulin, TSH excess
	Stupor, unresponsiveness	GHD
	Weakness	Adrenal insufficiency
Head	Large posterior and anterior fontanels	TSH deficit
	Poor head control	TSH deficit
	Decreased body hair	TSH deficit
	Dry hair	TSH deficit
	Lanugo	Adrenal excess
	Fine, silky hair	Hyperthyroidism
	Fine, wispy hair	GHD
	Hirsutism	Cushing's syndrome
	Low hairline	TSH deficit
Face	Dull or flat expression	Hypothyroidism
	Ovoid facies	Hypocalcemia
	Prominent forehead and jaw	Hypothyroidism
	Round or puffy face	Hypothyroidism, hypercalcemia, GHD
	Ruddy, plethoric face	Adrenal excess

(Continued)

TABLE 13–1. GUIDELINES FOR PHYSICAL ASSESSMENT OF ENDOCRINE SYSTEM FUNCTION (Continued)

Area of Assessment	Abnormal Finding	Possible Endocrine Problem
Eyes	Decreased blinking	Hyperthyroidism
	Cataracts	Hypocalcemia
	Loss of convergence	Hyperthyroidism
	EOM imbalance	Hyperthyroidism
	Exophthalmos	Hyperthyroidism
	Glassy eyes	Pituitary deficit
	Narrow palpebral fissures	Hypothyroidism
	Widened palpebral fissures	Hyperthyroidism
	Periorbital puffiness	Hypothyroidism
	Stellate iris (star-shaped)	Hypercalcemia
	Wide-set eyes	Hypercalcemia
Nose	Choanal atresia	GHD
	Depressed nasal bridge	Hypothyroidism
Mouth	Central incisor	GHD
	Cleft palate	GHD
	Delayed tooth eruption	GHD
	Hoarse or croaking voice	Hypothyroidism
Neck	Enlarged thyroid gland	Hyperthyroidism
Trunk	Buffalo hump	Adrenocortical excess
	Supraclavicular fat pads	Adrenocortical excess
	Truncal obesity	Adrenocortical excess
Secondary sexual characteristics	Change in size, symmetry, pigmentation, and presence of discharge in breasts	Adrenal excess
	Enlarged clitoris	Androgen excess
	Pubic hair: Distribution and amount	Hypogonadism
	Gynecomastia	Excess testosterone
	Striae in breast and abdomen	Adrenal excess
	Testicular size (enlarged) with secondary sexual hair	Androgen excess with excess glucocorticoids
Skin	Acne	Adrenal excess
	Bruising and petechiae	Adrenocortical hyperfunction
	Cool skin	Hypothyroidism
	Dry skin and hair	Hypothyroidism
	Facial hirsutism	Adrenal excess
	Increased pigmentation on the fingers, joints, elbows, knees	Primary adrenal decrease
	Jaundice	Hypothyroidism
	Pallor	Hyperinsulinemia
	Purple striae	Adrenal excess
	Sweating	Hyperthyroidism
	Thin, fragile skin	Adrenal excess
	Vitiligo on the face, neck, trunk	Secondary adrenal decrease

TABLE 13–1. GUIDELINES FOR PHYSICAL ASSESSMENT OF ENDOCRINE SYSTEM FUNCTION (Continued)

Area of Assessment	Abnormal Finding	Possible Endocrine Problem
Nails	Malformation and thickness or brittleness	Thyroid gland dysfunction
Musculoskeletal	Chubby limbs	GHD
	Limping	GHD
	Short fourth and fifth metacarpals	Hypocalcemia
	Muscles (atrophy)	Adrenal excess
	Muscles (decreased strength)	Androgen deficit
	Muscles (enlarged calf)	Hypothyroidism
	Muscles (poor control)	Hypothyroidism
	Muscles (poorly developed)	GHD
Neurological	Chvostek's sign (lip pursing)	Hypocalcemia
	DTR: Delayed relaxation phase	Hypothyroidism
	DTR: Hyperreflexive knee jerk	Hypocalcemia
	Hand and foot cramps	Hypocalcemia
	Trousseau's sign (carpal spasm)	Hypocalcemia

DTR = deep tendon reflex; EOM = extraocular movement; GH = growth hormone; GHD = growth hormone deficiency; TSH = thyroid-stimulating hormone.

Pituitary Excess: Growth Hormone Excess

Note any increase in height and weight. Growth hormone excess at an early age leads to gigantism. Children with growth hormone excess could grow up to be up to 8 feet tall and more than 300 pounds. This occurs when overproduction of growth hormone occurs before closure of the epiphyses of the long bones, so they are still capable of longitudinal growth.

TABLE 13–2. SIGNS AND SYMPTOMS OF GROWTH HORMONE DEFICIENCY

Appears younger than chronological age
Cherubic
Rounded face
Chubby limbs
Dimpling of the anterior abdominal fat
High-pitched, "reedy" voice
Increased height-to-weight ratio
Poorly developed muscle bulk
Fine and wispy hair
Delayed tooth eruption
Boys: Small penis (< 2.5 cm in length)
Growth velocity: < 5 cm/year from age 5 years through puberty

TABLE 13–3. PALPATION OF THE THYROID

Consistency of Thyroid Gland	Disorder
Soft	Normal
Soft firm, nontender	Graves' disease
Firm	Hashimoto's disease
Hard	Carcinoma
Goiter	
Soft to firm, nontender	Graves' disease
Diffusely swollen, tender	Subacute thyroiditis
One or more smooth, firm, round, or oval nodules	Toxic nodular goiter
Central rounded midline mass between thyroid and chin; moves upward when child sticks out tongue; not fixed	Thyroglossal duct cyst

Pituitary Deficit: Antidiuretic Hormone Deficiency

Diabetes insipidus results in polyuria up to 20 liters per day and polydipsia because the kidneys cannot reabsorb the water. Symptoms include irritability, mental dullness, coma, hyperthermia, hypovolemia, hypertension, tachycardia, dry mucus membranes, and poor skin turgor caused by inadequate water replacement. A 24-hour urine intake and output show increased serum osmalality, decreased urine osmalality, and specific gravity of 1.005 or less. A fluid deprivation test is indicated.

COMMON DISORDERS OF THE THYROID IN CHILDREN

Approach to the Thyroid Examination

Because most children are ticklish, touching the neck may elicit squirming, scrunching up the neck, and giggling. Therefore, sit the child on a chair or examination table and ask him or her to take a sip of water. Observe the area just above the sternal notch and the thyroid gland movement while the child is swallowing. Next have the child hyperextend the neck and observe for thyroid enlargement.

The thyroid gland cannot usually be palpated in newborns. If you can palpate it, then it is enlarged. The gland can be palpated in older children, but it should be soft and nontender. Problems are shown in Table 13–3.

Inspect the thyroid gland to see if it moves up and down during swallowing. Palpate the thyroid (see Chapter 5). Place your hand under the newborn's scapula and raise the baby's shoulders. Allow the newborn's head to fall back gently and observe the thyroid gland for enlargement. Palpate with one finger on either side of the gland. Table 13–3 shows the difference in consistency of the thyroid gland. A thyroglossal duct cyst may also be found as a midline mass between the thyroid and the chin. This cyst moves upward when the child sticks out the tongue. If distinct lumps are palpated on the thyroid, the child has a goiter.

Thyroid-Stimulating Hormone Excess: Graves' Disease

Thyroid disorders are classified as either hyper- or hypothyroidism. Children with hyperthyroidism are usually restless and irritable. They may have excessive sweatiness; loose, frequent bowel movements; tachycardia; and increased appetite without weight gain or possibly weight loss. Assess the eyes. The palpebral fissures are widened with decreased blinking (looks like child is staring), proptosis (eyes seem to bulge), exophthalmos (protrusion of the eyeballs), chemosis (injection and edema of the bulbar conjunctiva), loss of convergence, new onset of diplopia, and imbalance of extraocular muscle function.

Thyroid-Stimulating Hormone Deficit: Cretinism

Congenital hypothyroidism, or thyroid deficit, at an early age is the major cause of cretinism. Newborns should be screened for hypothyroidism to prevent irreversible mental retardation that occurs if left untreated. This problem manifests in newborns and infants as a low core body temperature; bradycardia; prolonged jaundice; dry skin and hair; low hairline; narrow palpebral fissures; wide-set eyes; depressed nasal bridge; puffy face; thick, protruding, enlarged tongue; dry skin; dull expression; large anterior (> 0.5 cm) and posterior fontanels; poor head control; poor muscle tone; hoarse cry; and poor feeding with resultant constipation.

Children with hypothyroidism have insidious changes that are barely noticeable or unrecognized by caregivers. The child is short for the age group with a puffy face and neck. Other physical findings include a decreased height-to-weight ratio; slow, thickened speech; croaking voice; bradycardia; cool, dry, scaly skin; decreased body hair; dry, lifeless hair; periorbital puffiness; constipation; enlarged calf muscles; and delay in the relaxation phase of deep tendon reflexes.

COMMON DISORDERS OF THE PARATHYROID GLAND IN CHILDREN

Parathyroid Dysfunction: Calcium Deficiency

Parathyroid dysfunction, or calcium deficiency, is caused by hypoparathyroidism, pseudoparathyroidism, or deficiency of vitamin D. Hypocalcemia caused by hypoparathyroidism presents as hyperreflexic knee jerk, delayed tooth development, Trousseau's sign (carpal spasm), Chvostek's sign (lip pursing), hand and feet cramps, parenthesis at the ends of the fingers, anxiety, and sometimes seizures. Cataracts are the result of long-term calcium deficiency.

Hypocalcemia caused by pseudoparathyroidism or vitamin D deficiency presents as moderate obesity and ovoid facies (i.e., long, thin face). Mild to moderate intellect deficit and short fourth or fifth metacarpals often occur.

Parathyroid Dysfunction: Calcium Excess

Hypercalcemia can be caused by hypersecretion of parathyroid hormone (PTH), but is usually caused by excessive amounts of vitamin D or A (or both). The child presents with symptoms of thirst, epigastric distress, irritability, lethargy, constipation, polyuria, and bedwetting. Infants have full cheeks, wide mouth, stellate iris (star-shaped) with supravalvular aortic stenosis. Mood changes (fussy and crying) and stomach pain associated with vomiting may also be present.

COMMON DISORDERS OF THE THYMUS IN CHILDREN

The thymus is located in the mediastinum, extending superiorly into the neck just below the thyroid. It is the central gland of the lymphatic system. Thymosin is the hormone that is produced. The thymus is largest at 2 years of age and involutes in adolescence. Problems with the thymus gland present as problems with the immune system.

COMMON DISORDERS OF THE ADRENAL GLANDS IN CHILDREN

The adrenal glands are located on the upper pole of the kidneys. Cortisol and aldosterone are essential for survival. Androgens are needed for initiating pubic and axillary hair development, skin and hair oiliness, and changes in the child's body build during preadolescent years.

Adrenal Gland Deficiency (Addison's Disease and Delayed Puberty)

Addison's disease is caused by an autoimmune process, infections (tuberculosis or fungal infection), neoplasm, or hemorrhage of the glands. Complete or partial adrenocortical failure may occur. Children may lose function of glucocorticoids, mineralcorticoids, and androgens. Onset is gradual. These children present with weakness, decreased endurance, hyperpigmentation of the skin and mucous membranes, anorexia, dehydration, weight loss, gastrointestinal disturbances, anxiety, depression, and emotional distress. They may also have intolerance to cold. Complications are caused by a decrease in extracellular fluid volume, hyperkalemia, and glucocorticoid deficit, which cause very high fever, psychotic behavior, and symptoms of shock.

Delayed puberty (failure along the hypothalamic-pituitary-gonadal axis) is characterized by absence of breast budding by age 13 years in girls or lack of testicular enlargement by age 14 years in boys. Causes of delayed puberty are outlined in Table 13–4.

TABLE 13–4. CAUSE OF DELAYED PUBERTY

Hypothalamus does not secrete GnRH
Pituitary tumor
Pituitary adenoma
Gonads unable to respond to LH
TSH deficit

LH = luteinizing hormone; GnRH = gonadotropin-releasing hormone; TSH = thyroid-stimulating hormone.

Adrenal Gland Excess: Cushing's Syndrome

Cushing's syndrome is caused by too much glucocorticoid and cortisol. It can also occur as a result of increased adrenocorticotrophic hormone (ACTH) producing a pituitary tumor. This problem manifests as recent weight gain, poor statural growth, fatigue, and mood changes. The weight gain is generally distributed evenly throughout the body but is very apparent in the face, trunk, and cervical region (i.e., buffalo hump). Lanugo (fine hair) may also grow downward from the forehead, from the occiput to the nape of the neck, and toward the lower lateral cheeks. The complexion is ruddy and plethoric. Growth may stop or slow. Muscle atrophy and decreased strength also occur. The skin and vasculature are thin, fragile, and susceptible to bruising. Adolescents may present with purplish striae of the skin, acne, and facial hirsutism. If there is an increase in androgens along with an increase of glucocorticoids, there will also be increased testicular size and secondary sexual hair. In addition, virilization may occur, causing deepening of the voice and enlargement of the clitoris or penis.

Adrenal Glands: Androgen Excess

Androgen excess can be classified as salt-losing or non–salt-losing excess. Salt-losing androgen excess presents as symptoms of shock, and non–salt-losing androgen excess presents as an unusual growth spurt and hyperandrogenism. Congenital adrenal hyperplasia is caused by a deficiency of 21-hydroxylase enzyme, which blocks the production of cortisol. This problem occurs *in utero* and presents in newborn girls as an enlarged clitoris, posterior labia fusion, and ambiguous external genitalia. Newborn boys with the disorder have a penis of normal or larger than normal size. Both boys and girls have a weak cry, lethargy, difficulty feeding, vomiting, and increased pigmentation anywhere on the body.

Precocious (premature) puberty occurs before a boy reaches age 9 years or a girl reaches age 8 years. In boys with testosterone excess, the testes enlarge and there is an increase in hair in the axillary and genitalia areas. They may also develop acne, oily hair, and adult-type body sweat odor. Girls who experience estrogen excess before age 9 years present with breast development, dark areolas, and nipple mounds. Also, the child may start menses, and the labia minora will enlarge and thicken. Leukorrhea, acne, oily hair,

TABLE 13–5. CAUSES OF PRECOCIOUS PUBERTY

Tumors: Brain, adrenal, gonadal
Hypothyroidism
Ovarian cysts
Genetic syndromes: McCune-Albright or Leydig cell hyperplasia
Exogenous sources: Viral or bacterial infection origination from the body or organ

axillary and genitalia hair, and adult-type body sweat odor may also occur. Table 13–5 outlines the causes of precocious puberty.

Hirsutism is hair growth in androgen-dependent areas under the chin; on the cheeks; between the breasts; and on the chest, shoulders, back, linea alba, abdomen, inner thighs, extremities, and digits.

Gynecomastia occurs in many teenage boys. It is caused by a temporary imbalance between estrogen and testosterone levels. The excess of estrogen causes breast and duct proliferation. It is a benign, reversible manifestation of puberty. Gynecomastia must be differentiated from a lipoma and from fatty tissue of obese patients.

Adrenal Glands: Androgen Insufficiency

Androgen insufficiency presents as fatigue, nonfading summer tan, listlessness, decreased muscle strength, dizziness, faintness on standing quickly, decreased appetite, salt craving, and weight loss.

Adrenal Glands: Excess: Aldosteronism (Conn's Disease)

Conn's disease is caused by a hypersecretion of aldosterone and is primarily a disease of the adrenal cortex. Primary aldosteronism is caused by adrenal hyperplasia or aldosterone-secreting tumors. Secondary aldosteronism is associated with plasma-renin activity and may be induced by nephritic syndrome, hepatic cirrhosis, congestive heart failure, trauma, burns, and stress. Symptoms, which are caused by sodium retention and potassium depletion, include hypertension, increased blood volume, alkalosis, muscle weakness, tetany, paresthesias, nephropathy, ventricle arrhythmias, polydipsia, and polyuria.

COMMON DISORDERS OF THE PANCREAS IN CHILDREN

Pancreas: Insulin Excess

Too much insulin leads to lowered blood sugar levels, resulting in hypoglycemic shock, symptoms of nervousness, sweating, chills, irritability, hunger, and pallor.

Pancreas: Insulin Deficiency (Diabetes Mellitus)

Diabetes mellitus is the hyposecretion of insulin with sudden childhood onset usually after a viral illness. Characteristics of diabetes mellitus are polydipsia, polyuria, overeating, weight loss, fatigue, and irritability.

TEST YOUR KNOWLEDGE OF CHAPTER 13

1. What history and review of system components are needed to assess the endocrine system?
2. What physical assessment findings would point you toward an endocrine diagnosis?
3. What physical findings are found with pituitary excess and pituitary deficiency?
4. What physical findings are found with thyroid excess and thyroid deficiency?
5. What physical findings are found with parathyroid excess and parathyroid deficiency?
6. What type of problems might be assessed in a child with a thymus deficiency?
7. What physical findings are found with adrenal excess and adrenal deficiency?
8. What physical findings are found with androgen excess and androgen deficiency?
9. Compare precocious puberty with delayed puberty.
10. What physical findings are found with insulin excess and insulin deficiency?

 ## BIBLIOGRAPHY

Algranati, P. S. (1992). The *pediatric patient: An approach to history and physical examination*. Baltimore: Williams & Wilkins.

Goldbloom, R. B. (1997). *Pediatric clinical skills*. Philadelphia: Churchill Livingstone.

Jarvis, C. (2000). *Physical examination and health assessment*. Philadelphia: W. B. Saunders.

Ruppert, S. D., Kernicki, J. G., & Dolan, J. T. (2000). *Dolan's critical care nursing*. Philadelphia: F. A. Davis.

Seidel, H. M., Ball, J. W., Dains, J. E, & Benedict, G. W. (2001). *Mosby's guide to physical examination*. St. Louis: Mosby.

Sierry, G. K., & Iannone, R. (2000). *The Harriet Lane handbook*. St. Louis: Mosby.

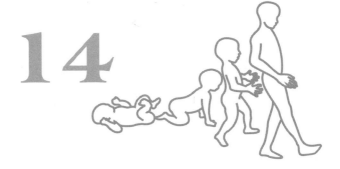

14

Assessment of the Genitourinary System

MARGARET R. COLYAR

OBJECTIVES
- *Develop appropriate techniques for examination of the genitalia in boys and girls.*
- *Ascertain age-appropriate gynecological examination of girls.*

Do not neglect examining the genitalia. Examination of the genitalia may reveal unsuspected abnormalities that may need treatment. The examination, whether on a boy or a girl, must be performed tactfully and skillfully to diffuse anxiety and tension

 HISTORY

Ask about the medical history of genitourinary problems. Determine if the child has had any surgical procedures in the genital or urinary system. Determine if the child is taking any medications that would affect the genitourinary system, what allergies the child has, and the immunization status. When taking the family history, include questions about cancer of the bladder, kidneys, uterus, cervix, ovaries, penis, testes, and prostate. In the review of systems, include questions about pain, lesions, and discharge from the vagina in girls and from the penis in boys. For adolescents, ask about sexual relations, sexually transmitted diseases, and menstrual history. The review of systems should also include questions about frequency; urgency; nocturia; dysuria; hesitancy; straining; urine color; and genital pain, lesions, and discharge.

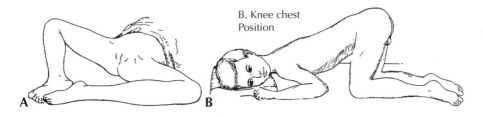

FIG. 14–1. Positions for female gynecological examination. (*A*) Frog-leg position. (*B*) Knee-chest position.

PHYSICAL EXAMINATION

GIRLS

Approach

Provide privacy and respect modesty. Using a soft, reassuring voice, chat about unrelated issues (e.g., school, sports, TV, friends, family, hobbies) during the examination. Demonstrate a matter-of-fact, confident, and relaxed attitude. Be unhurried but businesslike. Use a firm, deliberate touch and no stroking or soft touch.

Position

Infants and Toddlers: Frog-Leg Position Have the child in the semirecumbent position on the parent's lap with the hips flexed and abducted. Gently retract the labia majora laterally (Fig. 14–1).

Toddlers, Preschoolers, School-age Children: Knee-Chest Position Have the child in the knee-chest position with the knees 10 to 15 cm apart and the abdomen sagging on the anterior thighs. Gently retract the labia majora to one side. You should be able to see the entire length of the vagina and frequently the cervix. Use an otoscope to visualize. *Do not* let the otoscope touch the external genitalia or vagina.

External Genitalia

Note the condition of the labia majora, labia minora, mucocolpos, muscles, hymen, urethral meatus, and clitoris (Fig. 14–2). Look for labial adhesions (agglutination), which suggest chronic inflammation. Smegma and leukorrhea are common. If there is any unusual drainage present, obtain a culture.

Cultures in Prepubertal Girls

Moisten a swab with saline or sterile water. Have the child assume the knee-chest position or lie supine with the knees bent. Pass the swab into the vagina without touching the hymen (very sensitive) and send it to the laboratory for analysis.

159

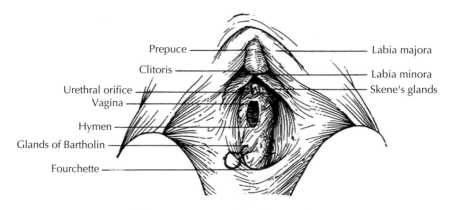

FIG. 14–2. External female genitalia.

Internal Genitalia

Vaginoscopy Perform vaginoscopy only if it is absolutely needed. The reasons for vaginoscopy are undiagnosed vaginal bleeding, refractory vaginal discharge, and suspected intravaginal foreign body. Apply 2% viscous lidocaine to the hymen. Lubricate the pediatric anoscope or otoscope speculum with warm water and gently insert it. The vagina is only 4 to 5 cm in length in prepubertal girls. Make sure that the child understands what you are doing and has seen the equipment. If the child is anxious, postpone the procedure.

Pelvic Examination

If this is the first gynecological examination, explain what you are going to do. Evaluate the child using the Tanner sexual maturity rating scale (see Chapter 3). Observe the external genitalia, keeping endocrine changes in mind (Table 14–1). Use a pediatric speculum of the appropriate size. Show the child the speculum and explain its use. Put the child in the lithotomy position with the knees loosely apart. Encourage relaxation and deep breathing. Lubricate the speculum with K-Y Jelly or warm water. Spread the labia to prevent pinching and insert gently in a downward path with posterior pressure to prevent compression of the urethra, which is very sensitive (Fig. 14–3). Visualize the vaginal walls and vault. Open the blades and bring the cervix into view. Inspect and swab if necessary. An endocervical specimen is best (see Fig. 14–4).

Vagina The vaginal vault should be pink, moist, and without lesions.

Cervix The cervical os (opening) should be round. After giving birth vaginally, the cervical os is slitlike. Many times, adolescents have reddened columnar epithelia around the cervical meatus. This is normal and does not suggest cervicitis.

160

TABLE 14–1. ENDOCRINE CHANGES ON THE FEMALE EXTERNAL GENITALIA

Androgen excess
- Axillary hair
- Sweat odor like that of adults
- Acne, oiliness of skin
- Hirsutism

Estrogen effect
- Mucosal appearance with secretions
- Thickening of the perihymenal tissue
- Increased development of the mons pubis, labia majora, and labia minora
- Leukorrhea

Bimanual Examination

Young Children The uterus should be located in the midline abdominal cavity in young girls. Using one finger lubricated with K-Y Jelly, lift the uterus upward toward the abdominal hand, which should be well above the suprapubic area. Check for size, shape, and position in the abdomen and mobility. The ovaries cannot be checked in the young girls because they are still high in the abdomen.

Adolescents The uterus should be down in the pelvis by this age. Using one finger lubricated with K-Y Jelly, lift the uterus upward toward the abdomi-

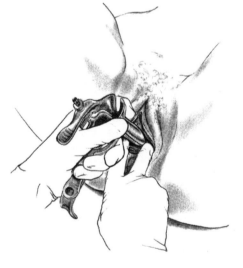

FIG. 14–3. Pelvic examination. Insert the speculum downward to decrease discomfort.

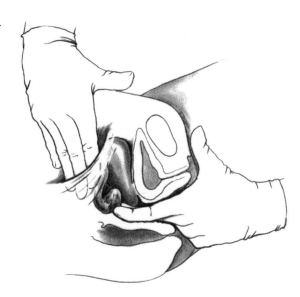

FIG. 14–4. Bimanual examination.

nal hand, which should be above the suprapubic area. Check for size (golf ball size if nulliparous), shape, and position in the pelvis; mobility; and degree of tenderness. Sweep the vaginal finger right and left and gently sweep the abdominal hand starting at the iliac crest downward. The normal ovary size is that of an almond. Figure 14–4 shows the bimanual examination.

Rectovaginal Examination

Insert one gloved finger in the vagina and one in the rectal vault. Gently sweep the two fingers to each side, checking for thickening or nodules on the septum. Do a stool hemoccult test if stool is obtained.

Documentation

Documentation of the pelvic and bimanual examination should include Tanner sexual maturity staging and the condition of the external genitalia, vagina, cervix, uterus, and ovaries, indicating the presence of lesions and discharge with size and location. Examples are as follows:

> Normal: Tanner 2. External genitalia without lesions. Vagina pink and moist, cervical os round without lesions or discharge, no cervical motion tenderness, uterus smooth, ovaries intact.

> Abnormal: Tanner 3. One-cm papule on left labia majora without erythema or tenderness. Vagina pink with thick white discharge adhering to vaginal walls. Cervical os round with grayish discharge; no lesions. Positive cervical motion tenderness. Left ovary larger than right and tender on palpation.

BOYS

Approach

Provide privacy and respect modesty. Using a soft, reassuring voice, chat about unrelated issues (e.g., school, sports, TV, friends, family, hobbies) during the examination. Demonstrate a matter-of-fact, confident, and relaxed attitude. Be unhurried but businesslike. Use a firm, deliberate touch and no stroking or soft touch.

Position

Newborns, Infants, and Toddlers Have younger children lie supine with the knees apart.

Preschoolers and Young School-Age Children Have older children sit cross-legged.

Older School-Age Children and Adolescents As the child reaches late school age and adolescence, have him or her sit on the examination table or stand with the legs apart.

Inguinal Lymph Nodes

Palpate slightly below the bend of the leg and hip. Nodes are usually less than 1 cm and are soft, discrete, and moveable.

Penis

Normally the penis is hairless and without lesions. Palpate the shaft between the thumb and two fingers. It should be smooth, semi-firm, and nontender. A ventral curved shaft in newborns is known as chordee and should have further evaluation. Chordee is often associated the hypospadias. If the child is uncircumcised, retract the foreskin if the boy is older than age 3 years (the foreskin is not fully retractable until age 3 years). The foreskin should move easily. Do not forget to return the foreskin to position to prevent paraphimosis. Palpate the glans, which should be smooth and without lesions. Compress the glans and note the urethral meatus. The urethral meatus edge should be pink, smooth, and without discharge. The urethral meatus should be positioned centrally on the glans. Hypospadias is a meatus on the ventral side of the penis, and epispadias is a meatus on the dorsal side of the penis. Both hypospadias and epispadias should be evaluated for surgical repair.

Pubic Hair

The presence or absence should be consistent with age. Check for any lice or nits.

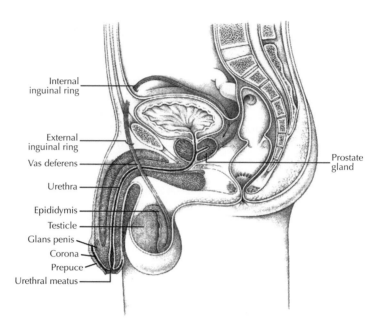

FIG. 14–5. External male genitalia.

Internal inguinal ring
External inguinal ring
Vas deferens
Urethra
Epididymis
Testicle
Glans penis
Corona
Prepuce
Urethral meatus
Prostate gland

Scrotum

Note the size of the testes. Use "testicle beads" for accurate measurement. Gently palpate the testes with the thumb and first two fingers from the top to bottom for size, shape, consistency, and tenderness. Identify the spermatic cord and vas deferens from epididymis to external inguinal ring. The epididymis is softer than the testes, smooth, and nontender. Note the presence of rugae and median raphe (line of union) (Fig. 14–5).

Palpate gently for masses. If a mass is present, include all of the following in your differential diagnosis: hernia, tumor, orchitis (inflammation of the testes), epididymitis (inflammation of the epididymis), hydrocele (accumulation of fluid in the scrotum), spermatocele (cystic swelling of the epididymis or testes), and varicocele (swelling of the spermatic cord).

In newborns, infants, and toddlers, check for undescended testicles. Retractile testes are normal. If you cannot move the testicle into the scrotum, it is undescended (cryptorchidism), which can lead to sterility. To check for undescended testicles, push down with one finger gently above the testes at the inguinal canal and palpate the scrotum between the thumb and forefinger for presence of the testicle. To check preschoolers and older boys, palpate for normal oval, firm, rubbery testes without lumps or lesions. If descent has not occurred by age 1 year, refer the child for possible surgical correction. If you are unsure, transilluminate the scrotum.

Transillumination When a mass other than testes or spermatic cord is suspected, transilluminate to determine if fluid, gas, or a solid mass is present.

164

Darken the room. Shine a light from behind the scrotum through the mass. Look for a light as a red glow. With fluid and gas, the red light will glow or show through. If blood or tissue is present, the red glow will not show through.

Inguinal Hernia

With a gloved hand, direct the forefinger up along the penis shaft into the external inguinal ring (feels like an indented area). Have the child shift his weight onto the other leg and turn his head away from the side being palpated and cough. If a hernia is present, a bulge will be felt. Large hernias invaginate the scrotal sac, and the sac will appear enlarged.

Femoral Hernia

Femoral hernias usually bulge outside the scrotum. Palpate the femoral area for a bulge. Usually there is none. If one is present, refer to a surgeon.

Documentation

Documentation of the male examination should include Tanner sexual maturity staging, report of all male genitalia structures, and all abnormalities with size and location. Examples are as follows:

> Normal: Tanner 2. Circumcised penis without lesions. Meatus midline on glans. External scrotum without lesions, no edema. Testes descended bilaterally, without nodules, nontender. Spermatic cord smooth; epididymus soft. No inguinal or femoral hernia palpable.

> Abnormal: Tanner 4. Uncircumcised penis with meatus midline on glans with purulent discharge. Scrotum twice as big on right as left. Testes descended bilaterally, without nodule, tender on right. Spermatic cord ropelike on right; smooth on left. Epididymis hard and tender on right; soft and nontender on left. Right inguinal hernia palpable. No femoral hernia palpable.

TEST YOUR KNOWLEDGE OF CHAPTER 14

1. What are the components of a history and review of systems for the gynecological system?
2. What are the appropriate positions for the gynecological examination by age group?
3. What external structures should be observed in the gynecological examination?
4. Describe how to do a pelvic and bimanual examination on a child.
5. What changes can be found in the adolescent cervix?

6. What are the appropriate positions for the male urogenital examination by age group?
7. What external structures should be observed in the male urogenital examination?
8. Describe how to perform inguinal and femoral hernia examinations.
9. What endocrine (androgen and estrogen) changes can be detected in the female external genitalia?

BIBLIOGRAPHY

Algranati, P. S. (1992). *The pediatric patient: An approach to history and physical examination.* Baltimore: Williams & Wilkins.
Emans, S. J., Laufer, M. R., & Goldstein, D. P (1998). *Pediatric and adolescent gynecology.* Philadelphia: Lippincott-Raven.
Goldbloom, R. B. (1997). *Pediatric clinical skills.* Philadelphia: Churchill Livingstone.
Jarvis, C. (2000). *Physical examination and health assessment.* Philadelphia: W. B. Saunders.
Sanfilippo, J. S. (2001). *Pediatric and adolescent gynecology.* Philadelphia:W. B. Saunders.
Seidel, H. M., Ball, J. W., Dains, J. E., & Benedict, G. W. (2001). *Mosby's guide to physical examination.* St. Louis: Mosby.

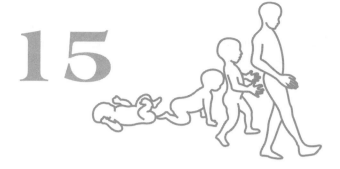

Assessment of the Integumentary System

Margaret R. Colyar

A child's skin is more reactive than an adult's skin. Assessment of a child's skin can give you clues about the child, both internally and externally. Good lighting is essential to do an adequate assessment of the skin. Both direct and tangential lighting are necessary for a complete skin examination. To begin, become aware of the common skin lesions in children (Table 15–1) so that when you observe them, you will not waste time considering many differential diagnoses.

HISTORY

Ask about the medical history of skin problems such as eczema, psoriasis, pityriasis, warts, molluscum contagiosum, melanoma, tinea, scabies, acne, herpes, birthmarks, or contact dermatitis. Ask if the child has had any skin lesion removed. In the family history, include questions about skin cancer and melanoma. Determine if the child is taking any medications that would affect the integumentary system. In the review of systems, include questions about changes in skin pigmentation, changes in moles (size or color), exces-

TABLE 15–1. COMMON SKIN LESIONS IN CHILDREN

Skin Lesions	Appearance
Acne	Plugged hair follicles • Open comedones (blackheads; caused by oxidation of the plugged material) • Closed comedones (whiteheads) • Papules, pustules, nodules, and cysts on the face, chest, back, and shoulders
Allergic drug reaction (wheals or urticaria)	Symmetric generalized erythematous papules; pruritic, red, raised patches of varying sizes with central paleness
Alopecia (traumatic)	Patches of hair loss caused by trauma from rollers, tight braiding, tight pony tails, and barrettes
Atopic dermatitis (eczema)	Pruritic erythematous papules and vesicles with weeping, oozing, and crusts on the scalp, forehead, cheeks, forearms, wrists, and flexor surfaces of the elbows and backs of knees
Café-au-lait spots	Large oval patch of light brown pigmentation; the presence of more than six spots is associated with neurofibromatosis
Chickenpox (varicella)	Small, tight, vesicular crops that first appear on the trunk and then spread to the face, arms, and legs (not palms and soles); becomes pustular, followed by crusting
Contact dermatitis	Local papular erythema sometimes with vesicles and weeping (poison ivy or poison oak) caused by an irritant in the environment or an allergy
Diaper dermatitis	Red, moist, macular patch with poorly defined borders
Herpes simplex (cold sores)	Vesicles and thin pustules that crust on lips
Intertrigo (candidiasis)	Scalding red, moist patches with sharply defined borders and satellite lesions
Impetigo	Moist vesicles and crusts with thin erythematous base and honey-colored drainage
Lice and nits	Live lice, tiny white ovoid eggs (nits) adherent to hair shafts
Measles (rubeola)	Red-purple maculopapular rash; starts behind ears, then spreads to face, neck, trunk, arms, and legs; does not blanch; Koplik's spots in mouth that are bluish-white, red-based elevations of 1 to 3 mm
Measles, German (rubella)	Pale pink papular rash that starts on the face and spreads to the arms and trunk; no Koplik's spots; presence of cervical adenopathy bilaterally
Pityriasis rosea	Herald patch with slightly scaling, pink, macular rash spreading over trunk and unexposed areas of the body
Psoriasis	Present during adolescence; erythematous patches covered by thick, dry, silvery, adherent scales; more common on extensor surfaces, bony prominences, scalp, ears, genitalia, and perianal area; arthritis in distal small joints may be present.

(Continued)

TABLE 15–1. COMMON SKIN LESIONS IN CHILDREN	
Skin Lesions	Appearance
Scabies	Faint linear tunnels in the superficial epidermis; if undetected for several months, they change to crusted nodules; in newborns and infants, they cover the entire body; in older children, the head is spared.
Seborrheic dermatitis (cradle cap)	Thick, yellow, greasy, adherent scales on the scalp and forehead; no pruritus
Scarlatina (scarlet fever)	Group A beta-hemolytic streptococcus; erythematous, dry, sandpaper-like diffuse rash on the entire body; strawberry tongue and Pastia's lines (darker red lines in flexor surfaces)
Tinea corporis (ringworm)	Fungal infection; circular erythematous patches; papular, annular scales with well-defined edge and central umbilication; appear anywhere on the body
Tinea pedis (athlete's foot)	Fungal infection; small vesicles and skin breaks between the toes and the sides of feet and soles
Tinea versicolor	Fungal infection; multiple oval macules with fine scales found on the neck, chest, upper back, shoulders, and upper arms of children and adolescents; color depends on skin pigmentation; on dark or tanned skin, lesions appear hypopigmented; in winter as the pigment fades, lesions appear tan or dark brown
Warts (verruca)	Viral epidermal neoplasms; hard and crusty or flat and smooth

sive dryness or moisture, pruritus, excessive bruising, rashes or lesions, medications, hair loss, changes in nails, environmental hazards, and self-care behaviors. Determine if the child has any medication, environmental, or food allergies.

PHYSICAL EXAMINATION

Observe the general condition of the skin, including the hair, nails, and mucous membranes. Hair should be shiny and even. The nails should be smooth, slightly curved, or flat. The mucous membranes should be moist. No edema should be present. Note birthmarks, scarring, and nevi. Look for abnormal abrasions, rashes, or cracking.

INSPECTION AND OBSERVATION

Location

Inspect the entire skin surface, including visible mucous membranes, hair, nails, and sweat glands. If a rash is present, determine if it is symmetrical, generalized, or localized.

TABLE 15–2. PRIMARY SKIN LESIONS		
Lesion	**Description**	**Example**
Macules*	< 1 cm in size, flat	Freckles, tinea versicolor
Patches*	Larger macules	Port-wine stain, vitiligo, café-au-lait spots
Papules†	< 1 cm, solid elevated	Wart, lichen planus, psoriasis, distinct borders
Plaques†	Solid elevated, > 0.5 cm	Flat top, indistinct borders
Nodules†	> 1 cm, elevated	Rheumatoid nodule
Tumors†	Large nodule	
Wheals or urticaria†	Palpable, red, circumscribed swelling	Hives
Vesicles‡	Raised, containing clear fluid	Blister, herpes simplex, herpes zoster
Bullae‡	Large vesicle	Bullous pemphigoid
Pustules‡	Vesicle with white cellular debris	Acne, folliculitis
Cyst‡	Sac contains fluid or semi-solid exudates	Sebaceous cyst, ganglion cyst
Comedo†§	Plugged hair follicle with keratin and sebum	Acne
Burrow†‡	Horizontal tunnel	Scabies
Telangiactasia*	Dilated small arterial or capillary	Rosacea, blood vessels on skin surface
Purpura*	Discoloration of skin caused by presence of vasculitis, trauma, of blood in tissue; will not blanch	Platelet deficiency
Petechia*	Tiny lesion of purpura	
Hematoma‡	Moderate-sized mass of purpura	Subungual hematoma
Ecchymosis	Large area of purpura	Bruise

* = Nonpalpable.
† = Palpable.
‡ = Fluid filled.
§ = Above skin surface.

Color

Determine the color of the rash. Describe exactly what you see. A rash or lesion may be one or more than one color.

Types of Lesions

Note the type of rash or lesion based on the accepted categories. Skin lesions are categorized as primary or secondary (Tables 15–2 and 15–3). Figures 15–1 and 15–2 illustrate some of the lesions.

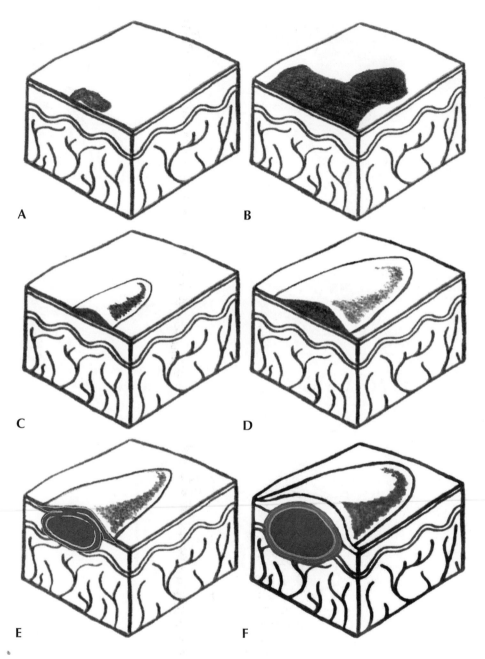

FIG. 15–1 (*A*) Macule. (*B*) Patch. (*C*) Papule. (*D*) Plaque. (*E*) Nodule. (*F*) Tumor.
Illustration continued on following page

171

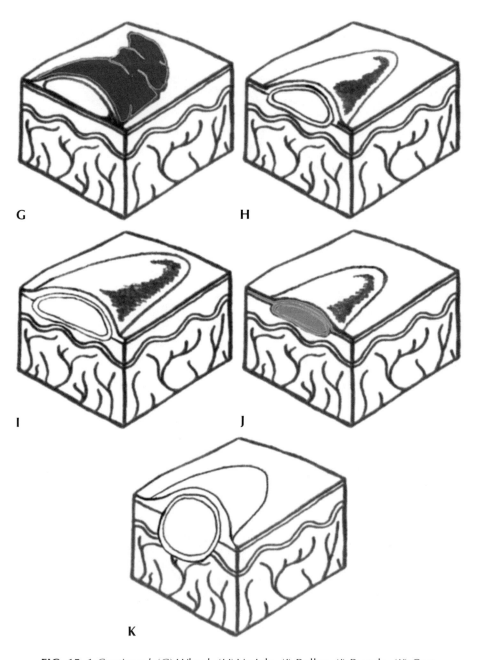

FIG. 15–1 *Continued* (*G*) Wheal. (*H*) Vesicle. (*I*) Bullae. (*J*) Pustule. (*K*) Cyst.

TABLE 15–3. SECONDARY SKIN LESIONS

Lesions	Description	Example
Scaling*	Flaking of the skin	Ichthyosis
Crusts*	Dried exudates	Impetigo, eczema
Lichenification*	Thickened and rough layers of skin	Chronic contact dermatitis caused by rubbing
Atrophy*	Thinning or wasting of tissue	Use of topical steroids
Epidermal atrophy	Decrease in epidermal tissue	Pigment changes, loss of skin lines
Dermal atrophy	Loss of dermal tissue	Skin depression
Excoriations	Loss of epidermal layers, exposing dermis	Abrasion
Fissures	Horizontal split in the skin	Surgical incision
Linear, wedged-shaped cracks	In vulva, as result of yeast infection	
Erosions or ulcers	Loss of epidermis	Chancre of syphilis, ruptured chickenpox
Scar	Fibrous connective tissue caused by healing	Keloid

* = Above skin surface.

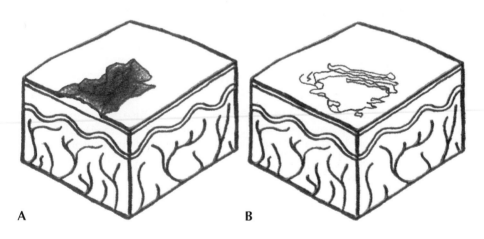

FIG. 15–2 (A) Crust. (B) Atrophy.

TABLE 15-4. PITTING EDEMA: SUBJECTIVE SCALE

1+ (mild edema)
4+ (deep pitting)

Documentation

Document the size, pattern or shape, color, elevation, location, temperature, moisture, and any exudates or edema. Be as descriptive as possible. An example is as follows:

> 1-cm irregular, two-toned brown papule on dorsal mid-right forearm, warm, dry, without edema or exudate.

PALPATION

Temperature

Check with the dorsal (back) of hand. Hypothermia is generalized coolness and is associated with circulatory shock. Hyperthermia can be caused by fever, exercise, infection, or inflammation.

Moisture

The mucous membranes should be moist if the child is well hydrated and dry if he or she is dehydrated. Palpate for elasticity by gently pinching the skin of the anterior chest or abdomen between the thumb and first digit. Release and note if immediate recoil or tenting is present. Tenting is associated with dehydration.

Edema

Fluid accumulation in the intercellular spaces can cause the skin to look puffy and tight. Edema may be pitting or nonpitting (Table 15-4). Unilateral edema is caused by local causes such as venous insufficiency, cellulitis, and trauma. Bilateral edema is caused by central causes such as congestive heart failure and kidney problems.

Hair and Scalp

Hair should be shiny and even (see Chapter 5). Common abnormalities in children include traumatic alopecia, lice or nits, seborrhea, tinea capitis, and hirsutism. Hirsutism that presents as male-pattern baldness in girls is caused by endocrine abnormalities.

Nails

Inspect and palpate. The nails should be smooth, slightly curved, or flat. Note the angle of the nail base, which should be approximately 160 degrees

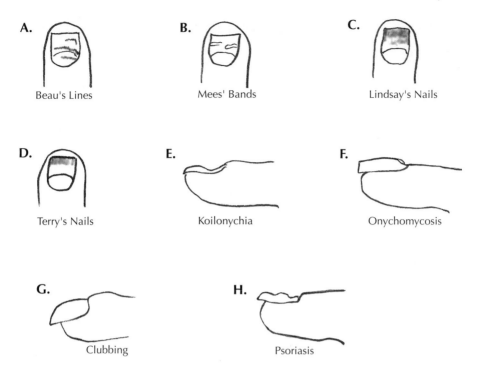

A. Beau's Lines

B. Mees' Bands

C. Lindsay's Nails

D. Terry's Nails

E. Koilonychia

F. Onychomycosis

G. Clubbing

H. Psoriasis

FIG. 15–3. Abnormal shapes of nails.

or curved 160 degrees or less (see Chapter 8). Clubbing is defined as a nail base greater than 180 degrees. The nail bed should be firm, not brittle or splitting as it is in early clubbing. Pits, grooves, or lines indicate nutritional deficiencies. Nails that are thickened with ridges indicate arterial insufficiency. Spoon-shaped nails (koilonychia) are seen in individuals with anemia. The nails are thin and depressed with the lateral edges tilted up. Paronychia is a red, swollen, tender inflammation of the nail fold. Onycholysis is separation for the nail from the nail bed, usually caused by fungus under the nail. Ingrown nails present as swelling and inflammation that occur at lateral nail folds. Subungual hematoma is trauma to the nail plate. Abnormal shapes of nails and disease processes (Fig. 15–3) are frequently noted in the well-child visit.

NEWBORN SKIN AND RASHES

Many rashes and lesions occur at birth or during the first few months of life. Become familiar with these so that you will be able to let the parents know what to expect (Table 15–5). Newborn skin color changes are shown in Table 15–6.

175

TABLE 15-5. NEWBORN SKIN RASHES, LESIONS, AND BIRTHMARKS

Lesions	Description
Lanugo	Fine hair covering body; more prevalent in premature infants; decreased with full-term and overdue infants
Vernix caseosa	Cheesy white substance that covers the entire body
Milia	Seen in 40% of newborns; white, opalescent pin-sized spots found mostly on the face and bridge of nose caused by obstructed sebaceous ducts; resolves within 1–2 weeks
Miliaria rubra	Obstructed sweat ducts caused by a warm, humid environment; looks like tiny, irritated papules or vesicles with erythematous base (prickly heat), usually resolve within 1 week
Vascular nevi (stork bite or angel kiss)	Capillary hemangiomas are seen in 50% of newborns; pink in color and blanch easily; usually found on the eyelids, nose, and nape of the neck
Port-wine stain or nevus flammeus	Dilated congested capillaries that do not go away; flat, red, purple or black in color; blanch only slightly; and are found usually on the face and scalp; if unsightly, require laser plastic surgery
Mongolian spots	Hyperpigmented areas anywhere on the body caused by an infiltration of the dermis by melanocytes; normal variant with no clinical significance; usually fade over the first 2 years of life; 90% of mongolian spots are found on the lower back of children of African-American, Asian, or Hispanic descent
Erythema toxicum neonatorum	Pinpoint, red-based macules caused by eosinophils; seen on the cheeks and trunk; disappear by the third day
Hemangioma simplex or strawberry mark	Soft, raised papules that usually enlarge in the first 6 to 10 months of life, then shrink and usually disappear by age 2 years; can appear anywhere on the body
Transient neonatal pustular melanosis	Occurs in 10% of newborns, usually African American; pus-filled vesicles that break down and make brown or black spots on the skin
Bruising	Occurs from birth trauma; note where it is located and the extent of the bruising; significant bruising causes a decrease in circulating blood

TABLE 15–6. COLOR CHANGES IN THE SKIN OF NEWBORNS	
Color	Indication
Red	Plethora or excess fluid in the blood vessels or total quantity of fluid in the body; polycythemia or hyperviscosity
Beefy red	Hypoglycemia
Red on one side, white on the other	Harlequin sign; 50% of the body (head to toe) pale, the other half dark pink or red; transient normal finding
White	Anemia, blood loss, vernix caseosa, or circulatory failure
Blue	Central cyanosis; acrocyanosis (feet and hands are blue); circumoral cyanosis (blue or pale discoloration around the mouth)
Yellow	Jaundice; hemoglobin in light-skinned children is 5 mg/100 mL; hemoglobin in dark-skinned children is < 5 mg/100 mL

TEST YOUR KNOWLEDGE OF CHAPTER 15

1. What are the components of the history and review of systems for the integumentary system?
2. What are the components of the physical examination of the integumentary system?
3. What are problems seen on the nails, and what is their etiology?
4. What are the common skin lesions in children? Describe them.
5. What are the types of primary skin lesions? Describe them.
6. What are the types of secondary skin lesions? Describe them.
7. What are the common skin rashes and birthmarks in children? Describe them.
8. When a skin lesion is discovered, what are the components of documentation necessary to describe the lesion?

BIBLIOGRAPHY

Algranati, P. S. (1992). *The pediatric patient: An approach to history and physical examination.* Baltimore: Williams & Wilkins.
Goldbloom, R. B. (1997). *Pediatric clinical skills.* Philadelphia: Churchill Livingstone.
Jarvis, C. (2000). *Physical examination and health assessment.* Philadelphia: W. B. Saunders.
Seidel, H. M., Ball, J. W., Dains, J. E., & Benedict, G. W. (2001). *Mosby's guide to physical examination.* St. Louis: Mosby.

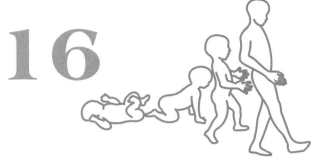

Assessment of Congenital Anomalies, Chromosomal Disorders, and Inherited Disorders

MARGARET R. COLYAR AND
GILLIAN TUFTS

OBJECTIVES
- *Differentiate between minor and major congenital anomalies.*
- *Understand how chromosomal disorders are transmitted.*
- *Recognize significant physical assessment findings in selected chromosomal syndromes.*
- *Ascertain relevant counseling that should take place regarding certain chromosomal syndromes.*

Certain physical findings seen in children can alert you to the potential of congenital anomalies and chromosomal disorders. Some of the congenital anomalies are minor and isolated. These are usually of no significance. Other congenital anomalies are major and occur in combination. *Congenital* means present at birth; however, some congenital anomalies do not become evident until later in life. In this chapter, a timetable of human prenatal development and overall assessment guidelines are presented along with minor and major congenital anomalies and chromosomal syndromes that occur frequently and that ambulatory care providers can manage. Syndromes that are very severe, resulting in death soon after birth or in the first year of life, are not included. The most common chromosomal disorders you will encounter include Down, fetal alcohol, Klinefelter's, Noonan's, trisomy 8, Turner's, and Waardenburg syndromes and neurofibromatosis. Inherited disorders by recessive transmission of Tay-Sachs disease, sickle cell anemia, and cystic fibrosis are also included (Table 16–1).

The entire process of growth, maturation, differentiation, and development occurs between conception and birth. When an egg is fertilized, it immediately begins the course to fetal maturity. Being aware of the fetal maturation timetable can help you determine when an abnormality occurred. Various viruses, malnutrition, trauma, mutations, teratogens, or maternal disease may affect the morphologic development of a rapidly differentiating structure or organ during the embryologic stage. After 14 weeks, when all organs, systems, and parts of the body have formed, any adverse effects are largely functional; major morphologic damage does not occur.

 # OVERALL ASSESSMENT GUIDELINES

When anomalies are found, always consider the parents. The trait may be familial but not indicative of a chromosomal syndrome. There are minor and major anomalies (Table 16–2). Single anomalies are common in the general population. Two anomalies are less common. More than two are usually associated with a chromosomal syndrome.

GENETIC TRANSMISSION OVERVIEW

The human has 23 pairs of chromosomes. Chromosomes are thread-shaped bodies contained within the nucleus of a cell that determine characteristics that will be passed on to offspring. The first 22 pairs of chromosomes are called autosomes, and the 23rd pair is made up of the two sex/gender chromosomes. Chromosomes carry genes, which are a section of codes on a deoxyribonucleic acid (DNA) strand. They are the smallest functional unit for transmission of a hereditary trait.

Alleles are different genes that can affect the same trait. For every allelic gene on one chromosome of a pair, a corresponding allele exists in the same position on the other chromosome of the pair. Homozygous alleles are alleles in a pair that are identical. Heterozygous alleles are alleles in a pair that are different.

 # INHERITANCE

There are three basic types of inheritance (Table 16–3): dominant, recessive, and X-linked. In addition, inheritance is affected by consanguinity, mosaicism, gene mutation, and teratogens.

Week	Development
	TABLE 16–1. TIMETABLE OF HUMAN PRENATAL DEVELOPMENT
1	Fertilization
	Zygote divides
	Early and last blastocyst formation
	Implantation begins
	Amniotic cavity development begins
2	Primitive yolk sac develops
	Blastocyst is completely implanted
	Primitive placental circulation established
	Embryo starts to develop
3	Embryo development continues; trilaminar embryo
	Neural plate and neural fold development
	Brain and thyroid development begin
	Heart tubes begin to fuse
4	Heart begins to beat
	Neural folds fuse
	Rudimentary gut, lungs, and kidneys form
	Heart bulges appear, neuropore closes, three pairs of branchial arches appear, otic pit appears
	Arm and leg buds appear, four pairs of branchial arches form
5	Nasal pits forming
	Hand plates (paddle shaped), lens pits, and optic cups form
	Brain has begun to grow rapidly, heart tube is divided into chambers
	Head much larger than trunk, cerebral vesicles distinct, leg buds (paddle-shaped)
6	Palate and upper lip form, arms bent at elbow, finger rays and auricular hillocks distinct, palate developing
7	Eyelids beginning, tip of nose distinct, toe rays appear, ossification begins, urogenital membrane and anal membrane appear; gender differentiation takes place
	Trunk elongating and straightening
	All essential systems are present
8	Upper limbs longer and bent at elbows, fingers distinct, anal membrane perforated, urogenital membrane degenerating, testes and ovaries distinguishable
	External genitals still in sexless state but have begun to differentiate
	Genital tubercle, urethral groove, and anus differentiate
	Beginnings of all essential external and internal structures are present
9	Beginning of fetal period—period of rapid growth
	Genitals continue to develop
10	Face has human profile; head is almost half of total length
	Genitals continue to develop
11	Rapid growth continues
12	Features of face have formed, and eyelids are present but not closed; palate is fusing; neck appears between large head and body; tooth buds and nail beds begin to form; identification of genitals is possible
13–16	Arms, legs, and trunk grow rapidly; fetus becomes active; scalp hair develops; skeleton is calcified; respiratory movements may be detected
17–20	First fetal movement is felt, eyebrows and tiny nipples form, sucks thumb and grabs umbilical cord
21–24	External ears are smooth and soft, skin is wrinkled and translucent, body is covered with lanugo and vernix
25–28	Subcutaneous fat begins to develop, fingernails and toenails are present, eyelids separate, eyes may open, scalp hair is well developed
29–term	Growth and elaboration occur

TABLE 16–2. MINOR AND MAJOR CONGENITAL ANOMALIES

Body Part	Anomalies

MINOR: Single anomalies are common in the general population and usually of no concern unless more than two occur together

Body Part	Anomalies
Face	Broad face
	Pinched face
Hair	Low-set posterior hairline
	Abnormal color
	Kinky, coarse, sparse, hypopigmented
	White forelock
	Widow's peak
	Male pattern baldness
	Upswept posterior hairline
	More than one whorl
	Electric hair
Eyes	Upper or lower slanting of the palpebral fissures
	Wide- or close-set eyes
	Nystagmus or strabismus
	Cataracts
	Lens: Stellate pattern
	Epicanthal folds
	Almond-shaped eyes
	Synophrys (fused eyebrows)
	Entropion
	Lacrimal duct stenosis
Ears	Small or low-set ears
	Round ears
	Ear tags or pits
	Punched-out grooves at back of ears
	Darwinian tubercle
	Indented upper helix
	Attached lobes, absent lobes, unattached lobes
	Creased earlobes
	Cleft or perforated earlobes
	Hairy ears
Nose	Flat nasal bridge
	Low nasal bridge
	Bulbous nose
	Short nose
	Downturned nasal tip
Mouth	Lip pits
	Full lower lip with depressed angles of the mouth (carp mouth)
	Long, smooth philtrum
	Asymmetry
	Geographic tongue
	Furrowed tongue (scrotal tongue)
	Short frenulum

(Continued)

TABLE 16–2. MINOR AND MAJOR CONGENITAL ANOMALIES (Continued)

Body Part	Anomalies
Thorax	Funnel chest (pectus excavatum)
	Pigeon chest (pectus carinatum)
	Harrison's groove
	Shield chest (broad and short upper thorax)
	Widely spaced nipples
	Accessory nipples
	Bifid or protuberant xyphoid
Abdomen	Diastasis recti
	Umbilical or ventral hernia
	Skin umbilicus (results in "outie" for life)
	Membranous umbilicus (membranes of cord extend out onto the surrounding skin, resulting in a very flat, smooth umbilicus)
	Single umbilical artery
	Unusual umbilical position
Skin	Milia
	Miliaria
	Capillary hemangiomas
	Mongolian spot
	Lipomas
	Café-au-lait spots
	Nevi
	Freckles
	Port-wine stain
	Telangiectases
	Supernumerary nipples
	Skin dimples
Back	Hair tufts or dimples at base of spine
	Bifid spinous process
Extremities	Simian palmar creases
	Longitudinal plantar crease
	Tapered fingers
	Clinodactyly (incurving of the fifth finger)
	Syndactyly (fused digits)
	Polydactyly (extra digit)
	Camptodactyly (permanent flexion of digit)
	Brachydactyly (short digits)
	Adducted thumb in palm of hand
	Hairy elbows
	Tibial bowing
	Femoral bowing
	Intoeing or out-toeing
	Pes planus (flatfoot)
	Genu varum (bowleg)
	Genu valgum (knock-knee)
	Overriding toes

(Continued)

TABLE 16–2. MINOR AND MAJOR CONGENITAL ANOMALIES

Body Part	Anomalies
Genitalia	Hypospadias
	Epispadias
	Large phallus
	Micropenis
	Hydrocele
	Cryptorchidism
	Micro- or macro-orchidism
	Hymenal remnants
	Adhesions between labia minora
Anus	Anal tags
	Rectal polyps
	Hemorrhoids
	Anal stenosis

MAJOR: Major anomalies are of greater concern than minor anomalies and usually need intervention

Head	Anencephaly
Hair	Alopecia
	Sparse hair
	Hypopigmentation
	Hypertrichosis (hairy body)
	Elongated sideburns
	White forelock
	Straight lashes
	Tangled lashes
	Hair fragility
	Very curly hair (if not a family trait)
	Low hairline (Turner syndrome)
Face	Facial clefting
	Hypoplastic midface
	Lateral facial hypoplasia (malar eminence and zygoma are flat)
Eyes	Colobomas
	Asymmetry of the orbits
	Exophthalmos
	Hypertelorism or hypotelorism
	Ectropion
	Telecanthus
	Shortened palpebral fissures
	Anophthalmos (absence of the eye)
	Microphthalmos (very small eye)
	Eyelid clefts, absent, or fused
Ears	Deformed pinna
	Cauliflower ear
	Upward or forward displacement
	Microtia (small ear)
	Triangular ears
	Absence of ear

(Continued)

TABLE 16–2. MINOR AND MAJOR CONGENITAL ANOMALIES (Continued)

Body Part	Anomalies
Nose	Choanal atresia
	Deviated septum
	Deficient nasal tip
	Widely separated nares
	Nasal pits
	Encephalocele (bulge over nasal bridge)
Mouth	Cleft lip or palate
	Asymmetry of lips or mouth
	Distorted dental arch
	Microglossia or macroglossia
Neck	Webbing
	Short neck
	Thyroglossal duct cyst or sinus
Thorax	Absence of clavicles
	Absence of pectoralis major muscle
	Beaded ribs
	Short sternum
	Cleft sternum
	Ectopia cordis (entire central chest wall is deficient)
Abdomen	Gastroschisis (defect of abdominal wall not at umbilicus)
	Duodenal atresia
	Imperforate anus
	Omphalocele
	Hernia into the umbilical cord
	Inguinal hernias
	Meckel's diverticulum
Skin	Redundant abdominal skin
	Callus formation
	Hyperelasticity
	Thick skin
	Thin skin
	Ichthyosis
	Hypopigmentation
	Absence of skin
	Neurofibromas
	Giant pigmented nevi
	Dark, flat, pigmented nevus over midthoracic spine
	Hypopigmented ash-leaf spots
	Vitiligo

(Continued)

DOMINANT INHERITANCE

Dominant inheritance is the expression of a characteristic that is controlled by only one gene of a pair. The other controls suppression of the characteristic. When a single copy of an abnormal dominant gene is transmitted, the child will have the genetically transmitted problem. An example of dominant inheritance is neurofibromatosis. Dominant inheritance is expressed in capital letters (S).

184

TABLE 16–2. MINOR AND MAJOR CONGENITAL ANOMALIES

Body Part	Anomalies
Extremities	Hypoplastic or absent clavicles
	Hypoplasia of pectoralis muscles
	Disproportionately long or short limbs
	Missing limbs
	Asymmetry of limbs
	Club foot
	Thumb and radial hypoplasia
	Joint contractures
	Joint webbing
	Monodactyly
	Arachnodactyly
	Macrodactyly
	Ectodactyly (split hand or foot or lobster-claw deformity)
Back	Spina bifida occulta
	Meningocele
	Myelomeningocele
	Winged scapulas
	High scapulas
	Scoliosis
	Pilonidal sinus
Genitalia	Ambiguous genitalia
	Absence of phallus
	Hermaphroditism
	Duplication of external genital structures
	Epispadias
	Exstrophy of the bladder (bladder herniated)
	Severe hypospadias with chordae
	Double meatus
	Bifid scrotum
	Transposition of penis and scrotum
	Imperforate hymen
	Absence of vagina
	Shallow vagina
	Duplicate vagina
Anus	Imperforate anus
	Rectal agenesis (very high, blind-ending rectum)

RECESSIVE INHERITANCE

Recessive inheritance requires that both allelic pairs of a given trait be recessive. When both parents donate the recessive gene, the recessive trait will be expressed. If both copies of the gene are abnormal, the abnormal trait will be transmitted. When both parents carry the same abnormal recessive gene, there is a 25% chance of the child inheriting two copies of the abnormal gene and subsequently developing the genetically transmitted problem. Examples of recessive inheritance are cystic fibrosis and sickle cell disease. Recessive inheritance is expressed in lower-case letters (s).

185

TABLE 16–3. INHERITANCE TABLES

Mother and father both carry only dominant genes:

Mother (SS)   Father (SS)

	(S)	(S)
(S)	SS	SS
(S)	SS	SS

All offspring have the trait.

Mother carries dominant genes; father carries a recessive gene:

Mother (SS)   Father (Ss)

	(S)	(s)
(S)	SS	Ss
(S)	SS	Ss

All offspring have the trait.

Mother carries a recessive gene; father carries a recessive gene:

Mother (Ss)   Father (Ss)

	(S)	(s)
(S)	SS	Ss
(s)	Ss	ss

25% chance of having the trait.

Mother carries only recessive genes; father carries only recessive genes:

Mother (ss)   Father (ss)

	(s)	(s)
(s)	ss	ss
(s)	ss	ss

100% chance of having the trait.

Mother carries a hemophilic gene (X) and a normal gene (X); father carries hemophilic genes (XY):

	(X) Hemophilic	(Y) Hemophilic
(X) Hemophilic	XX Girl (Carrier)	XY Boy (Hemophilic)
(X) Normal	XX Girl (Normal)	XY Boy (Normal)

25% chance of having a hemophilic boy.

X-LINKED (SEX-LINKED) INHERITANCE

X-linked inheritance is even more complicated than dominant or recessive inheritance (see Table 16–3). The sex chromosomes are X and Y. Men have an X and a Y chromosome on the 23rd pair. Females have two X chromosomes on the 23rd pair. The X chromosome carries more genes than the Y. If a woman inherits a defective gene on the X chromosome from her mother and the second X sex chromosome that comes from the father is not defective, the woman will be a carrier of the disorder but will not have the disorder. In X-linked recessive inheritance, males are affected and females are carriers. Occasionally a female carrier shows mild signs of the disease. Sons of a female carrier have a one in two chance of being affected. Daughters of a female carrier have a one in two chance of being a carrier. Daughters of affected men are carriers. Sons of affected men are not affected. In the general population, there are at least 250 X-linked disorders. Examples of X-linked disorders are color blindness, Duchenne muscular dystrophy, fragile X syndrome, and hemophilia.

CONSANGUINITY

It is thought that we all carry at least one abnormal recessive gene. In addition, the sexual partner or parent usually carries a different abnormal recessive gene. However, when cousins or other relatives conceive, the chance of a couple carrying the same abnormal recessive gene increases. The risk of having a child with a recessive disorder increases with consanguinity. These inherited conditions often involve metabolic disorders resulting from enzyme deficiencies and are often life threatening.

MOSAICISM

Mosaicism is a condition in which an individual who develops from a single egg or sperm has two or more cell populations that differ in genetic constitution. Most commonly, there is a variation in the number of chromosomes in the cells. Mosaicism is caused by gene mutations or nondisjunction (i.e., failure of the chromosome pair to separate during meiosis) of the chromosomes during early embryogenesis, causing a variation in the number of chromosomes in the cells. Nondisjunction can occur during the first or later mitotic divisions of the zygote. Monosomic cells are nonviable, so mosaic conditions represent a mixture of normal and trisomic cells. The degree of clinical involvement depends on the type of tissue containing the abnormality and may vary from near normal to full manifestation of a syndrome.

MUTATION

A mutation is an unusual change in genetic material that occurs spontaneously. The alteration changes the expression of the gene. A mutant gene has undergone a change such as a loss, gain, or exchange of genetic material, which affects the normal transmission and expression of a trait. Mutant genes can be amorph (inactive), antimorph (inhibits the normal influence of its allele in the expression of a trait), hypermorph (increased activity in expression of a trait), or hypomorph (level too low to result in abnormal expression of a trait). Genes are stable units, but when mutation occurs, the abnormality is often transmitted to future generations.

TERATOGENS

A teratogen is any substance, agent, or process that interferes with normal prenatal development, causing the formation of one or more developmental

TABLE 16–4. COMMON TERATOGENIC AGENTS

Teratogens	Abnormalities
Radiation	CNS, Skeletal
MICROBES	
Rubella	Congenital heart defects, severe vision and hearing loss, microcephaly, mental retardation, cerebral palsy
Cytomegalovirus	CNS, ophthalmic
Herpes simplex virus	Growth delay, skin lesions, retinal abnormalities, micro-cephaly
Toxoplasma gondii	Blindness, microcephaly, hydrocephaly, mental retardation, seizure disorder
CHEMICALS	
Alcohol	FAS
Antibiotics (tetracycline)	Tooth defects
Antiepileptics	Cleft lip and palate, congenital heart disease, micro-cephaly, abnormalities of nails and fingers, growth retardation
Aspirin	Decreased amniotic fluid, fetal growth restriction, premature closure of the ductus arteriosus
Cancer chemotherapy	CNS, growth retardation, finger and cardiovascular malformations
Potassium iodide	Congenital goiter
SEX HORMONES	
Progesterone	Masculinization of female fetus; hypospadias in males
Estrogen	Structural defects in the genital tract in females
TRANQUILIZERS	
Thalidomide	Absence of upper portion of one or more limbs
Vitamin A	Cranial and facial malformations

CNS = central nervous system; FAS = fetal alcohol syndrome.

abnormalities in the fetus. Teratogens act directly on the developing organism or indirectly, affecting such supplemental structures as the placenta or some maternal system. The type and extent of the defect are determined by the specific kind of teratogen and its mode of action, the embryonic process affected, genetic predisposition, and the stage of development at the time of exposure. The period of highest vulnerability in the developing embryo is from the third through the twelfth weeks of gestation. Differentiation of the major organs and systems occurs during this time period. Later periods of gestation are concerned with growth and elaboration of the fetus; thus, susceptibility to teratogenic substances decreases. Common teratogenic agents are noted in Table 16–4.

TABLE 16–5. PREVALENCE OF SELECTED GENETIC DISORDERS	
Disorder	**Approximate Prevalence**
Down syndrome	1/700–1/l000
Klinefelter's syndrome	1/1000 males
Noonan's syndrome	1/1000–1/2500
Trisomy 8	1/25,000–1/50,000
Turner's syndrome	1/2,500–1/10,000
Neurofibromatosis (von Recklinghausen's syndrome)	1/3000–1/3500
Waardenburg syndrome	1/20,000–1/40,000
Tay-Sachs disease	1/3,000 in Ashkenazi Jews
Sickle cell disease	1/500 in people of India, Caribbean, Mediterranean, African descent
Cystic fibrosis	1/2,000 in people of European descent
Fetal alcohol syndrome	1/200–1/1000

 INCIDENCE AND PREVALENCE

Incidence is the number of new cases in a particular period of time. Incidence is expressed as a ratio, in which the number of cases is the numerator and the population at risk is the denominator. Prevalence is the number of all new and old cases of a disease or occurrences of an event during a particular period of time. Prevalence is expressed as a ratio, in which the number of events is the numerator and population at risk the denominator. Prevalence of the disorders discussed in this chapter is shown in Table 16–5.

 KARYOTYPING

Karyotyping, the study of chromosome constitution, is important in determining the extent of the chromosomal abnormality. An example of a karotype is 47,XY+21 for Down syndrome. The first number is the total number of chromosomes. The second letters are the sex chromosomes. Then the chromosomes that are missing, extra, or abnormal are added. A normal female would be expressed as 46,XX, and a normal male would be expressed as 46,XY. Examples of karotyping for certain genetically transmitted diseases are presented in Table 16–6.

 GENETIC COUNSELING OVERVIEW

The main goal of genetic counseling is to inform individuals, couples, and families about hereditary disorders so that they understand what it means to have the disorder, their risk of developing or transmitting the disorder, and

TABLE 16–6. KAROTYPING: GENETICALLY TRANSMITTED PROBLEMS	
Problem	**Karotype**
Down syndrome	46,XY+21
Klinefelter's syndrome	47,XXY
Extra Y or X	48,XXXY; 49,XXXXY; 48,XX,XY; 49,XXX,XY
Turner's syndrome	45,XO
Single X	Mosaics: XO/XX or XO/XXX

measures to treat or prevent the disorder. With information, they are prepared to make informed decisions about reproduction. Counseling should be nondirective, timely, and compassionate. Providers need to be aware of psychological issues such as denial, grief, and anger as well as ethnic, cultural, social, religious, and educational factors. Follow-up to assess understanding and offer support is essential, particularly after a termination for a fetal abnormality. The elements of genetic counseling are noted in Table 16–7. A list of resources for families is outlined in Table 16–8. Competencies for the public health workforce are provided by the Centers for Disease Control and Prevention at their Web site, Genetics and Disease Prevention, *www.cdc.gov/genetics/training/competencies/comps.htm.*

TABLE 16–7. ELEMENTS OF GENETIC COUNSELING	
Element	**Procedures**
Establishing the correct diagnosis	Chromosome analysis
	Autopsy and photographs of malformations
	Radiographs of structural abnormalities
	Blood and tissue samples
Risk estimation	Pedigree of three generations
Communication	Information on inheritance and transmission
Discussion of risk to offspring	Discussion of the options
	Not having (more) children
	Ignoring the risk
	Artificial insemination by donor
	Ovum donation
	Antenatal diagnosis and termination of pregnancy
Discussion of testing	Discussion of the appropriate tests
	Chorionic villus sampling
	Amniocentesis
	Percutaneous umbilical blood sampling
	Carrier detection

TABLE 16–8. RESOURCES FOR FAMILIES	
Resource	Web Address
Alliance of Genetic Support Groups	www.geneticalliance.org
American Society of Human Genetics	www.faseb.org/genetics
MAGIC Foundation for Children's Growth	www.magicfoundation.org
March of Dimes Birth Defects Foundation	www.modimes.org
Mountain States Genetics Network	www.mostgene.org
MUMS National-Parent-to-Parent Network	www.waisman.wisc.edu/mums/home.html
National Newborn Screening and Genetics Resource Center	http://genes-r-us.uthscsa.edu
National Organization for Rare Disorders	www.NORD/rdb.com/orphan
Tyler for Life Foundation, Inc.	www.savebabies.org

Genetic counseling also includes informing the parents of the testing options available. They include chorionic villus sampling, amniocentesis, percutaneous umbilical blood sampling, and carrier detection.

HISTORY

PREPREGNANCY

Determine the mother's medical history, surgical history, and family history (see Pedigree Plotting). Note any medications (prescribed, over-the-counter, herbals, recreational) that the mother was taking at the time of conception. Determine nutritional status before conception. Ask about ingestion of alcoholic beverages and tobacco use. Ask about the home environment, including the type of housing, factories or industries close to the home, chemical use in the home, and other teratogen exposure.

PREGNANCY

Obtain a thorough prenatal and perinatal history. Ask if any prenatal care was obtained, nutritional patterns, weight gain, prenatal tests conducted and results, accidents, illnesses, unusual medications or dental procedures, all potentially harmful environmental exposures (radiation, chemical fumes), excessive heat (hot tubs, saunas, fever), tobacco, alcohol, home remedies, and recreational drugs (marijuana, cocaine, methamphetamines, heroin). Check previous pregnancy history for previous spontaneous abortions, stillbirths, and problems conceiving. Note the mother's age. There is an increased risk of chromosomal problems as the mother ages. Occurrence is 1 case in 200 births at age 35 years, 1 in 65 at age 40 years, and 1 in 20 at age 45 years.

LABOR AND DELIVERY

Ask about the labor and delivery experience of the mother and baby. Note the presentation (breech birth is associated with many syndromes), difficulties that occurred, length of labor, and whether any asphyxia occurred. Ask about the Apgar score.

FETAL FACTORS

Ask if the baby grew consistently throughout the pregnancy or if the growth was too slow or too fast. When did the mother first feel the baby move? Was there any point when movement stopped or became unusually strong? Were the baby's movements always felt in just one part of the abdomen?

NEONATAL STATUS

Gather data about the child's progress during the first few weeks of life. Note any problems with feedings; weight gain; development; and complications such as infections, jaundice, seizures, floppiness, apnea, fever, or bowel or bladder problems.

PEDIGREE PLOTTING

Pedigree is the line of descent, lineage, or ancestry of a family. In genetics, pedigree is a chart that shows the genetic makeup of a person's ancestors. Pedigree plotting is used to analyze inherited characteristics or disease in a particular family. Figure 16–1 gives a key to symbols for pedigree notation. Shaded circles or squares indicate the family members who are affected by the disease or trait and those who are carriers. The generations are divided by a dotted line, with the most recent generation at the bottom. Members of each family are arranged from left to right according to age, with the eldest on the left. A pedigree should include three generations if possible.

✺ COMMON CHROMOSOMAL SYNDROMES

There is a wide variation in the presentation of anomalies of any chromosomal syndrome. They may present with varying levels of severity.

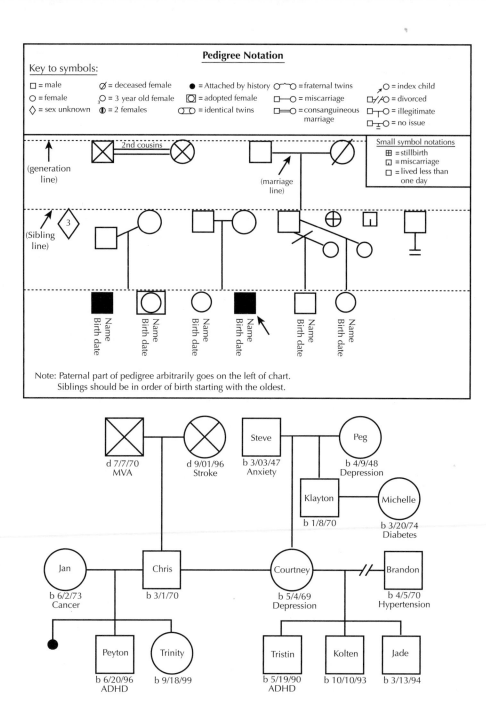

FIG. 16–1. Pedigree plotting.

193

1 in 1445 at age 20 years
1 in 800 at ages 29 to 34 years
1 in 270 at ages 35 to 39 years
1 in 100 at ages 40 to 44 years
1 in 25 to 50 at ages > 45 years

Chromosomal syndromes that occur frequently and that the ambulatory care provider can manage are included. Syndromes that are very severe, resulting in death soon after birth or in the first year of life, are not included.

DOWN SYNDROME (TRISOMY 21)

Down syndrome, or trisomy 21, is the most common genetic disorder in childhood. It is a condition of excess chromosomal material, an extra chromosome 21, passed to the fetus from the parents. The overall incidence of trisomy 21 is 1 in 660 of all live births, with about 1 in 150 first-trimester spontaneous abortions also attributed to the disorder. The risk of a child being born with this disorder increases as the mother ages. Not only does it seem that chromosomal disorders occur more frequently as the parents age, but older mothers may also be more tolerant of an affected fetus. The risk figures are presented in Table 16–9.

Transmission

Down syndrome is the result of an extra chromosome 21. The majority of cases of trisomy 21 (90% to 95%) are caused by nondisjunction, or failure of the chromosome pair to separate during meiosis. This produces an ovum or sperm with two copies of the same chromosome, instead of the expected one chromosome. With Down syndrome, the child has three copies of chromosome 21.

The remaining cases of trisomy 21 are caused by chromosomal translocation, in which a segment of one chromosome is transferred onto the end of another chromosome. Down syndrome may be caused by a 14/21 translocation. In about 90% of children with Down syndrome, the chromosomal defect for both translocation and nondisjunction is maternal; the remaining 5% to 10% percent are paternal in origin. In 1% to 3% of those with Down syndrome, the chromosomal defect is mosaic and the individual has a mixture of normal and trisomy cells. The physical and mental signs and characteristics are milder in mosaic individuals.

Clinical Features

There is not one single anomaly that characterizes Down syndrome (Fig. 16–2). Suspicion is raised by the presence of several minor anomalies along

194

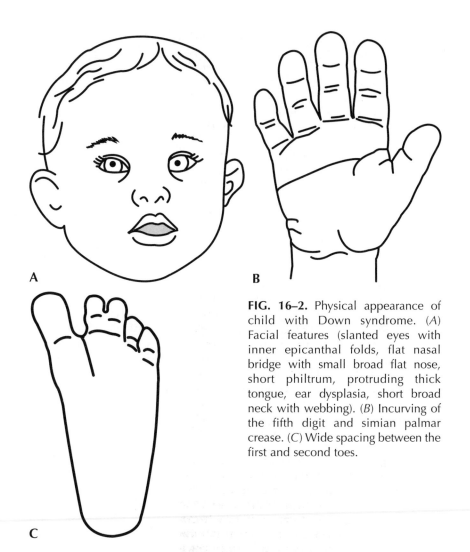

A

B

FIG. 16–2. Physical appearance of child with Down syndrome. (*A*) Facial features (slanted eyes with inner epicanthal folds, flat nasal bridge with small broad flat nose, short philtrum, protruding thick tongue, ear dysplasia, short broad neck with webbing). (*B*) Incurving of the fifth digit and simian palmar crease. (*C*) Wide spacing between the first and second toes.

C

with a few major anomalies. The major and minor anomalies found in Down syndrome are summarized in Table 16–10. There are several significant medical problems that the Down syndrome individual can develop. Forty percent of infants with Down syndrome are born with structural cardiac defects. Hypothyroidism is common and should be screened for annually. Respiratory infections are also common. The risk of developing leukemia is 15 to 20 times higher in this population than in the general population. Hearing and vision problems are common. Males are nearly universally sterile. Females can reproduce, but most experience ovulatory failure and enter menopause early. Overall, developmental milestones are reached but, depending on the severity of the mental retardation, attainment is often delayed.

TABLE 16–10. MAJOR AND MINOR ANOMALIES FOUND WITH DOWN SYNDROME

Major	Minor
Congenital heart disease	Slanted eyes with inner epicanthal folds
Atrioventricular shunts	Flat nasal bridge with small, broad, flat nose
Ventricular septal defects	Protruding, thick tongue
GI defects	Ear dysplasia
Duodenal atresia	Short, broad neck with webbing
Celiac disease	Brachycephaly
Thyroid disorders	Brushfield spots
Conductive hearing loss	Wide spacing between the first and second toes
Mental retardation	Short and stubby fingers
	Incurving of the fifth digit
	Simian palmar crease

Physical appearance of the child with Down syndrome includes: (1) facial features (slanted eyes with inner epicanthal folds; flat nasal bridge with small, broad, flat nose; short philtrum; protruding, thick tongue; ear dysplasia; short, broad neck with webbing); (2) incurving of the fifth digit and simian palmar crease; and (3) wide spacing between the first and second toes.

Counseling

The clinical diagnosis may be made first on the basis of the appearance of the infant. A chromosomal study should then be done to confirm the diagnosis. Analysis of the chromosomes also clarifies the type of chromosomal defect present. This information is then used to determine the likelihood of the same parents conceiving another child with Down syndrome. The risk of having another child with Down syndrome depends on the maternal age when the child with trisomy 21 was born. Mothers with late maternal age continue to have the same age-related risk. However, younger mothers, under age 30 years, have an increased risk (sixfold) compared with their own age peers. The risk of having a child with Down syndrome is correlated with maternal age, not paternal age. Overall, the parents of a child with Down syndrome do have a generalized increased risk for having another child with congenital anomalies. This risk is 1% to 2%; 50% of that is the risk of having a second child with Down syndrome. For the parents of a child with Down syndrome caused by chromosomal translocation, it is important to have chromosomal studies performed because the various types of translocations have differing risks for another Down syndrome child, varying from no risk to 100 percent.

Children born with Down syndrome can lead happy, healthy lives. An important factor in the productivity and longevity of their lives is based on the environment in which they are raised. A nurturing, stimulating environment aids the child in meeting his or her physical and intellectual potentials. Institutionalization of these children robs them of the opportunity to develop to their maximum potential because of individual stimulation. The intelligence quotient (IQ) of children with Down syndrome is between 20 and 80. Many of these individuals are able to work and live semi-independently to independently. Individuals with Down syndrome have survival rates into their 50s and 60s. Just over half die by age 60 years, and nearly 90% die by age 70 years. Some succumb to problems caused by sudden infant death syndrome, congenital heart disease, or respiratory infections during their first 5 years. From ages 5 to 39 years, the survival rate parallels that of the general population. Higher rates of stroke and accelerated senility may play a role in the reduced survival rate seen as the person grows into the 50s and 60s.

Regular, routine well-child visits are important. As with nonaffected children, monitoring growth and development, physical assessment, immunizations, and anticipatory guidance for the family are necessary. For children with Down syndrome, assessing and anticipating development needs allows early intervention and developmental management, which gives the child the optimum chance for meeting his or her potential.

FETAL ALCOHOL SYNDROME

Fetal alcohol syndrome (FAS) is the result of exposure to elevated blood alcohol (teratogen) levels by the developing fetus during pregnancy. There is no known alcohol level that leads to the syndrome, but research indicates FAS to be dose related. FAS was first recognized in the late 1960s. The pathogenesis of the syndrome is not known, but it appears that the breakdown product of ethanol, acetaldehyde, is the most likely factor. Acetaldehyde crosses the placental membrane and the fetal blood–brain barrier, causing decreased protein synthesis, impaired cellular growth and migration, neuronal cell death, decreased production of neurotransmitters, increased free radical formation, and inhibition of myelination of axons. It is estimated that some FAS effects are seen in one in 200 to 1000 live births. The incidence is equal across the sexes.

Transmission

The amount of alcohol ingested and the resulting severity of the syndrome are variable. Ingestion during the first trimester seems to put the child at more risk for being born with the signs of FAS. Infants exposed to elevated alcohol levels in the last trimester tend to have problems with growth delays, low birth weight, and behavioral abnormalities. Miscarriage and stillbirths are more common for mothers of FAS children. A total of 30% to 50% of children whose mothers consumed heavy amounts of alcohol during the pregnancy exhibit signs of FAS. These are women who are taking over seven

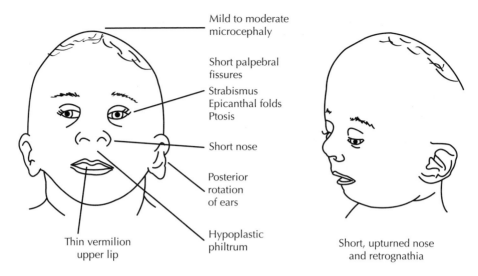

Mild to moderate microcephaly

Short palpebral fissures

Strabismus
Epicanthal folds
Ptosis

Short nose

Posterior rotation of ears

Hypoplastic philtrum

Thin vermilion upper lip

Short, upturned nose and retrognathia

FIG. 16–3. Physical features of fetal alcohol syndrome.

drinks of alcohol per day. For more moderate drinkers who take four to six drinks per day, more subtle signs of FAS are seen. Prematurity and low birth weight for gestation can result with the ingestion of as little as two to three drinks per day. Binge drinking has a more adverse effect on the fetus than does steady drinking of the same volume of alcohol. There is some evidence that the father's alcohol intake at the time of conception may also have some teratogenic potential. It is not clear why some children are affected by a mother's heavy alcohol consumption and others are not. It may be the differences in the mother's or child's ability to metabolize the acetaldehyde.

Clinical Features

The diagnosis of FAS is made clinically based on prenatal and postnatal growth retardation, central nervous system (CNS) abnormalities, and craniofacial malformations (Fig. 16–3). Genetic testing can be done to rule out other genetic disorders that physically present in similar manners, such as Noonan's syndrome, trisomy 18, de Lange's syndrome, or Smith-Lemli-Opitz syndrome. These disorders share many of the same features as FAS in newborn infants.

In general, infants with FAS are born small for gestational age, tend to have problems with catch-up growth, and tend to stay thin. As infants, children with FAS are hypotonic and irritable. When they grow older, these children may have problems with hyperactivity and various developmental delays, especially speech, language, and motor delays. On entering school, children with FAS exhibit low-average intelligence. They exhibit problems with poor judgment, oppositional and defiant behavior, lying, stealing, inap-

TABLE 16–11. PHYSICAL AND DEVELOPMENTAL SIGNS IN CHILDREN WITH FETAL ALCOHOL SYNDROME

MOST COMMON, PRESENT IN > 80%

Microcephaly
Mild to moderate mental retardation
Fine motor control disability
Irritability in infancy
Poor sucking ability
Persistent growth retardation—in length
Narrow palpebral fissures
Shallow, flat, poorly formed philtrum
Thin, smooth upper lip

LESS COMMONLY NOTED, 30 TO 80%

Hypotonia
Hyperactivity, as older child
Strabismus
Epicanthal folds
Cardiac anomalies, such as atrial or ventricular septal defects
Short nose
Sacral dimple
Hypoplasia maxilla
Hemangiomas

LESS COMMONLY NOTED, < 25%

Ptosis
Cleft lip or palate
Some limited joint mobility
Hypoplasia of the nails and digits, especially the fifth digit
Small, rotated kidneys
Hypospadias

propriate response to social cues, absence of reciprocal friendships, social withdrawal, mood lability, bullying, and anxiety. Ethanol appears to be neurotoxic. Structural changes occur within the brain when a fetus is exposed to elevated ethanol levels. Ethanol can cross the placenta at any time during the pregnancy and may interrupt normal neuronal development. Table 16–11 summarizes the physical and mental stigmata found in children with FAS. Congenital cardiac anomalies, renal defects, and cranofacial abnormalities are frequently observed.

Counseling

There is no genetic defect in this syndrome; FAS is a congenital anomaly. The cause is external and is preventable. Early identification and education of women who may be using alcohol is extremely important for healthcare providers. Ensuring that the woman's contraceptive needs are met may help to prevent a child from being born with FAS.

Mild to moderate mental retardation is frequently seen in children with FAS. Attention problems, learning disabilities, and poor social skills are common in this group and may continue into adulthood. Early recognition and intervention, as with other congenital disorders, may help the child to develop to his or her fullest potential.

KLINEFELTER'S SYNDROME

In Klinefelter's syndrome, which affects males only, extra X chromosomes have been passed from the parents to the child. This syndrome is often not recognized until puberty, when the effect of having the additional X chromosomes becomes apparent. The number and severity of the abnormalities associated with Klinefelter's syndrome increases with greater numbers of X chromosomes present. The most common abnormality is a 47,XXY karyotype. Men with only one additional X chromosome usually have little mental impairment and few physical signs but do experience sexual disorders. These men often have infertility and libido problems. Men with three or more X chromosomes tend to show more marked congenital malformations and mental retardation. Twenty percent of males with Klinefelter's syndrome are aspermic.

Transmission

The karyotype seen in Klinefelter's syndrome in the majority of cases is 47,XXY, accounting for more than 50% of males with this disorder. The majority of the remaining males affected have a 46,XY/47,XXY mosaic pattern. More rarely, those affected have additional X chromosomes, such as 48,XXXY or 49,XXXXY. The genetic defect may come from either parent. In approximately 60% of Klinefelter's syndrome cases, the defect is caused by problems during oogenesis, with the remaining 40% of cases caused by errors in spermatogenesis. Nondisjunction of the X chromosome during meiosis is thought to be the underlying cause of the extra chromosome, or X chromosome aneuploidy, in Klinefelter's syndrome.

Clinical Features

Typically, no physical manifestation of Klinefelter's syndrome is seen until the child reaches puberty, although a tall, slim stature with long limbs may be noted before the syndrome is recognized and diagnosed. Puberty is often delayed or progresses poorly once begun. At that time, because of the presence of the additional X chromosome, subnormal testosterone levels, small testicles, reduced libido, and sterility are seen. Spermatogenesis is blocked by the additional X chromosome; thus, these men are infertile because there is no sperm production. Mental capacity is normal compared with that of the general population, but there is a higher rate of learning disabilities. There is a tendency toward delayed motor or language milestones. Shyness, assertiveness, lack of judgment, and immaturity are personality traits seen in adolescents and young adults with Klinefelter's syndrome. Antisocial behaviors may be more common. Up to 40% of men with Klinefelter's syndrome have problems with gynecomastia.

Counseling

Predisposing factors for the syndrome are not known. It is considered a sporadic or accidental genetic occurrence. There is an increased risk for parents to have a second child with congenital disorders. This risk is 1% to 2%, and the parents should be advised to seek genetic counseling before further pregnancies.

Men with Klinefelter's syndrome can lead healthy, normal lives. The small percentage with two or three extra X chromosomes may require additional social support. Their longevity equals that of the general population. Testosterone treatment can reverse the libido issues and helps prevent gynecomastia. If not recognized early and prevented, gynecomastia may require surgical correction. Therapy with testosterone should be started in the early teen years.

NOONAN'S SYNDROME

Noonan's syndrome appears to be an autosomal dominant genetic disorder. It may affect either gender and appears not to have an ethnic or racial predilection. The initial characteristics of the newborn may be similar to those of Turner's syndrome or FAS. Thus, Noonan's syndrome must be differentiated from these conditions. A chromosomal study is needed to confirm the diagnosis. Then more accurate information can be given to the family as to the cause of the congenital anomalies and the prognosis for the child. The average age at diagnosis is 9 years.

Transmission

Noonan's syndrome is an autosomal dominant, single-gene disorder. The genetic defect resulting in Noonan's syndrome is unknown. Chromosomal studies show normal karyotyping. There have been several documented familial cases, but most cases appear to be random. Transmission of the affected gene seems to be increased in women; a 3:1 ratio of females to males has been noted.

Clinical Features

Noonan's syndrome includes many clinical features (Fig. 16–4). There are several facial characteristics, congenital heart disease, skeletal abnormalities, and genital dysfunctions found in individuals with this disorder. Mild retardation occurs in up to 30% of children with Noonan's syndrome. Developmental milestone delays and learning disabilities may also be present. Failure to thrive is common in infancy, and the growth spurt during ado-

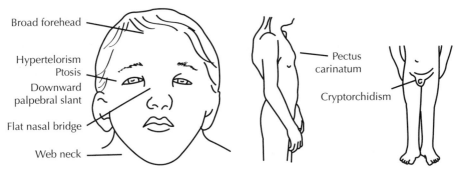

FIG. 16–4. Physical features of Noonan's syndrome.

lescence may be absent. Table 16–12 summarizes the physical anomalies that characterize Noonan's syndrome. Heart disease occurs in about 80% of children with this syndrome. The most common cause is pulmonary stenosis, leading to right-sided heart dysfunction. There are many anomalies involving the face, including the eyes, nose, and neck. The characteristic shield chest (broad, flat chest with widely spaced nipples) is present. Lymphedema of the feet occurs in about 15%. Many people with Noonan's syndrome may have a delayed onset of puberty. Affected women have regular menses and are fertile. Men have more problems: approximately 75% of men with Noonan's syndrome have undescended testes, with 50% experiencing sterility.

Counseling

Parents are advised to undergo genetic counseling and screening before conceiving another child. The parent affected with Noonan's syndrome has a 50% risk of passing the abnormal gene to each child. Fertility is normal in women but may be reduced in men because of the common problem of cryptorchidism. This may account for the increased transmission seen from women to their children.

TABLE 16–12. CHARACTERISTICS OF CHILDREN WITH NOONAN'S SYNDROME	
Short stature	Deep philtrum
Mild retardation	Low-set fleshy ears
Low posterior hairline	Micrognathia
Triangular-shaped face	Pterygium colli
Broad forehead	Flat, shield-like chest with widely
Epicanthal folds and ptosis	spaced nipples
Downslanting palpebral fissures	Cardiac anomalies: Pulmonary stenosis
Hypertelorism	Cubitus valgus
Flat nasal bridge	Lymphedema

The life span of most individuals with Noonan's syndrome is the same as that of the general population. The degree and number of congenital anomalies may lead to a poorer prognosis, such as the presence of pulmonary stenosis with resulting pulmonary hypertension. Typically, the degree of mental retardation is mild and social skills are adequate.

TRISOMY 8

Trisomy 8 is similar to trisomy 21 in that an extra number 8 chromosome is present. This genetic defect is the most common defect after the trisomies 21, 18, and 13.

Transmission

Genetic screening shows a third chromosome 8. Most cases of trisomy 8 are thought to result from nondisjunction of chromosome 8. Most children with this syndrome are mosaic, accounting for 85% of the cases. A mosaic child has some normal cells interspersed with the cells having the trisomy 8 genetic makeup. When low-frequency mosaicism is present, accounting for about two-thirds of patients with trisomy 8, the diagnosis can be easily missed. A smaller percentage of children are partially mosaic. Partially mosaic children have part of the extra chromosome 8 missing and present with only slight clinical manifestations. If partial mosaic trisomy 8 is present, the additional part of the extra chromosome includes only the long or short arm of the chromosome. Differing physical and developmental findings are seen, depending on which part of the arm is present. The syndrome seems to affect male children at a higher rate, with a 5:1 male to female ratio.

Clinical Features

The appearance of these infants is characteristic, and a clinical diagnosis can usually be readily made. Children with mosaic trisomy 8 may have many physical anomalies. Table 16–13 summarizes the physical and developmental characteristics found in this group. Up to 90% of these infants are mildly to moderately retarded. Scaphocephaly (i.e., a skull that is abnormally long and narrow) is present in many of these infants. The eyes may be widely spaced and deep set, or an abnormally increased interpupillary distance may be present. Many of the infants have abnormalities of the ears. About 50% of them have strabismus and scoliosis. Many experience problems with joints as they age, with contractures that require treatment. Deep furrows at the hands and soles are noted in about 75% of affected infants. Several organs show congenital anomalies. Hydronephrosis, ureteral obstruction, congenital heart disease, or cryptorchidism have been noted in 25% to 50% of individuals with trisomy 8.

TABLE 16–13. CHARACTERISTICS OF CHILDREN WITH TRISOMY 8	
Mental retardation	Thick, everted lower lip
Expressionless face with deep-set eyes	Highly arched palate
Hypertelorism	Micrognathia
Low-set, deformed ears	Deep furrows at palms and soles
Broad, up-turned nose	Contractures of the digits

Counseling

Life expectancy is normal for these individuals. The mortality rate of children with trisomy 8 is low. The quality of life is related to the degree of mental retardation present. Lack of language development can be a major stumbling block for many individuals with trisomy 8. When contractures are present, surgery may be indicated.

TURNER'S SYNDROME

Turner's syndrome, which affects females only, is a condition of too few chromosomes and is one of the most common monosomies seen in infants. Instead of the normal 46 chromosomes present in each cell of the body, there are only 45. The second sex chromosome is missing, resulting in the karyotype 45,XO. It appears that approximately 20% of spontaneously aborted fetuses have Turner's syndrome.

Transmission

Turner's syndrome may be caused by complete or partial absence of the second sex chromosome. About 60% of females with Turner's syndrome have a complete monosomy, with a karyotype of 45,XO. Mosaic Turner's syndrome accounts for 20% of females with Turner's syndrome. Mosaicism results in several karyotypes; XO/XX, XO/XY, or XO/XX/XXX patterns may be seen. The remaining 10% to 20% percent have 46 chromosomes, but one of the X chromosomes is abnormal. The abnormal X chromosome may have a deletion in a portion of the long or short arm of the X chromosome. The chromosomal disorder is usually the result of disjunction during meiosis or after mitosis within the egg or sperm. The chromosome defect may occur in either the mother or father. Females with one normal and one abnormal X chromosome present are more likely to exhibit more serious congenital anomalies or mental retardation. The differences in the karyotype determine the physical characteristics, congenital anomalies, and potential problems that the individual will experience.

Clinical Features

The physical characteristics (Fig. 16–5) of children with Turner's syndrome may be mild enough that diagnosis of the syndrome is delayed. This is par-

TABLE 16–14. CONGENITAL ANOMALIES OF INFANTS WITH TURNER'S SYNDROME	
Small stature	Short metacarpals
Webbing of the neck	Exostosis of the tibia
Low posterior hairline	Lymphedema of the hands and feet
"Shield chest" with widely spaced nipples	
Cubitus valgus	Genital hypoplasia

ticularly true of girls with a mosaic pattern. The first sign of a possible problem may be discovered during a workup for short stature during childhood, when the adolescent fails to develop secondary sex characteristics, or when the child does not have the expected growth spurt at puberty. Some girls may present with sufficient anomalies to allow diagnosis early in life. Girls with one normal X chromosome and one abnormal X chromosome tend to display more of the physical signs at birth, such as the presence of a webbed neck or lymphedema. The physical anomalies of Turner's syndrome are summarized in Table 16–14. The intelligence level is typically normal, but these children may have spatial disorientation and moderate degrees of learning disorders. In addition, they have congenital ovarian failure and cardiovascular anomalies. Abnormalities of the neck and various skeletal abnormalities are common. Lymphedema of the hands and feet may be present at birth, but this sign decreases with age. Congenital anomalies of various organs may also be present. Coarctation of the aorta and hypertension occur about 25% of these individuals. Renal anomalies such as horseshoe kidney may be present in up to 40% of children with this syndrome. Dysgenesis (failure) of the ovaries occurs in about 90% of girls with Turner's syndrome, which requires external hormones to initiate puberty. The uterus andvagina are frequently intact but small. Occasionally, women with mosaicism may be fertile. Women with Turner's syndrome with any partial piece of theY chromosome are at risk for developing gonadoblastoma in any remaining gonadal tissue. Screening should be obtained, and any remaining gonadal tissue should be removed. Hypothyroidism is common in affected individuals.

Counseling

Turner's syndrome should be differentiated from Noonan's syndrome, which shares many of the same physical characteristics at birth. Genetic screening is important to determine Noonan's syndrome and to determine the karyotype of the chromosomal abnormality. The parents of a Turner's syndrome child have a 1% to 2% percent increased risk for having a second child with a congenital anomaly. Additionally, these parents should be genetically screened themselves. If one of the parents carries a structurally abnormal X chromosome, the risk increases.

A small number of women with Turner's syndrome do become fertile. This group most likely has 46, XX/XO mosaic, in which some cells have a

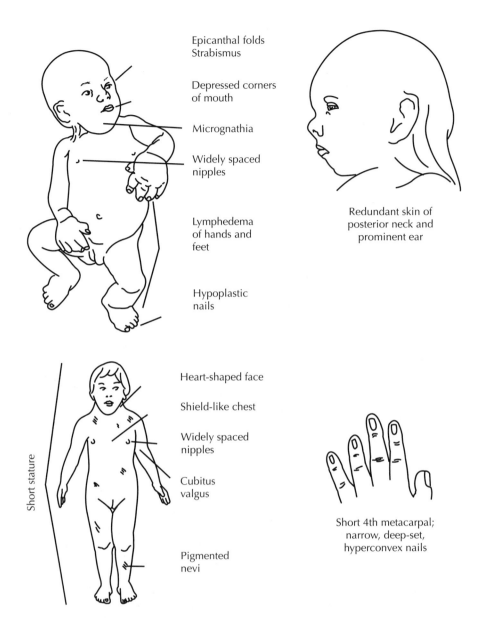

Epicanthal folds
Strabismus

Depressed corners
of mouth

Micrognathia

Widely spaced
nipples

Lymphedema
of hands and
feet

Hypoplastic
nails

Redundant skin of
posterior neck and
prominent ear

Short stature

Heart-shaped face

Shield-like chest

Widely spaced
nipples

Cubitus
valgus

Pigmented
nevi

Short 4th metacarpal;
narrow, deep-set,
hyperconvex nails

FIG. 16–5. Physical features of Turner's syndrome.

normal chromosomal cell line. A small number of pregnancies have occurred in women with the syndrome. The risk of spontaneous abortion, trisomy 21, and sex chromosome aneuploidy is increased. Although a small number of pregnancies have occurred, most women with Turner's syndrome should be considered infertile.

Individuals with Turner's syndrome can live happy, full lives. Surveillance for problems should be done throughout childhood and into the adult years, such as monitoring for cardiac anomalies or hypertension. Correction of the cardiac anomalies or webbing at the neck may be necessary. The majority of affected women are infertile. An infantile uterus may be present, with only streaks of gonadal tissue for ovaries. Most of the girls and women with Turner syndrome need cyclic hormone replacement until menopause, starting at age 10 years.

FRAGILE X SYNDROME

Fragile X syndrome results from a single-gene mutation on the X chromosome. The genetic problem is an abnormal repetition in the DNA sequence. The genetic instructions for making FMR-1, a protein required for normal functioning of the brain, is located on the X chromosome. In normal individuals, the DNA sequence for the FMR-1 repeats itself 5 to 50 times. Individuals with 50 to 200 repetitions are said to be in a premutation carrier state. The premutation state can be present in either males or females because both carry the X chromosome. In individuals with 200 or more repetitions, a full mutation state is present. The number of repetitions present is important when providing genetic counseling to parents and in establishing the prognosis of the individual child. Depending on the number of repetitions present, an individual with fragile X syndrome may exhibit various physical signs and varying degrees of mental retardation, learning disabilities, or other emotional problems. Approximately one in 250 females and one in 700 males carry the premutation defect.

Transmission

The genetic code resulting in fragile X syndrome is carried on the X chromosome. If a father carries the premutation gene, only the daughters will be affected. The sons remain unaffected because only the father's Y chromosome is transmitted. All daughters are typically affected only as carriers of the genetic defect and do not exhibit symptoms clinically. These daughters are referred to as heterozygotes, carrying one normal X chromosome and one abnormal X chromosome. Each daughter will have a 50% chance of passing the premutation gene to her children. Typically, the gene is transmitted in the premutation state, but with each successive transmission, risk increases for mutation to expand from the permutation to the full mutation state. The risk of transmitting the full mutation gene increases as the number of repetitions on the mother's X chromosome increases. If 60 to 80 repetitions of the mutation for the FMR-1 protein are present, the chance of transmitting the full mutation increases to 30%. However, if 90 or more repetitions are present, the risk of transmitting the full mutation becomes closer to 100%.

TABLE 16–15. CHARACTERISTICS SEEN IN FRAGILE X SYNDROME

Physical Features	Mental Impairments and Disabilities
Large head	Mental retardation (borderline to moderately severe)
Long face	
Wide, protuberant ears	Hyperactivity
Flat nasal bridge	Short attention span
Loose joints	Learning disabilities
Large testicles (seen after puberty)	Language delays; <10% of boys may be non-verbal at age 5 years
	Autism or autistic characteristics
	Anxiety
	Temper tantrums
	Poor eye contact
	Oversensitivity to tactile or environmental stimuli
	Hand flapping and biting

Clinical Features

The severity of symptoms seen in fragile X syndrome is dependent on the number of repetitions of the genetic code responsible for the FMR-1 gene present. In individuals with full mutation, more than 200 repeats of the gene code, a range of mental impairments and physical features may be present. Table 16–15 lists the physical and mental characteristics seen in individuals with fragile X syndrome. Fragile X syndrome is the most common inherited cause of mental retardation. This impairment may be seen to varying degrees in up to 90% of fragile X males. The signs and symptoms listed are seen more frequently in males. Females, even when full mutation is present, are usually less clinically affected than males because they have a second normal X chromosome that continues to produce the FMR-1 protein. The physical characteristics and mental impairments are seen much less commonly than in males. Mental and emotional problems may be present, but overall, females with fragile X syndrome develop normally. Mental retardation, when present, is mild to borderline. Learning disabilities, shyness, and mood disorders can plague females with fragile X syndrome. As children, both boys and girls may initially present with behavioral and developmental problems. Language delays, hyperactivity, and temper tantrums can be present early in childhood. These early signs can be subtle.

To confirm the diagnosis of fragile X syndrome, a sample of blood is necessary. The laboratory test performed is done through molecular genetic techniques. The test can be performed as prescreening before pregnancy, during pregnancy, or after birth, when fragile X syndrome is suspected on a clinical basis. Screening women of childbearing age may be cost effective because of the large number of women who are carriers of the fragile X syndrome gene mutation. Diagnosis can be made as early as 18 to 24 months for boys, based on when physical or emotional signs or symptoms were first noted. In girls, the diagnosis is typically later. An advantage of early diagnosis is early intervention.

Counseling

Genetic counseling is important for the families of individuals with fragile X syndrome. Parents should be referred to a genetic counselor to assess the risk of other family members having or carrying the faulty FMR-1 gene. If the mother is a carrier, counseling should include her sisters because they also may be in the premutation state.

Recognition of fragile X syndrome early in life is important. Early entry into various programs, depending on amount of disability present, aids the child in developing to his or her potential. Children diagnosed with the disorder before age 3 years may take advantage of the Individuals with Disabilities Education Act and begin intervention early. Speech therapy, behavioral programs and counseling, and psychopharmacology are a few of the treatment options available to individuals with fragile X syndrome.

NEUROFIBROMATOSIS

Neurofibromatosis (formerly known as von Recklinghausen's disease) is the most common type of neurocutaneous syndrome. In infants and children, multiple hyperpigmented macules or freckling may be seen. In adults, the syndrome disorder may be more easily recognizable. Multiple small and large soft tissue tumors may occur on every part of the body. The "Elephant Man" in 19th-century England is the most famous case. The tongue, stomach, intestines, kidney, bladder, and heart may be affected. Abnormalities in the skeletal system may also be present.

Transmission

The syndrome is an autosomal dominant disorder in about 50% of cases. The remaining cases are sporadic and represent new gene mutations. There are two types of neurofibromatosis, NF-1 and NF-2. NF-1 is by far the more common type. A defect in chromosome 17 leads to the underlying pathology of neurofibromatosis. The NF-1 gene contains the genetic codes for the protein neurofibromin. Neurofibromin appears to function as a tumor suppressor. The NF-1 gene is large, which may explain the high rate of spontaneous mutations seen in neurofibromatosis. The genetic disorder leading to NF-2 is located on chromosome 22. NF-2 is also autosomal dominant. This gene is responsible for the encoding of a different protein. Although the two conditions share a common name, overlap between the two conditions is minimal. One condition does not lead to the other.

Clinical Features of Neurofibromatosis-1

The two disorders of neurofibromatosis are clinically distinct (Fig. 16–6). The clinical signs and symptoms and prognosis differ. In NF-1, skin and neural tumors, ocular manifestations, bony abnormalities, and mental handicaps are seen. The mental retardation is mild and occurs in 4% to 8% of patients with the disorder. Learning disabilities, speech problems, and attention-deficit disorders are found at a higher rate among children with NF-1. A total of 40% to 60% of patients with neurofibromatosis exhibit these signs. Seizures may be a common complication, occurring in about 20% of patients. Table 16–16 summarizes the clinical characteristics of patients with NF-1. The initial signs may be present at birth or appear shortly after. More than 50% of patients with NF-1 show signs during the second year of life. Lisch nodules are present in over 90% of children with NF-1, especially those older than age 6 years. Lisch nodules, or hematomas, are pigmented lesions within the iris. These hematomas do not cause symptoms, but because they are not present in normal individuals, they can be used to confirm the diagnosis of NF. The skin manifestations of the syndrome are the most common finding in patients with NF-1. They include café-au-lait spots, freckling in the intertriginous areas, and neurofibromas. The café-au-lait spots (i.e., irregular, variably shaped, pale yellow to light brown macules) often precede the appearance of the more complex tumors, the neurofibromas. Neurofibromas involve the skin and underlying peripheral nerve endings and appear as a diffuse thickened and hyperpigmented area. They can overgrow and involve the adjacent bone if they are present on an extremity. They can also be found within the gastrointestinal (GI) tract. Occasionally, neurofibromas are found at birth, but they tend to become more apparent at puberty or during pregnancy. A small, rubbery, purplish skin lesion or the more complex lesion of the plexiform neurofibromas may also be present. Plexiform neurofibromas can be present at birth; these lesions tend to be more highly pigmented and are thicker. The diagnostic criteria are listed in Table 16–17. Two or more of the criteria are needed to make the diagnosis of NF-1.

Clinical Features of Neurofibromatosis-2

Neurofibromatosis-2 is less common. This syndrome accounts for about 10% of those with neurofibromatosis. NF-2 involves the eighth cranial nerve. Typically, bilateral acoustic neuromas are found. The initial symptoms usually appear during the teen years or in the early 20s. As the tumor grows and expands, pressure is placed on the acoustic nerve, resulting in progressive hearing loss, tinnitus, unsteadiness, or facial weakness. Schwann-cell or glial tumors and meningiomas are also common in patients with NF-2. Although café-au-lait spots and neurofibromas may be present, these skin findings are much less common in those with NF-2 than in those with NF-1. When the café-au-lait spots are present in persons with NF-2, they tend to be less than

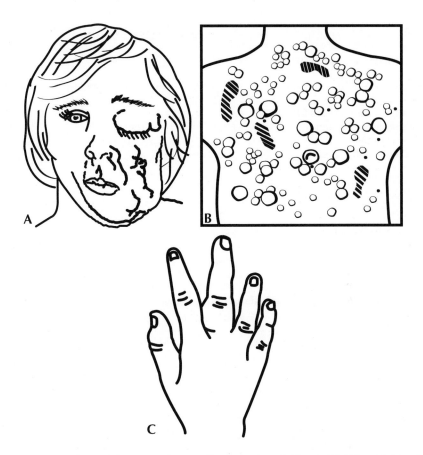

FIG. 16–6. Physical features of neurofibromatosis. (*A*) Head. (*B*) Skin. (*C*) Hand.

6 cm in size and are more plaquelike. The ocular Lisch nodules and axillary freckling are not found in patients with NF-2.

Counseling

Counseling should be provided for parents with neurofibromatosis. As with other autosomal dominant conditions, parents have a 50% chance of passing the affected gene to their children. Mosaicism does occur in neurofibromatosis. It is important to identify those with mosaicism because their risk of transmitting the affected gene to their offspring is often less than the expected 50%. For these individuals, estimating the percentage of affected cells may alter their risk of transmission. The genetic defect in NF-2 is thought to be caused by a somatic mutation; therefore, the risk of transmission is negligible. However, some cases of genetic transmission have occurred.

TABLE 16–16. CHARACTERISTICS OF NEUROFIBROMATOSIS-1

SKIN MANIFESTATIONS
Café-au-lait spots
Axillary or inguinal freckling, multiple 2- to 3-mm hyperpigmented macules
Neurofibromas
OCULAR MANIFESTATIONS
Lisch nodules, hematomas located within the iris
Optic gliomas
SKELETAL LESIONS
Macrocephaly
KYPHOSCOLIOSIS
Dysplasia of the sphenoid wing
Spina bifida
Pseudoarthrosis
NEUROLOGIC COMPLICATIONS
Mild mental retardation
Seizures
Learning disabilities
Attention-deficit disorders
NEOPLASMS, INCREASED RISK FOR:
Neurofibrosarcoma
Rhabdomyosarcoma
Leukemia
Wilms' tumor

There is no specific treatment for neurofibromatosis. Prognosis of the syndrome is dependent on the location and size of the skin lesions. Surgical intervention may be needed. Detection of other complications, such as skeletal or kidney abnormalities and various neuronal tumors, should be performed periodically. Psychological counseling may be necessary for some patients.

WAARDENBURG SYNDROME

Waardenburg syndrome is associated with congenital deafness. Several congenital anomalies are seen in individuals with this syndrome. There are two types of Waardenburg syndrome, type I and type II, and each has differing clinical features. Type I is the more common syndrome and may account for 2% of all incidence of congenital deafness seen. A type II has been suggested to exist as a separate disorder, but it may really represent a variation of type I.

Transmission

Both type I and type II are autosomal dominant genetic transmission disorders. The chromosomal abnormality for type I is located on chromosome 2, and the genetic mutation for type II is found on chromosome 3. It is possible

TABLE 16–17. DIAGNOSTIC CRITERIA FOR NEUROFIBROMATOSIS-1*

Café-au-lait spots
　At least 5 spots > 5 mm in prepubertal patients
　At least 6 spots > 15 mm in postpubertal patients
　These are present in nearly 100% of patients
Axillary or inguinal freckling
The presence of two or more neurofibromas or the presence of one plexiform neu-
　rofibroma
Two or more Lisch nodules present within the iris of the eye
　These are present in > 90% of patients
The presence of an optic glioma
　These are present in approximately 15% of patients with NF-1
The presence of a distinct skeletal lesion
Having a first-degree relative who meets the criteria for NF-1

* Two need to be present for the diagnosis.
NF = neurofibromatosis.

that older age in men may account for a new mutation. This is a condition of autosomal dominance with complete penetrance, meaning that the genotype of the offspring will have the genetic mutation. But there is variable phenotypic expression of the mutation seen in the different individuals with the syndrome.

Clinical Features of Type I

The facial features of type I are apparent at birth (Fig. 16–7). More than 80% have dystopia canthorum and a broad nasal root. In dystopia canthorum, the medial canthi of the eyes are located more laterally. The interpupillary and outer canthal distances remain normal. Deafness occurs in approximately 25% of children with type I Waardenburg syndrome. Several other anomalies are noted in these patients (Table 16–18). Physical anomalies include patchy, depigmented hair. A white forelock is the dominant feature, occurring in about 40% of patients. Premature graying of the hair, eyebrows, and eyelashes may occur by the third decade.

Clinical Features of Type II

Type II Waardenburg syndrome shares some of the same congenital features, with a few differences. In type II, the medial canthi are located in the normal position. A higher percentage of people with type II experience deafness, which affects up to 50%.

Counseling

This syndrome is not life threatening. Early recognition of deafness is important. Early intervention promotes adequate speech and learning. Any child thought to have this syndrome needs to have audiometric studies performed early in life.

213

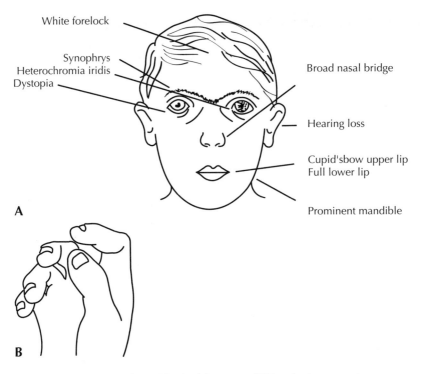

White forelock

Synophrys
Heterochromia iridis
Dystopia

Broad nasal bridge

Hearing loss

Cupid'sbow upper lip
Full lower lip

A

Prominent mandible

B

FIG. 16–7. (A) and (B). Physical features of Waardenburg syndrome.

🎱 INBORN ERRORS OF METABOLISM

The next several disorders are inborn errors of metabolism. Three common problems are presented: Tay-Sachs disease, cystic fibrosis, and sickle cell anemia. These types of disorders may be common in the general population or may have a tendency to occur within certain ethnic groups. Inborn errors of metabolism may involve the functioning of many types of proteins (e.g., cell receptor function or an enzyme defect). They may also be caused by problems with a particular protein's presence or absence.

TAY-SACHS DISEASE

Tay-Sachs disease is one of several disorders that involves lysosomal lipid storage. Tay-Sachs disease is also known as GM-2 gangliosidosis I. Gangliosides, made up of sphingolipids, simple sugars, and a sialic acid, are located within all cell membranes. They are complex molecules and are a normal constituent of the neuronal and synaptic cell membranes. As part of their natural course, recycling occurs by the enzymes present within the lysosomes. If a deficiency of the enzymes exists, the gangliosides build up, resulting in Tay-Sachs disease. There are several steps in the degradation

214

TABLE 16–18. CHARACTERISTICS OF WAARDENBURG SYNDROME

White forelock	Heterochromia of the irides
Premature graying of hair, eyebrow, eyelashes	Upturned upper lip (Cupid's bow)
	Full lower lip
Deafness	Possible cleft lip or palate
Laterally placed medial canthus (not seen in type II)	Prominent mandible
	Hypopigmentation of the skin

process of the gangliosides and the enzyme deficiency in Tay-Sachs disease that occur along the process. There are several other lysosomal storage disorders with enzyme deficiencies at other points along the pathway. The basic enzyme defect in Tay-Sachs disease is lack of β-hexosaminidase A. Two isoenzymes are needed for total β-hexosaminidase enzyme activity. The various mutations may affect one or both of the isoenzymes.

The storage disorders may involve the peripheral tissues, the CNS, or both. Tay-Sachs disease involves storage problems only within the cells of the CNS. There is no peripheral tissue, organ, or bony involvement, as may be seen with other lysosomal storage disorders. Tay-Sachs disease has the most devastating effects of the lipid storage disorders.

There are two forms of Tay-Sachs disease. The infantile and juvenile (late-onset) forms differ in their time of onset, severity of symptoms, and prognosis. The juvenile form is also called GM-2 gangliosidosis III; when this form begins later in life, it is referred to as adult GM-2 gangliosidosis. Tay-Sachs disease occurs most frequently in Ashkenazi (central or eastern European) Jews. The carrier rate in this population is 1 in 30.

Transmission

Various genetic mutations result in the enzyme defect seen in Tay-Sachs disease. The genetic defects are located on chromosome 15. The mutation may occur in different points within the gene. Mutations that result in partial or reduced enzymatic activity may produce less severe forms of the disease. The mutation that leads to the infantile form of the disease also differs from that causing the juvenile-onset form. An autosomal recessive defect is responsible for both forms of Tay-Sachs disease.

Clinical Features: Infantile Onset

The onset, progression, and ultimate prognosis vastly differ between the two forms of Tay-Sachs disease. The onset of the infantile form begins during the first year of life. The child develops normally until about age 5 or 6 months. Then alterations in neurological status are noted. Initially, decreased eye contact and focusing are seen along with an exaggerated startle reflex at a time when the startle reflex should have disappeared. By the first birthday, the infant may be severely hypotonic and blind and may interact very little with the surrounding environment. Seizures may develop as well as an enlarged head size, up to twice the normal size. The increased head size is caused by the ganglioside material deposited within the brain. Cherry red spots within the macula are nearly universally seen in these infants. Children with infantile Tay-Sachs typically die between age 2 and 4 years.

Clinical Features: Juvenile Onset

The onset in the juvenile form of Tay-Sachs may be at 2 years or may be as late as the second or third decade of life. Initially, the family may note clumsiness followed by ataxia, choreoathetosis (i.e., slow, writhing, continuous, involuntary movements), and dysarthrias. Cherry red spots within the macula are not associated with the juvenile or adult forms. As with the infantile form, only the CNS is involved. There is no organomegaly or bony changes, which may be seen in other lysosomal storage disorders. Blindness, spasticity, and seizures may occur before death. Death typically occurs in the second decade of life.

The disorder is confirmed through blood testing. A detection test for the hexosaminidase A isoenzyme is available. The test is inexpensive and accurate. The test can be performed to screen for the carrier state and may be used for diagnosis of the disorder during the first trimester via chorionic villus sampling.

Counseling

Screening for the carrier state is accurate and cost effective in populations in which the prevalence is high, such as in Ashkenazi Jews. Depending on whether a heterozygote state exists in the individual, the risk of transmission for individual couples can be calculated. Screening during pregnancy can be done, especially for couples who both possess the heterozygote state. There is no cure for Tay-Sachs disease.

CYSTIC FIBROSIS

Cystic fibrosis is an inheritable, autosomal recessive trait. The disorder is caused by a deletion of a single amino acid code from the gene for the protein cystic fibrosis transmembrane conductance regulator (CFTR). This regulator protein contains 1480 amino acids. Alteration of one amino acid may result in a functional change of the protein. The CFTR protein functions as a chloride channel. The change in the regulatory function of CFTR causes an alteration in chloride ion and water movement across epithelial cells. The tissues affected are those of the respiratory tract, sweat glands, gallbladder, and pancreas. Inhibition of the channel caused by the altered protein results in a thick, viscous secretion. The thick secretions within the bronchioles of the lungs lead to obstruction with frequent lung infections; bronchiolectasis; and eventually, reduced pulmonary function. This is the most common cause of chronic lung disease in children. In the pancreas, the viscous secretions also lead to duct obstruction. Reduced capacity to break down and metabolize fats and proteins is seen. The blockage and retention of secretions within the pancreas result in autodigestion, inflammation, and scarring. Pancreatic insufficiency is likely over time.

Cystic fibrosis is seen most commonly in children of European descent. The type of mutation differs among ethnic groups. Interestingly, it has been supposed that one reason why the gene mutations for cystic fibrosis have endured over the years, even with potentially fatal outcomes, is the resistance of the patient to cholera. The intestinal epithelium does not respond when exposed to the cholera bacterium, and the patient survives.

Transmission

Cystic fibrosis is inherited as an autosomal recessive disorder. The cystic fibrosis gene is located on chromosome 7, which includes the genetic codes for the 1480 amino acids that make up the CFTR protein. A single gene mutation, resulting in deletion of a single amino acid, is the underlying cause of the symptoms seen in patients with cystic fibrosis. Ethnic origin plays a role in which genetic mutation is seen. The majority of children with cystic fibrosis have a single deletion of genetic code for phenylalanine at amino acid position 508. The protein that is then produced by the offspring is the CFTR protein minus the phenylalanine. The deletion of this amino acid is the most common and is seen in approximately 70% of patients of North European ancestry who have cystic fibrosis. Other mutations also occur, but less frequently. A total of 540 different mutations within the cystic fibrosis gene have now been identified. In other ethnic groups, different mutations are found. In up to 60% of Ashkenazi Jews, the mutation is at amino acid position 1282. A mutation at position 542 is commonly found in patients from Spain. The differing genotype and phenotype result in the variability of clinical manifestations seen in patients with cystic fibrosis.

Clinical Features

Cystic fibrosis involves several body systems. Symptoms are seen involving the respiratory tract, GI tract, pancreas, and sweat glands. The initial symptoms of cystic fibrosis often involve the GI tract or the lungs. Approximately 10% of patients present at birth with meconium ileus. As the child grows, digestion problems and failure to thrive or to gain weight begins. Without the pancreatic exocrine hormones, digestion of fats, protein, and fat-soluble vitamins is impaired. Pancreatic insufficiency occurs in 80% to 85% of children with cystic fibrosis. Greasy, bulky stools; gas; bloating; and abdominal pain are frequent GI complaints. Rectal prolapse may occur.

There are numerous respiratory symptoms of cystic fibrosis. Cough, recurrent pneumonia or bronchiolitis, atelectasis, hemoptysis, and clubbing are a few of the clinical signs and symptoms seen in individuals with cystic fibrosis. Chronic sinusitis and nasal polyps are common. Nasal polyps are seen in about 20% of patients some time during the course of the illness.

Other systems are involved also. Sexual maturation is delayed in both genders. Only about 5% of men have sperm production; the rest are infertile. In women, intermittent amenorrhea and reduced fertility are seen. In women with good pulmonary function, pregnancy is well tolerated.

Diagnosis is made through performing the sweat test. Sweat is collected, and chemical analysis of the sodium and chloride content is obtained. A level of greater than 60 mEq per liter of chloride present in the sweat is diagnostic for cystic fibrosis. Levels lower than 40 mEq per liter are considered normal. With levels in-between, the analysis should be repeated. A positive sweat test result is considered diagnostic of cystic fibrosis when either clinical symptoms consistent with the syndrome are present or there is a family history of the disorder.

Counseling

Carrier status and prenatal detection of cystic fibrosis are now possible. Because this is an autosomal recessive trait, both parents must be carriers of the trait, meaning that they are heterozygotous, or that they have one normal gene and one abnormal gene for the trait. Although both parents are unaffected by the disorder, they are at risk for transmitting the cystic fibrosis gene to their offspring. For each child of the heterozygous carriers, there is a 25% risk of being affected by the disorder and a 50% risk of being a carrier of the trait. Prenatal diagnosis of cystic fibrosis can be made through chorionic villus sampling at 8 to 10 weeks' gestation or an amniocentesis obtained at 12 to 16 weeks. This type of testing, along with testing potential carriers, is best done at a cystic fibrosis center for detailed genetic counseling.

Treatment of children with cystic fibrosis should be initiated early and should be aggressive. Care is best done by a multidisciplinary team or through referral to a cystic fibrosis center. The goal is to maintain pulmonary function and nutritional status to lengthen survival and provide for quality of life. Much progress has been made in the treatment of persons with cystic fibrosis, and the median age of survival has increased dramatically. Forty years ago, the average life span was 4 years; the average life span has increased to more than 30 years.

SICKLE CELL ANEMIA

Sickle cell anemia results in intermittent chronic hemolytic anemia. It is caused by premature destruction of brittle and poorly deformable red blood cells. Sickle cell anemia is one of many disorders that occur from a defect in the hemoglobin molecule. More than 600 structural mutations in hemoglobin have now been identified; sickle cell anemia is one of them. The hemoglobin S molecule behaves much like normal hemoglobin A when underoxygenated states occur. When the hemoglobin S is exposed to a deoxygenated state, the abnormal hemoglobin molecules interact, forming polymers within the red blood cell. Distortion of red blood cells and damage to the cell membrane then occur. The resulting sickle shape of the red blood cell is more rigid and friable. The life span of these cells is about 10 to 20 days, resulting in chronic anemia. Sickle cell disease is seen in individuals from India, the Caribbean, and the Mediterranean area, as well as those of African descent, in whom it is a common genetic disorder, especially in America. In the United States, 1 in 12 individuals of African descent carries the sickle cell trait, and 1 in 600 shows clinical signs of sickle cell anemia. It is possible that the gene defect for sickle cell anemia has lasted over the years because it protects against certain types of malaria.

Transmission

The gene for sickle cell anemia is inherited in an autosomal recessive pattern. For the disease manifestations to be seen, each parent must carry one gene for the abnormal hemoglobin S. Normal hemoglobin is made up of two pairs of globulin subunits, two α and two β, and is referred to as hemoglobin A. Sickle cell anemia is caused by a single substitution of an amino acid. The resulting hemoglobin molecule is hemoglobin S. Glutamic acid, an amino acid located at position 6, has been replaced by valine with the β subunit.

Clinical Features

Sickle cell anemia is manifested by chronic anemia and periodic acute painful episodes. Chronic hemolytic anemic may be present by age 4 months. By this time, the fetal hemoglobin is nearly gone, and the more fragile hemoglobin S predominates. The signs and symptoms of sickle cell anemia result from vaso-occlusive episodes caused by the sickled red blood cells. As the blood circulates throughout the body and enters the slower capillary circulation, the red blood cell sickles because of the local hypoxia and acidosis. The sickling–unsickling process repeats itself until the normal red blood cell becomes permanently sickled for the duration of its life span. These sickled red blood cells cause vascular occlusion in the tiny capillaries, resulting in ischemia and necrosis. Pain then occurs. Any part of the body can be affected. Pain in infants and young children usually involves the extremities. In older children, pain is usually felt in the head, chest, abdomen, and back. Splenic infarcts are common. Pulmonary infarction and cerebrovascular occlusion may also occur.

Diagnosis is made by electrophoresis of the hemoglobin. Hemoglobin S behaves differently from the normal hemoglobin A. Anemia is present when a complete blood count is drawn. The reticulocyte and white blood cell counts are typically elevated.

Counseling

Sickle cell anemia is an autonomic recessive disorder. Carriers of sickle cell anemia are referred as having the sickle cell trait. Rather than having the normal genotype hemoglobin AA, they have hemoglobin AS. When each parent carries the AS genotype, they have a 25% chance of having a child with sickle cell anemia and a 50% chance of having a child who has the sickle cell trait. They also have a 25% percent chance of having a normal child with hemoglobin AA. Prenatal diagnosis is available for at-risk couples.

There is no cure for sickle cell anemia, although bone marrow transplant is a possible future treatment. Supportive care during crisis and measures to prevent complications are the treatment for the disease.

TEST YOUR KNOWLEDGE OF CHAPTER 16

1. What are the components of the history for a child with genetic problems?
2. Describe the components of pedigree plotting.
3. Discuss inheritance.
4. What are the components of genetic counseling?
5. What is karyotyping?

 ## BIBLIOGRAPHY

Aase, J. M. (1990). *Diagnostic dysmorphology*. New York: Plenum Publishing.

Able, E. L., & Hannigan, J. H. (1995). Maternal risk factors in fetal alcohol syndrome: Provocative and permissive influences. *Neurotoxicology and Teratology, 17,* 445–462.

Batshaw, M. L. (1997). *Children with disabilities*. Baltimore: Paul H. Brookes Publishers.

Cassidy, S. B. (2001). *Management of genetic syndromes*. New York: Wiley-Liss.

Centers for Disease Control and Prevention. (2001). Genetics and Disease Prevention. Available at: *http://www.cdc.gov/genetics/training/competencies*

Goldbloom, R. B. (1997). *Pediatric clinical skills*. Philadelphia: Churchill Livingstone.

Goodman, R. M., & Gordin, R. J. (1983). *The malformed infant and child*. New York: Oxford University Press.

Jackson, P. L,. & Vessey, J. A. (2000). *Child with a chronic condition*. St. Louis: Mosby.

Jones, K. L. (1997). *Recognizable patterns of human malformations*. Philadelphia: W. B. Saunders.

Jorde, L. B., Carey, J. C., Bamshad, M. J., & White, R. L. (2000). *Medical genetics*. St. Louis: Mosby.

Lissauer, T., & Clayden, G. (1997). *Illustrated textbook of paediatrics*. London: Mosby.

Mullins, N. L. (Ed.) (2000). *Mosby's medical & nursing dictionary*. St Louis: Mosby.

Nelson, W. E. (Ed.) (2000). *Textbook of pediatrics*. Philadelphia: W. B. Saunders.

Warkany, J., Lemire, R. J., & Cohen, M. M. (1981). *Mental retardation and congenital malformation of the central nervous system*. Chicago: Year Book Medical Publishers, Inc.

West, J. R., Chen, W. J. A., & Pantazis, N. J. (1994). Fetal alcohol syndrome: The vulnerability of the developing brain and possible mechanisms of damage. *Metabolic Brain Disease, 9,* 291–322.

Zittelli, B. J., & Davis, H. W. (1997). *Atlas of pediatric physical diagnosis*. St. Louis: Mosby.

Assessment by Age Grouping and Special Issues

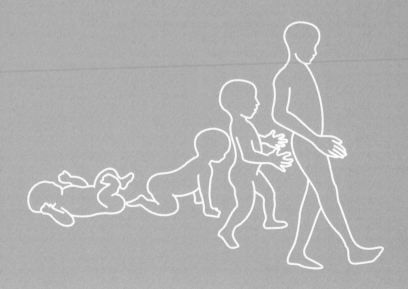

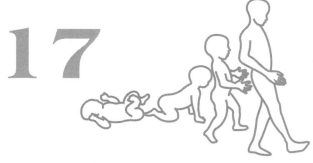

Premature Infants

GILLIAN TUFTS

OBJECTIVES
- *Understand the common problems exhibited by premature infants.*
- *Determine when premature infants catch up both developmentally and physically.*
- *Gain an understanding of the differences that families of preterm infants encounter versus those of term infants.*
- *Identify developmental lags early to promote early intervention.*

Up to 7% of all babies born each year are born preterm, or before 37 weeks' gestation. The weight of these infants is less than 2500 g or 5.4 lb. These babies are called low birth weight or preterm infants and account for approximately 50% of all newborn intensive care unit (NICU) admissions. Approximately one third of preterm infants are born before 32 weeks' gestation and are referred to as very preterm or very low birth weight infants. Typically, these infants weight less than 1500 g or 3.2 lb. This group of infants accounts for approximately 25% of NICU admissions, with approximately 1% being those infants who weigh less than 1000 g. The earlier the gestational age at birth, the higher the risk of neurologic and developmental sequelae.

Although the survival rate for infants born at less than 28 weeks' gestation or with birth weights under 1000 g is now reaching 90%, the survival may come at a high cost for these infants and their families. The possible long-term effects of preterm birth are many: major neurologic sequelae, such as hydrocephalus, cerebral palsy, sensory deficits, and cognitive delays; increased risk for respiratory problems, including reactive airway disease, respiratory infection, and sudden infant death syndrome (SIDS); and possibly behavioral problems, such as hyperactivity or various learning disabilities.

For many years after the preterm birth, routine well-child care plays an important role in identifying developmental delays. The delays may be subtle changes or impairments in motor or cognitive development or in behavior. These disabilities may affect the child long after the infant period and may lead to lifelong problems. Early detection and intervention may improve the overall quality of life. The primary care provider may well serve as the coordinator of various medical and social services needed to optimize the infant's health.

This chapter focuses on assessment in ambulatory care settings of the child born at 32 weeks' gestation or beyond. However, some issues of very low birth weight infants are included because these infants, along with the low birth weight group, eventually enter the primary care setting for well-child or episodic care.

INITIAL OR INTERVAL HISTORY

During the initial office visit, it is important to review the entire hospital course with the parent or parents. Ask about problems during the pregnancy and about the cause of the preterm delivery. Review the events surrounding the birth. Ask about the hospital course, including the length of stay, medications given, and any complications the infant experienced. Complications may include neurologic insult, respiratory distress, anemia or other nutritional deficiencies and necrotizing enterocolitis.

Obtain the birth weight of the infant and the most recent measurements of length, weight, and head circumference. Be sure to obtain the gestational age of the infant. The group of infants who are small for their gestational age—infants with intrauterine growth retardation—may be at additional risk. Infants whose birth weight is at or below the tenth percentile for gestational age are considered small for gestational age. This group is not included in this chapter. Many factors are known to lead to premature birth (Table 17–1). These factors may be fetal, maternal, placental, or uterine in nature. It is optimal if the primary healthcare provider has a grasp of these factors to aid in prevention of future premature births.

Begin the visit by asking the parents about their concerns and if they have any questions regarding the infant's care. Then review the feeding, sleeping, and elimination patterns of the infant. For preterm infants, it is important to assess the amount and timing of the feedings, as well as whether the infant is breast or bottle fed. Review what the infant was fed in the hospital, such as parenteral feedings, supplementation with breastfeeding, or special formulas. Ask if the infant has any feeding problems, such as reflux or vomiting; if the infant tires easily when feeding; and what type of nipple is being used.

Ask about any vitamin or mineral supplements given to the infant. Review the number of wet diapers and the number of stools per day. Ask

TABLE 17-1. FACTORS KNOWN TO CAUSE PRETERM BIRTH			
Fetal	**Maternal**	**Placental**	**Uterine**

Multiple gestation
Fetal distress
	• Infection
	  ○ Bacterial vaginosis
	  ○ Chlamydia
	• Urinary tract infection
	• Group B strep vaginitis
	• Chorioiamnionitis
	• Preeclampsia
	• Chronic illness
	• Drug abuse
		• Placenta previa
		• Abruptio placentae
			• Bicornate uterus
			• Incompetent cervix
			• Premature rupture of membranes
			• Polyhydraminos

the parent to briefly describe the infant's day, including the amount of awake time and the number of hours spent sleeping. Premature infants often have irregular sleep–wake patterns, which may be discouraging to the parents.

Next complete the review of systems, covering HEENT (head, eyes, ears, nose, and throat), the respiratory and musculoskeletal systems, and the skin, in addition to the gastrointestinal and genitourinary areas already covered. Ask specifically about any respiratory distress the infant may have experienced during the hospitalization to assess the risk for future respiratory problems. Questions regarding the nervous system can be asked when assessing the gross and fine motor development. Review with the parents what they have noticed the infant doing in terms of gross motor, fine motor, and language skills. It is very important to include this part of the assessment of preterm infants because they are at more risk for developing subtle neurologic deficits. Ask if the infant has been back to the emergency room since discharge or if there has been any illness. Obtain a list of the medications the infant is taking.

Ask if the infant received any immunizations before discharge from the hospital. Table 17–2 summarizes the information to obtain at the well-child visit. If this is the initial visit, additional information regarding the birth events and hospital course are also important to obtain and record in the chart.

FAMILY ASSESSMENT

A vital part of any infant visit is assessment of the family. It is important to assess the amount of stress the primary caregiver is experiencing because it directly affects his or her ability to care for the child. The amount of stress experienced by the family caring for a healthy preterm infant is less than that experienced by those caring for an infant with continuing medical problems.

TABLE 17–2. SUBJECTIVE INFORMATION TO OBTAIN AT A ROUTINE WELL-CHILD VISIT FOR A PREMATURE INFANT

GENERAL PARENTAL CONCERNS

Feeding
- Breast, bottle, or both
- Problems with breastfeeding, such as sore nipples, trouble latching on
- If formula-fed:
  - Type
  - Iron fortified?
- Number of feedings over 24-hour period
- Intervals of feedings
- Amount per feeding; for breast-fed infants, how long each side
- Problems noted, such as fatigue, reflux, vomiting, cyanosis
- Vitamin use

SLEEP
- General pattern of awake versus sleep periods
- Number of nighttime awakenings
- Hours of sleep during the day
- Position of sleep
- Location of sleeping
- Comfort measures

REVIEW OF SYSTEMS
- Crying or fussiness
- Tearing at eyes or discharge
- Nasal symptoms
- Cough
- Gastrointestinal: Vomiting or spitting-up pattern; frequency and consistency of stools
- Genitourinary: Number wet diapers; color of urine
- Equal use of extremities
- Skin rashes

FAMILY ASSESSMENT
- Changes in:
  - Living arrangement
  - Job situation
  - Finances
  - Marital status
- For primary caregiver:
  - Sufficient rest
  - Support system
  - Return to work
- Birth control method

Are the parents getting enough rest? Any there problems with finances, jobs, or living arrangement? Problems in these areas can increase familial stress. Ask the primary caregiver if he or she works or is planning to return to work soon. What child-care arrangements have been made? Ask about the other siblings. What birth control method is being used? Have the parents had a chance to get out without the child? It is important for the parents to have

226

time to themselves. Strain from an early delivery or from caring for an infant with medical problems can produce problems between the parents. Lack of time together, a disorganized lifestyle, or additional financial burdens put a strain on even the best of relationships.

PERIODICITY TABLE

Preterm infants may need more frequent office visits than full-term infants. It may be necessary to more closely monitor the growth parameters and the developmental milestones of these infants. Inform parents of the need for more frequent and potentially longer visits, especially during the first few months of life. The goals of these visits are much the same as for healthy term infants: to provide health assessment and maintenance in a continuous and comprehensive manner.

It is vitally important for the infant and their families that the healthcare provider establish an effective relationship with the parents, gain an understanding of the child's cultural background, and assess for family stressors to identify early families at risk. Periodic visits to the office also aid in the early detection of disease processes and detection of developmental or behavioral problems.

As with full-term infants, health maintenance is important, such as receiving the recommended immunizations or fluoride treatments. Because preterm infants are potentially different from other infants to which the parents may have been exposed, anticipatory guidance specific to their infant is of the utmost importance.

SCREENING

GROWTH PARAMETERS: ADJUSTED AGE

Adequate growth can be monitored through measuring the infant's length, weight, and head circumference at regular intervals. Use of the standard growth curve for plotting and monitoring growth measurements is recommended for preterm infants but should be done using the adjusted age, not chronologic age. Adjusted age is the postnatal age minus the number of weeks the infant was delivered early. For example, a child whose gestational age at birth was 32 weeks would have 8 weeks subtracted from his or her chronologic age. At 42 weeks, this infant would physically and developmentally be considered age 34 weeks. Adjusted age should be used until 18 months for the head circumference, until 24 months for weight, and until 42 months for the child's length.

CATCH-UP GROWTH: HEAD

Catch-up growth begins with head growth. A preterm infant's head may seem disproportionately large when compared with his or her weight and length. A growth in head circumference more than 2 cm/week raises con-

TABLE 17–3. DESIRED GROWTH RATES IN PRETERM INFANTS	
First 3 Months:	**Months 3 through 12:**
• Weight 20–30 g/day	• Weight 10–15 g/day
• Height 0.7–1.0 cm/week	• Height 0.4–0.6 cm/week

cerns for possible neurologic compromise. This is especially true in infants with a history of intraventricular or intracranial hemorrhage or hydrocephalus. The catch-up growth rate is highest between 36 and 44 weeks postconception or 4 weeks before and after the date when the child was to be born.

WEIGHT AND LENGTH

For premature infants, a growth rate of 20 to 30 g/day for weight and 0.7 to 1.0 cm for length per week is desirable for the first 3 months after birth. For the following 9 months, or until 1 year of adjusted age has been reached, the desirable weight and length gains are halved (Table 17–3).

VISION

Infants born prematurely are at risk to develop various eye and visual problems. Retinal vascularity is usually completed around 40 weeks postconception in normal full-term pregnancies. Premature birth interrupts the normal pattern of growth, resulting in progressive, poorly regulated blood vessel growth within the retina. This is termed retinopathy of prematurity. The disorder occurs almost exclusively in infants born before 32 weeks' gestation or whose birth weight is less than 1500 g. Ninety percent of infants who weigh less than 750 g experience some degree of retinopathy. The incidence drops to 47% for infants who weigh 1000 to 1250 g. The risk of developing retinopathy also depends on exposure to supplemental oxygen and other conditions, such as anemia, intraventricular bleeding, or necrotizing enterocolitis.

Any infant with risk factors must be referred to an ophthalmologist. For an infant weighing less than 1500 g at birth or who was born before 30 weeks' gestation, a screening ophthalmic examination should be done at approximately 6 weeks of chronologic age and repeated as recommended by the specialist. For infants who weigh 1500 to 1800 g or who were born between 30 and 35 weeks' gestation and were exposed to oxygen, a screening ophthalmic examination should be obtained.

Preterm infants are also at greater risk for developing strabismus, myopia, and amblyopia. Strabismus is up to four times more common in premature infants. Management of these problems is the same as with full-term infants. During each well-child visit, careful assessment of the eye needs to be completed.

228

HEARING

Preterm infants, especially very preterm infants, may be exposed to many potential ototoxic agents that can harm the developing auditory system. Drugs (e.g., gentamicin or furosemide), infection, hypoxia, and elevated bilirubin levels are some of the frequent causes of ototoxicity. There is a relatively high incidence of hearing loss in premature or ill infants. Rates as high as 2% to 4% have been found. Testing of the brainstem auditory evoked response (BAER) should be obtained before the infant is discharged home and should be repeated between the third and sixth month for very premature infants. The BAER testing screens for unilateral or bilateral hearing loss or for conductive or sensorineural loss, and can classify the loss as mild to profound.

PHYSICAL EXAMINATION

A complete head-to-toe physical examination should be performed at each visit. Use the same guidelines, based on the age of the child, as done at the well-child visits for the term infant. Normal physical signs of prematurity may be found on examination. Table 17–4 outlines normal physical findings and potential complications found in preterm infants.

DEVELOPMENT

The developmental milestones are used by the parents and the provider to determine the progress of the infant. For the parents, milestones of when the baby smiles, sits independently, or begins to walk are viewed in relationship to other infants. For the provider, the timing of when the various developmental milestones are reached can be used to screen for mild to severe developmental impairment.

Gross and fine motor skills, language, cognition, and social skills need to be monitored. It is often easier to obtain the history regarding the development while performing the physical examination. Ask the parents what they have noted at home and what concerns they have regarding the infant's development. A high percentage of parental concerns turn out to be accurate. It is important to listen to and address parents' worries. It is also important to point out the child's advancements to the parents.

For very low birth weight infants, routine developmental screening in the office may not be sensitive enough to pick up subtle abnormalities. This group of infants may be better served by a formal assessment through various community agencies with programs in place to serve preterm infants. There is a federal mandate for states to provide early intervention programs for high-risk preterm infants. The Disabilities Education Act, a law that provides for all individuals with developmental disabilities, has been extended to include early intervention for infants and toddlers. Primary healthcare providers who will potentially care for preterm infants, especially very

TABLE 17-4. PHYSICAL ASSESSMENT OF PRETERM INFANTS: POTENTIAL FINDINGS ON PHYSICAL EXAMINATION

HEENT
- Abnormal head growth
- Dolichocephaly (head is long and narrow in appearance)
- Abnormal facies (long face, narrow forehead, deep-set eyes) typically change with maturity
- Strabismus, amblyopia
- Routine ear examination findings but increased risk for otitis media
- Palatal groove and high-arched palate
- Abnormal teeth formation, malformation, enamel defects, discolorations

RESPIRATORY
- Presence of chronic lung disease, defined as supplemental oxygen use at 36 weeks
- Elevated respiratory rate or heart rate, presence of retractions, presence of wheezing, poor color, poor feeding tolerance

CARDIOVASCULAR
- Routine examination

GASTROINTESTINAL
- Gastroesophageal reflux: Occurs more frequently in preterm infants
- Short bowel syndrome; after bowel resection for necrotizing enterocolitis, may see diarrhea or failure to thrive
- Constipation: Occurs more frequently in preterm infants

GENITOURINARY TRACT
- Inguinal hernias, preterms with increased risk, especially with birth weight under 1250 g
- Presence of hydrocele

SKIN
- Scars of the posthospitalized infant
  - Posttracheostomy
  - Chest tube: May cause deformity in the adult breast (not common)
  - Pinpoint scars at dorsum of hands: Fade but may stay visible in the older child
  - Multiple heel sticks from blood sampling – fade but may be visible in the older child
  - Hemangiomas

HEENT = head, eyes, ears, nose, and throat.

---

preterm infants, should become familiar with the various programs in their communities that provide services and support for preterm infants and their families.

Ultimately, the goals of development are the same for premature infants as for full-term infants. For gross motor skills, gradual cephalocaudal development is expected, beginning with head and trunk control to the development of locomotion. At the same time, there is a progressive loss of the primitive reflex responses and the emergence of the postural responses as equilibrium balance develops, which demonstrates the integration of the motor and sensory systems within the brain. An infant with central nervous system damage may exhibit sustained primitive reflexes and a slow appearance of the postural reflexes.

Fine motor control is exhibited through the development of the pincer grasp. The skill of the infant improves over the first year of life from batting at objects to the ability to pick up small objects with the fingertips.

Language develops, both in the ability to understand what is spoken and to express what is thought or needed. Social and emotional development describes how infants learn to trust and interact with their environments. Preterm infants may initially respond differently than full-term infants, especially infants who spent time in the NICU. For many preterm infants, normal cognitive development is possible. Some preterm infants, especially very preterm infants, may have suffered neurologic insults, and their cognition, as well as other areas of development, may be impaired. It is important to identify these infants early for timely referral and intervention.

When assessing the infant's development, the milestone progression should be based on the infant's adjusted age rather than chronologic age. At each visit, it is important to remind the parents of the infant's current adjusted age. The adjusted age should be used until 2 to 3 years of age for infants born under 1500 g. For infants who weigh more, it may be necessary to use the adjusted age for only the first 12 months. A formal screening can be performed in the office using the Denver Developmental II screening instrument. An informal assessment can also be done, but the provider must be sure to screen for development in the areas of gross and fine motor control, language, cognition, and social skills. For older infants and children, it is important to ask the parents about behavioral problems at home and school. When faced with a developmental delay, be sure to look at the total picture. For example, for an infant who has been ill, mild delays can be expected.

Guidelines have been developed for the premature infant developmental milestone attainment. These guidelines help primary healthcare providers decide when to refer infants to specialists for more formal evaluation and intervention. Table 17–5 summarizes the red flags for development in preterm infants.

When the infant is on the parent's lap or on the examination table, the various maneuvers to test gross and fine motor skills can be performed. For example, after performing the abdominal examination or examination of the hips, you can check for head lag, the ability of the infant to sit with adequate head control or to sit independently. To screen fine motor control, place an object in the infant's hand and watch how he or she handles the object. Assessment of how the child handles the object should be done in relation to the adjusted age. For example, a 6-month-old infant born at 32 weeks' gestation (adjusted age equals 4 months) may reach and hold the object in one hand or put the object to his or her mouth. This is appropriate for a 4-month-old full-term infant but is delayed for a 6-month-old child if the child's age has not been adjusted by 2 months because of the prematurity.

In general, for healthy premature infants, use the developmental milestones for the adjusted age to assess if the infant is on track for that infant's situation. Each preterm infant's situation is different because of the number of weeks premature, whether there have been medical complications, or if there is any persisting illness. With the latter, a delay in the infant's devel-

TABLE 17–5. DEVELOPMENTAL RED FLAGS IN PRETERM INFANTS

Healthcare providers can use the following screening guidelines to decide when it is warranted to refer preterm infants for formal developmental testing. Adjusted age is used for each age category.

At 6 months adjusted age, the infant:
- Is not sitting, even with support
- Makes no effort to reach or bat at objects
- Does not localize to sound
- Only momentarily grasps
- Keeps hands fisted
- Does not mouth objects

At 12 months adjusted age, the infant:
- Sits but does not crawl
- Does not search for a hidden object
- Does not vocalize consonant and vowel combinations
- Does not attend to books
- Does not respond to simple familiar directions such as "pat-a-cake"

At 18 months adjusted age, the infant:
- Does not walk
- Does not imitate sounds or motor actions
- Cannot build a tower with blocks
- Is most interested in putting toys in mouth at play
- Knows fewer than eight words

At 24 months adjusted age, the infant:
- Does not put two words together in speech
- Has play skills that remain primarily imitative
- Has gross motor skills that are lacking in balance and control
- Cannot complete a simple puzzle or shape sorter
- Cannot identify basic body parts

At 36 months adjusted age, the infant:
- Does not follow simple commands, including "give me"
- Does not use prepositions in speech
- Cannot copy a circle
- Has such poor articulation that it is impossible for others to understand
- Does not jump with both feet off the ground

At age 4 years, the child:
- Still uses phrases instead of sentences
- Does not know color names
- Cannot give first and last names
- Cannot pedal a tricycle

opment may be expected. If there are unexpected delays, further evaluation is needed.

PARENT–CHILD INTERACTION

Observe the parent–child interaction throughout the visit. Note how the parent holds and talks to the child. Does the parent hold the infant loosely with disinterest, or does the parent appear overprotective or overly responsive to the infant? How does the infant respond to the parent? Ask the parent how he or she comforts the infant. Lack of interest by either party may indicate parental depression or a lack of bonding. These signs are potential indicators of a family at risk. Early intervention promotes overall well-being for the family. There are special issues for the families of preterm infants, which are covered later under anticipatory guidance.

EGO DEVELOPMENT

The goal for ego development of preterm infants is the same as for term infants and children. Preterm infants follow the same stages of Erikson's psychosocial theory of ego development as in other children, but some experiences of preterm infants may make it difficult during the first weeks to months. If the infant is born with physical problems and hospitalization is required, attending to the nurturing of the infant can be difficult. If the infant is preterm but healthy, a hospital stay can interfere with the normal bonding and attachment that takes place after birth. The positive effect of human touch and skin-to-skin contact with preterm infants in the NICU has been well documented. The initial lack of response and possible avoidance of interaction by the infant in the NICU can make parenting difficult. This self-protective behavior, learned to keep out intrusive stimuli, may make the infant seem distant and not interested in the parents. This behavior may continue long after discharge. Helping parents learn to read the cues of their infant as they grow and develop will aid the parents in being more effective in supporting the emotional development of their infant.

LEAD SCREENING

The American Academy of Pediatrics (AAP) recommends that lead screening be performed as part of routine health supervision at about age 9 to 12 months and again at about age 24 months. Early detection can prevent the resulting neurotoxicity of the developing child. In areas where universal lead screening is not warranted, testing should be completed on those children who are at risk. The following are considered risks for elevated lead levels:

- Living in a dwelling built before 1950
- Regularly visiting dwellings built before 1950, such as daycare facilities
- Having a sibling or playmate with elevated blood lead levels
- Living with an adult whose job or hobby involves the use of lead
- Living near an industry using lead in production

HEMATOCRIT

A complete blood count (CBC) and reticulocyte count should be obtained. Eventually, nearly every preterm infant becomes anemic because their iron stores, which are typically laid down during the last weeks of pregnancy, are inadequate. Frequent blood tests during the NICU stay may also contribute to the low blood count. The CBC and reticulocyte count are usually checked on discharge from the hospital and should be checked again at ages 2 and 4 months. The blood count in a premature infant is lower than that of a term infant, reaching the lowest value at about 2 months chronologic age. Iron supplementation should be given. The doses and length of treatment are reviewed in the Nutrition section of this chapter.

IMMUNIZATIONS

The AAP recommends that infants born prematurely receive routine immunizations and, in most cases, at the usual time. For preterm infants, chronologic age rather than adjusted age is used to determine when the vaccines are given. There is some concern, however, regarding the immature immune system of premature infants and their ability to mount adequate antibody response to the vaccine.

The diphtheria, tetanus, and acellular pertussis vaccines should be given at the usual recommended 2, 4, 6, and 12 months chronologic age. Diphtheria and tetanus toxoids appear to be highly immunogenic in preterm infants, and levels of antibody for both appear to be comparable with those of full-term infants. The immunogenic effect of pertussis is not as well known.

Injectable, inactivated polio vaccine (IPV) is given at the usual chronologic ages of 2, 4, and 12 months. The first dose may be given while the infant is still hospitalized.

For preterm infants, the hepatitis B vaccine is given at the usual recommended ages of birth, 2 months, and 6 months. The exception to this rule is based on the infant's weight. The first hepatitis B injection is delayed until the infant's weight has reached 2000 g or more. Infants who weigh less than 2000 g may not seroconvert, and thus may not be adequately protected. Infants born to mothers who are positive for hepatitis B should receive the first hepatitis B vaccine within 12 hours of birth, similar to the treatment for full-term infants.

The pneumococcal conjugate vaccine (PCV7) is recommended for all children 23 months and younger and is given at 2, 4, 6, and 12 to 15 months of age. Infants of very low birth weight (less than 1500 g) can be immunized at the time that they attain a chronologic age of 6 to 8 weeks.

The *Haemophilus influenzae* type b (HIB) vaccine should be given at the routine recommended ages. Use chronologic age, not adjusted age, for preterm infants. Measles, mumps, and rubella (MMR) and varicella vaccines can be given as for full-term infants.

As each new vaccine becomes available, the efficacy in preterm infants needs to be evaluated. In general, it is recommended that the routine vaccines be given in the usual time schedule, but this may not be true for each individual preterm infant. Table 17–6 summarizes the usual immunization schedule for preterm infants.

The AAP Committee on Infectious Diseases and Committee on Fetus and Newborn recommend that immunizations against respiratory syncytial

TABLE 17–6. RECOMMENDED IMMUNIZATIONS FOR PRETERM INFANTS*

Immunization	Schedule
DtaP	2, 4, 6, and 12-15 months chronologic age
Polio (IPV)	2, 4, 6-18 months chronologic age
HIB	2, 4, 6, and 12-15 months chronologic age
Hepatitis B	All infants with mothers who are hepatitis B positive
	After 2000 g has been attained or birth, 2 and 6 months chronologic age
Pneumococcal conjugate	2, 4, 6, and 12-15 months chronologic age
MMR	12-15 months
Varicella	After 12 months with no history of varicella infection

* Check the Centers for Disease Control and Prevention's Website for updates.
DtaP = diphtheria, tetanus, acellular pertussis; HIB = *Haemophilus influenzae* type b; IPV = inactivated polio vaccine; MMR = measles, mumps, and rubella.

virus (RSV) be given for infants born at 35 weeks' gestation or less. Palivizumab (Synagis), a recombinantly produced monoclonal antibody, is used monthly throughout the RSV season. The rationale for palivizumab use is based on a large, randomized study that found a 55% reduction in hospitalization rates for RSV in the high-risk pediatric population.

Palivizumab is given to those infants with risk of developing severe RSV. The risk of developing severe RSV depends on the number of weeks premature, the presence of chronic lung disease, or both. High-risk infants are given a monthly injection during the RSV season to reduce the risk of serious illness or hospitalization. Outbreaks of RSV generally occur from October to December and the end of March to May. Regional differences do occur, and each provider needs to be aware of the RSV season in his or her community. The criteria for palivizumab use are summarized in Table 17–7. There are a large number of children born between 32 and 35 weeks' gestation. Because of the cost of palivizumab, the drug should be reserved for infants with additional risk factors. Other aspects of the infant's life may influence the decision of palivizumab prophylaxis, rather than just the presence or absence of lung disease. Other underlying conditions that may predispose infants to respiratory complications, including neurologic disease,

TABLE 17–7. PRETERM INFANTS AT RISK FOR RESPIRATORY SYNCYTIAL VIRUS: INDICATIONS FOR MONTHLY PROPHYLAXIS*

- Infants younger than age 2 years with chronic lung disease who have received treatment for lung disease less than 6 months before the onset of RSV season
- Infants born at 28 weeks gestation or less who are younger than age 1 year
- Infants born at 29 to 32 weeks gestation who are younger than age 6 months
- Infants born at more than 32 weeks: Not used except in those infants with RSV risk factors, including chronic lung disease or social factors

* Note: Synagis dosing: 15 mg/kg intramuscular injection monthly during respiratory syncytial virus season.

young siblings, child-care center attendance, exposure to tobacco smoke in the home, or availability of emergent hospital care for severe respiratory illness, may be considered in the decision of whether or not to administer palivizumab.

 # ANTICIPATORY GUIDANCE ISSUES

GROWTH AND DEVELOPMENT

After an infant has arrived at home, the parents may turn their attention away from the medical issues of having a premature baby to concerns of how the baby is growing and developing. The milestones of the first smile, rolling over, sitting independently, and taking the first steps may be of great concern. It is important for the parents and their families to understand that preterm infants may develop differently from full-term infants. When parents understand the differences, they can adjust their expectations to be more in line with the capabilities of the infant. They should not be discouraged when the infant does not develop in the same manner as their other children or as a friend's child. Preterm infants may follow a different developmental schedule, but this does not prevent the infant from developing into a normal, healthy child. Encourage the parents to compare their infant only with himself or herself and to focus on month-to-month growth and progress.

When determining the expected developmental age for the various milestones, adjusted age should be used rather than chronologic age. The adjusted age is calculated by subtracting the number of weeks born early from the chronological age. This adjusted age in weeks should be used until the child attains 24 months of age for very low birth weight babies. For low birth weight infants (i.e., those with birth weights greater than 1500 g) the adjustment may be necessary only for the first year of life. Remind the parents that the infant has lost growth and development time because he or she was not allowed to complete maturation in utero. The time lost may be only 1 or 2 weeks, but it may be as much as 10 to 12 weeks for very preterm infants. In infants with medical complications, such as persisting respiratory distress, development may seem to lag even further behind the adjusted age during the first year.

STIMULATION

The interaction between the infant and parents is vital to the infant's overall growth and development. Preterm infants may respond differently than full-term infants and have different needs. It is important for the parents to understand the infant's body language, including when interaction is desired and when the infant is saying, "No more. I've had enough." Table 17–8 summarizes the various behaviors that an infant may express to invite or avert social interaction. Clues of readiness indicate that the infant is ready to handle social interaction. Signs of distress indicate that the interaction is

TABLE 17–8. BEHAVIORS OF PRETERM INFANTS FOR READINESS AND CESSATION OF INTERACTION

SIGNS OF READINESS
- Relaxed posture
- Flexion of the extremities
- Looking attentively with quiet body movements
- Eye contact (even momentarily)
- Mouthing or sucking motions

SIGNS OF DISTRESS
- Yawning
- Averting gaze
- Arching back or extending extremities
- Furrowed brow, worried look
- Increased spitting up, gagging, hiccups
- Irregular breathing, cyanosis, or pallor
- Extending fingers
- Limpness

becoming overwhelming or adversely affecting the infant. When signs of distress occur, the parent should stop the current activity. These behaviors can be confusing to some parents. Review techniques to calm the baby. Advise the parents to decrease overall visual and auditory stimulation by turning down the lights or using soothing music. Gently rocking, swaddling, or talking to the infant can also soothe a distressed baby. Caution parents that too many soothing activities at once can also result in overstimulation of the infant.

Stimulation of the infant in various manners aids growth and development. As the infant grows, the parents can provide many of the same activities as with the full-term infants. For gross motor control, the parent can exercise the infant's arms and legs while bathing or help the infant roll from front to back. For older infants, encourage the parent to provide opportunities for play and experimentation. To encourage fine motor development, the parents can provide toys such as rattles or items of various textures for the infant to handle. Mirrors and colorful mobiles (be cautious of the strings) are aids for visual stimulation. Encourage the parents to talk and sing to the infant. Reading to the infant or child aids auditory and language development. Playing music also promotes auditory development and can be soothing. Encourage parents to hold, rock, and cuddle the infant frequently.

SAFETY

Many of the safety issues for preterm infants are similar to those for full-term infants. There are a few additional issues to keep in mind.

- Infants and toddlers should always be in a car seat, never held in a parent's lap. Infant car seats are made for infants who weigh more than 7 lb. Many preterm infants weigh less than this when they are discharged to home. A rolled towel or sheet placed along the sides of the car seat helps to support the head and trunk. An adult should be seated next to the infant in the rear seat to monitor for respiratory distress if the head becomes bent to the side. Oxygen saturation can be checked while the infant is seated in the car seat before leaving the hospital.

- When bathing the infant, the parent should always check the water temperature with an elbow before placing the infant in the water. In general, tap water temperature should be less than 120°F to prevent accidental burns.
- Infants should never be left alone in the bath.
- Recommend that the primary caregiver become comfortable with giving infant cardiopulmonary resuscitation (CPR). Some preterm infants are at more risk for apneic spells or SIDS.
- Always encourage parents to have a smoke alarm in the household. Encourage parents to have a fire strategy with an escape plan that includes the infant.
- Limit the number of people handling the infant; avoid crowds.
- If possible, avoid daycare until the infant is at least 6 months of age or up to 12 months with higher-risk infants.
- Avoid cigarette smoke around the infant.

DENTAL ISSUES

The American Academy of Pediatric Dentistry recommends that infants' gums be cleansed every day. Encourage the parent to gently massage the gums with a soft washcloth wrapped around a finger. As with any infant, discourage the practice of bottle propping. Remind parents that feeding is a time of closeness. Much of the infant's early social interaction revolves around feeding. Fluoride is instituted in the same manner as with full-term infants.

Occasionally, an infant with a history of hyperbilirubinemia may show discoloration of the teeth. This does not affect the permanent teeth. Enamel defects from pressure by an endotracheal tube also may be seen. There is increased risk of dental caries if there are defects in the enamel, but again, this will not affect the permanent teeth.

NUTRITION

There are several criteria that preterm infants must meet before discharge from the NICU. Included in the criteria are the ability of the infant to take an adequate amount of milk by nipple and to gain weight adequately. This is typically met at about 35 to 36 weeks' postconceptual age. Infants who weigh less than 1500 g or are less than 34 weeks' gestation may not be able to coordinate breathing, sucking, and swallowing, and they may require tube feedings. The effort of sucking may be a limiting factor in the success of breastfeeding. The use of bottle-feeding expressed breast milk may be temporarily needed. Larger preterm infants who weigh 1500 to 1800 g often tolerate oral feedings well. For these infants, a higher caloric supplementation may be necessary only initially.

Preterm infants may be difficult feeders. At each visit, it is important to review with the parent how the feedings are progressing and to provide support. Infants who have experienced prolonged periods of tube feedings with a lack of nonnutritive sucking may need much patience and coaching from parents. For infants and parents, feeding should be a time for closeness and social interaction, not frustration or anxiety. It is important for the healthcare provider to recognize when problems arise and to support and listen to the parents.

The AAP states that all infants benefit from human milk and recommends that breastfeeding be promoted in all infants, including ill, preterm infants. Nutritive and non-nutritive advantages have been shown for both full-term and preterm infants. The advantages include higher developmental outcomes over those for formula-fed infants. Because preterm infants are at a higher risk for developmental delays, breastfeeding may have an additional benefit. Premature infants ideally need 120 to 130 kcal/kg per day.

During the first weeks after premature birth, infants may need fortification of the breast milk or formula. In the case of a chronically ill infant (e.g., those with chronic lung disease or malabsorption disorders), the need may be as high as 150 kcal/kg per day. Breast milk or formula provides approximately 20 kcal/oz.

For those born before 34 weeks' gestation, breast milk may not provide sufficient nutritive support. A more calorically dense formula may be needed, one that provides 24 to 27 kcal/oz. If the infant is breastfeeding, supplementation may be needed. Supplementation of breast milk is recommended until the infant weighs 2000 g or more.

The use of the higher concentration formulas may put infants at risk for untoward gastrointestinal or renal side effects. Dehydration, diarrhea, flatus, lactose intolerance, edema, and delayed gastric emptying with regurgitation are possible. Typically, fortification is needed only during the hospitalization. For a 34- to 36-week infant, fortification of breast milk or the use of specialized premature formula should be used with caution as hypercalcemia may develop. Usually, after 34 to 36 weeks' postconceptual age or a weight of 2000 to 2500 g has been reached, breast milk or standard-strength formula is adequate. It is recommended that an assessment of the nutritional status be made before and after the infant is discharged to home. For infants born between 34 and 37 weeks' gestation with a birth weight greater than 1800 g, only growth measurements are needed.

Parents may wonder and ask about when to start solids. Timing for the introduction of solid foods remains the same as with the full-term infant, but adjusted age is used. As with the full-term infant, waiting until the infant has adequate head control and oral-motor control for the swallowing of solid food is advised.

Preterm infants may be at risk for anemia, lower bone density, and failure to thrive. Supplemental vitamin intake is recommended. During hospitalization, preterm infants may have received vitamin E, calcium, phosphorus,

TABLE 17–9. SUMMARY OF THE NUTRITIONAL ISSUES OF
PRETERM INFANTS

- Most preterm infants require 120–130 kcal/kg/day; in some situations, up to 150 kcal/kg/day or more may be used
- Before 34 wk gestation or under 2000 g, high-calorie formulas or supplementation of breastfeeding is necessary
- Supplementation of vitamins A, B, C, and D is recommended for infants who are breastfeeding
- Iron supplementation is recommended in all preterm infants, starting at 2 months of age:
  - 2 to 3 mg/kg/day for 6 months in those with birth weight > 100 g
  - Up to 4 mg/kg/day for those weighing < 1000 g at birth until the first birthday
  - Solids may be initiated at 4–6 months adjusted age, when motor skills permit
- Feeding issues may arise in very preterm infants, so they need frequent assessment

or folate supplementation to reduce the risk of hemolytic anemia, rickets, or osteopenia. These supplements are generally discontinued at discharge. Once home, a multiple vitamin containing vitamins A, B, C, and D should be used in those infants who are breastfeeding. Most formulas contain enough of these vitamins and do not need supplementation; however, for the infant who takes in less than 450 mL of formula each day, vitamin supplementation is also recommended.

Iron stores in preterm infants are depleted at around 2 months of chronologic age. Frequent blood sampling may be an additional risk factor for anemia. Iron is given at a rate of 2 to 3 mg/kg per day in the low birth weight infant. Iron supplementation in the formula-fed and breastfed infants should be started at 6 to 8 weeks of age and should be continued until 6 months of age unless otherwise indicated. For those infants weighing less than 1000 g at birth, supplementation of iron at 4 mg/kg per day should be used. The recommendation is to continue iron supplementation until the infant's first birthday. Table 17–9 provides a summary of the nutritional issues of preterm infants.

DISCIPLINE AND PARENTING

Toward the end of the visit, review age-appropriate parenting skills. As with full-term infants, discipline is not needed for the first several months. At approximately 6 months adjusted age, preterm infants may be more aware of and experiment with their environment. Encourage the parents to learn simple discipline techniques. For example, if the infant reaches for an electric cord or bites while breastfeeding, a simple, stern "no" followed by distraction or physical removal is all that is needed. Encourage parents to structure a safe home environment. Remind parents that frequent holding or cuddling of the infant will not result in spoiling. Meeting the infant's needs, reducing frustration, and providing stimulation help to establish an infant's trust in his or her world, just as with full-term infants.

Last, encourage the primary caregiver to take time for himself or herself. This may be additionally important for parents of premature infants who have spent time in the hospital. Also encourage the caregiver and the partner to take time together, such as occasional brief times away from the child. Encouraging time spent away from the infant depends on the stability of the infant and the capability of the person caring for the infant in the absence of the parent.

Parenting a preterm infant has additional challenges. The parents have become parents prematurely. The infant's expected date of birth may have been weeks away, and the early birth may have caught the parents unprepared. If the infant required an extended hospitalization, time away from work, home, or other children can greatly increase the stress the parents experience. Depending on the events surrounding the birth and any postnatal complications, the parents may have gone through the various stages of grieving by the time of the first office visit. This may be more evident in parents of infants with illness.

BONDING

There are several problems unique to preterm infants. Bonding and attachment issues are important during the first months of life, and premature delivery may disrupt the bonding and attachment processes. Early delivery to parents who are not yet prepared, the fragile appearance of the infant, or the lack of responsiveness of the infant may lead to an abnormal bonding or attachment process, which may affect the parent–child interaction and relationship for months and years to follow.

Bonding is the relationship the mother forms with the infant shortly after birth. Physical closeness, such as eye contact and skin-to skin contact, between the mother and the infant aids in establishing the bond. Premature infants are often separated from their mothers after birth, which may disrupt this process.

Attachment by the infant to the parent is a process that takes place over the next months to a year. Talk with the parents about these issues. Encourage parents not to be concerned about missing the early bonding period and point out to them the ways the infant is responding to them. Anxious parents may easily overlook the subtle gaze of the infant or the calming effect they have on the infant.

VULNERABLE CHILD SYNDROME

Vulnerable child syndrome stems from alterations in parenting styles that can have long-lasting developmental and behavioral outcomes in a child. An infant or child is reviewed as fragile or vulnerable even when physical and developmental growth is normal. There is usually a history of infertility or miscarriages, prematurity, or a life-threatening illness in the infant. The parent continues to fear that the infant or child is at risk for further illness or death.

TABLE 17–10. VULNERABLE CHILD SYNDROME: BEHAVIORS EXHIBITED BY PARENTS

- Difficulty in separating from the child
- Not allowing other trusted adults to care for the child
- Sleep problems: Bedtime refusal, nighttime awakening, or cohabitation
- Overprotective behaviors by the parent, such as limiting the child's activity or involvement with other children or adults
- Overpermissiveness, in which a lack of discipline or limit setting may be seen

There are several features of the vulnerable child syndrome. By recognizing the symptoms, intervention may be started early. Behaviors exhibited by parents are outlined in Table 17–10. The long-term effects of the vulnerable child syndrome are behavior and developmental issues that may affect the child throughout toddler years and into the school-age years. Early recognition and intervention may help in preventing these problems from becoming lifetime issues for the child.

TEST YOUR KNOWLEDGE OF CHAPTER 17

1. What is the difference between a preterm infant and a very preterm infant?
2. What are some of the problems preterm infants encounter?
3. Describe the components of the initial history in the ambulatory care setting.
4. Why is a family assessment necessary with the evaluation of preterm infants?
5. What is the difference between the chronologic age and the adjusted age?
6. Discuss how to arrive at an adjusted age for preterm infants.
7. How long is adjusted age used to evaluate preterm infants?
8. Describe the parameters of catch-up growth for head circumference, weight, and length.
9. What type of visual and hearing problems can be expected in preterm infants?
10. Describe the physical examination in preterm infants.
11. How are developmental milestones evaluated in preterm infants?
12. How do ego and emotional development progress in preterm infants?
13. What screening tests are needed in preterm infants? When should they be done?
14. What is the immunization schedule for preterm infants?
15. Why is RSV prophylaxis recommended in preterm infants?

16. What cues do preterm infants exhibit that alert parents of the infants' readiness for or need for cessation of interaction?
17. What safety issues and dental concerns are necessary for preterm infants?
18. What special needs for nutrition are found in preterm infants?
19. Describe the parenting and discipline needed with preterm infants.
20. What behaviors are exhibited by parents with vulnerable child syndrome?

 BIBLIOGRAPHY

American Academy of Pediatrics, Committee on Environmental Health. (1998). Screening for elevated blood lead levels. *Pediatrics*, 101: 1072–1078.

American Academy of Pediatrics, Committee on Infectious Diseases. (2000). Recommendations for the prevention of pneumococcal infections, including the use of pneumococcal conjugate vaccine (Prevnar), pneumococcal polysaccharide vaccine, and antibiotic prophylaxis (RE9960). *Pediatrics*, 106, 362–366.

American Academy of Pediatrics, Committee on Infectious Diseases and Committee on Fetus and Newborn. (1998). Prevention of respiratory syncytial virus infections: Indications for the use of palivizumab and update on the use of RSV-IGIV (RE9839). *Pediatrics*, 102, 1221–1216.

American Academy of Pediatrics, Committee on Injury and Poison Prevention and Committee on Fetus and Newborn. (1996). Safe transportation of premature and low birth weight infants. *Pediatrics*, 97, 758–760.

Berkowitz, C. D. (2000). *Pediatrics: A primary care approach*. Philadelphia: W.B. Saunders.

Bernbaum, J. C., & Hoffman-Williamson, M. (1991). *Primary care of the preterm infant*. St. Louis: Mosby.

D'Angio, C. T. (1999). Immunization of the premature infant. *Pediatric Infectious Disease Journal*, 18, 824–825.

Dixon, S. D., & Stein, J. T. (2001). *Encounters with children*. St. Louis: Mosby.

Hall, R. T. (2001). Nutritional follow-up of the breastfeeding premature infant after hospital discharge. *Pediatric Clinics of North America*, 48, 453–460.

Hoekelman, R. A. (2001). *Primary pediatric care*. St. Louis: Mosby

Johnson, C. P., & Blasco, P. A. (1997). Infant growth and development. *Pediatrics in Review*, 18, 224–242.

Mills, M. D. (1999). The eye in childhood. *American Family Physician*, 60, 907–916.

Trachtenburg, D. E., & Miller, T. C. (1995). Office care of the small, premature infant. *Primary Care*, 22, 1–21.

Zitelli, B. J., & Davis, H. D. (1997). *Atlas of pediatric physical diagnosis*. St. Louis: Mosby.

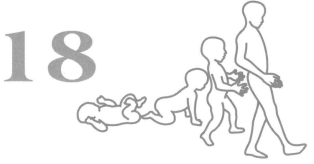

Assessment of the Newborn

Margaret R. Colyar

Assessment of newborn infants encompasses the neonate at the time of birth and up to age 2 weeks. This is a period of fast growth and change. Healthcare providers must be well versed in techniques of physical assessment to discover underlying problems and be able to dispel new parents' fears. Areas of emphasis for this age group include determining if congenital anomalies, birth trauma, and neonatal medical problems exist. Also, the gestational age of the child is determined at this time (see Chapter 3).

GENERAL APPROACH

Assessment of a newborn should be performed in front of the parents. This is a good time to educate the parents and answer specific questions. You must be very flexible and adapt the examination to the temperament of the child. Be sure to keep the child warm during the examination because newborns have difficulty maintain their body temperature. Comparing sides is a must. One side of the child should look like and do the same as the other side of the child. For example, the child's arms should flex and extend equally;

TABLE 18–1. SCREENING INFORMATION FOR PROVIDERS	
Organization	Web Address
National Adrenal Disease Foundation	www.medhelp.org.nadf/
Endocrine Web	www.endocrine.com
American Thyroid Association	www.thyroid.org
Thyroid Foundation of America	www.tfaweb.org/pub/tfa
Cystic Fibrosis Foundation	www.cff.org
Cystic Fibrosis Index of On-Line Resources	www.vmsb.csd.udu/
Parents of Galactosemic Children	www.galactosemia.org
Georgia Comprehensive Sickle Cell Center	www.emory.edu/peds/sickle
Maple Syrup Urine Disease Family Support	www.msud-support.org
National PKU News	www.pkunews.org

otherwise, suspicion of nerve or muscle damage is in order. If observation reveals areas of concern, you should make repeated observations to determine the extent of the problem.

Any deviations from what is expected should be kept in context. For example, the discovery of a heart murmur may be problematic or just a normal variation. If, along with a murmur, central cyanosis, substernal retractions, and nasal flaring are seen, the deviation should be referred.

All abnormal findings should be evaluated objectively. That is, laboratory tests, vital signs, and diagnostic procedures should be accomplished before a final diagnosis is made. Some features can be evaluated subjectively. For example, you may find unusual ear placement or slanted eyes. Look at the parents and siblings for familial traits before determining that a major problem exists.

HISTORY

For this age group, maternal history, including prenatal, perinatal, and obstetrical history, should be elicited (see Chapter 4).

SCREENING

Screening includes measurement of vital signs, height, weight, head and chest circumference, newborn adaptation, gestational age, and maturity. Further information on newborn screening can be obtained easily in ambulatory clinic through various organizations that have developed informational Websites (Table 18–1).

VITAL SIGNS

Temperature, heart rate, respiratory rate, and blood pressure should be measured in newborns immediately after birth (see Chapter 3). A typical newborn has trouble maintaining his or her body temperature because of an immature hypothalamus. The first temperature should be measured rectally and, if it is within normal range, it can then be measured by the axillary method. Newborns usually have a lot of debris in the ear canal because of the birth process; therefore, tympanic temperatures are contraindicated. In addition, tympanic thermometers are not accurate because they vary with ambient temperature and are affected by debris in the ear. If the child is under a warmer, skin temperature probes should be used.

Newborns may have irregular and fast heart rates that vary between 120 and 160 beats per minute. The heart rate should be measured by auscultation of the apex of the heart for 1 full minute.

Newborns may also have irregular respiratory rate and rhythm. Therefore, the respirations should also be counted for 1 full minute. While taking the respiratory rate, observe the newborn for signs of respiratory distress such as nasal flaring, grunting, intercostal or substernal retractions, and central cyanosis.

The blood pressure should be measured using a right arm and a right thigh measurement to rule out coarctation of the aorta. If the first blood pressure is within the normal range and there is no suspicion of disease risk, then one measurement is usually acceptable.

HEIGHT, WEIGHT, AND CIRCUMFERENCE OF THE HEAD AND CHEST

Height, weight, and occipital-frontal circumference (OFC) must be plotted on the appropriate charts at the time of birth and each succeeding well-child examination (see Chapter 2). Newborns must be measured in the supine position. Measure from the top of the skull to the heel. Because newborns have been in cramped positions for several months, it may be difficult to get an accurate measurement. Average height for newborns is 20 in.

Weight is measured with newborns unclothed. Make sure the scale to be used has been calibrated to 0 before using. The average weight for newborns is 3.6 kg.

Head circumference, or OFC, is measured using a flexible paper tape measure. A paper tape measure is optimal because it will not stretch. Measure around the largest circumference of the cranium (just above the ears and eyes) and record in centimeters. Repeat the measurement three times and take the average. The average OFC is 32 to 36 cm for normal newborns. If the OFC is less than 32 cm, which may indicate microcephaly, or greater than 36 cm, which may indicate macrocephaly, refer the child to a pediatrician.

Chest circumference is also measured using a flexible paper tape measure. Measure the chest circumference at the nipple line. Chest circumference is usually 2 cm smaller than the OFC at birth. Between age 6 months and 1 year, they become equal; after that time, the chest circumference is larger than the head circumference.

GESTATIONAL AGE

Gestational age is the approximate age of a newborn infant based on flexibility of joints and condition of the skin. To determine the gestational age, the Dubowitz or Ballard scale is used (see Chapter 27). An infant is considered premature if the gestational age is assessed to be 37 weeks or less. Full term is considered to be 38 to 42 weeks' gestation, and postmature is 42 or more weeks' gestation.

APGAR SCORING

Apgar scoring (see Chapter 3) is an assessment of newborn adaptation. Screening begins at birth and is usually measured at 1 minute and 5 minutes. The Apgar score (which has five parameters) is part of the respiratory assessment of a newborn, and it measures successful transition to extrauterine life. The five parameters are A (appearance: skin, color), P (pulse), G (grimace: irritability), A (activity: muscle tone), and R (respiratory effort). The Apgar score at 1 minute indicates the status of the fetus *in utero*. It indicates cord pH and intrauterine asphyxia. The 5-minute Apgar score reveals how the child is reacting to out-of-utero life. A 10-minute Apgar score should be done if the child had a poor score (< 6) at 5 minutes. A score of 8 to 10 is excellent, a score of 4 to 7 is worrisome, and a score of 0 to 3 is critical.

EGO DEVELOPMENT: TRUST VERSUS MISTRUST

During the newborn period, the child is in the ego development stage of trust versus mistrust, as discussed by Erikson (Table 18–2). Parents who attend to the child's needs of food, rest, and hygiene assist the child's ego development. A child who feeds well and gains weight appropriately exhibits a positive resolution of hope and trust. When basic needs are not met, a negative resolution of fear develops.

COGNITIVE DEVELOPMENT

Newborns are in the sensorimotor stage of cognitive development, as discussed by Piaget (see Table 18–2). During this stage, development of primitive reflexes indicates normal cognitive processes. Knowing which primitive reflexes should be exhibited is essential when assessing newborns.

 EXAMINATION SEQUENCE

Before examining newborns in the nursery, you must wash your hands and forearms and remove jewelry to prevent injury to the infant. In some nurs-

TABLE 18–2. EGO AND COGNITIVE DEVELOPMENT IN NEWBORNS		
Theory	Stage of Development	Expectations
Ego	Trust vs. mistrust	Positive resolution: Hope and trust Feeds well Gains weight appropriately Negative resolution: Fear
Cognitive	Sensorimotor	Normal development of reflexes Crying Rooting Sucking Grasping

eries, a gown must be worn. Examine newborns in a well-lit area that is free of drafts. Have all equipment needed to complete the examination nearby for easy access. Special care must be taken to keep the infant warm because newborn infants are unable to regulate their body temperature well at birth. Therefore, undress the infant only as needed to assess various body systems. Use of a radiant heat warmer during the examination assists the child in temperature regulation.

If the child is crying, it is difficult to auscultate accurately. Techniques that may be used to console the child are to insert a pacifier or a gloved finger in the child's mouth. Giving the child a bottle, burping, and changing the diaper also may be used to settle the infant. Talking in a soothing voice is also helpful. Be sure to ask for the parents' permission before giving a bottle or pacifier because some breastfeeding mothers prefer for their child to not have an artificial nipple.

ORDER OF PHYSICAL EXAMINATION

Observation or inspection should be done first while the child is resting and alert. Because normal newborns sleep 20 h/d, this may be difficult. Observation or inspection is 90% of the examination of a newborn. Note the child's transition from sleep to alertness. Note the quality, strength, and pitch of the cry. Auscultation is done next, and palpation and percussion are done last. The examination should be done in a logical manner from head to toe anteriorly, then head to toe posteriorly. The neurologic assessment may be done during the examination or at the end.

SKIN

Check the appearance of the skin for color (Table 18–3), thickness, petechiae, purpura, edema, and hair distribution. Assess for unusual peeling, cracking, rashes, or abrasions. Normal findings include birthmarks, drying and peeling, and other skin findings (Table 18–4). Also observe the skin for elasticity as an indicator of dehydration. Do this by noting any loose extra skin at the

TABLE 18–3. COLOR OF NEWBORNS' SKIN AND INDICATIONS

Color	Indication
Red	Plethora: Polycythemia or hyperviscosity (overfullness of blood vessels OR excess total quantity of fluid in body)
Beefy red	Hypoglycemia
Red/white	Harlequin sign (50% of body red; 50% of body white); caused by changes in circulation; considered normal
White	Anemia, blood loss, vernix caseosa, circulatory failure
Blue	Central cyanosis (circumoral or earlobes); hemoglobin in white children should be 5 mg/dL; for dark-skinned children, it should be < 5 mg/dL
Blue	Acrocyanosis (hands and feet); should disappear by day 3
Yellow	Jaundice; best seen in sunlight; blanch tip of nose or gum line to detect (bilirubin must be > 5 mg/dL)

calf or lower abdomen. Although this is an indicator of dehydration, it can also indicate that the baby is premature but is sometimes normal in newborns.

TABLE 18–4. SKIN FINDINGS IN NEWBORNS

Name	Presentation	Location on Body
Café-au-lait spot	Pale tan macule	Entire body
Cavernous hemangiomas	Large, blood-filled, cystic papules	Scalp, face, and head
Erythema toxicum neonatorum	Pinpoint, red-based macules	Cheeks and trunk
Lanugo	Fine hair covering body	Entire body
Milia	White dots	Face and bridge of nose
Miliaria	Tiny, red, irritated lesions	Face and over any sweat gland
Mongolian spots	Hyperpigmented macules: gray, blue, or black	Lower back, buttocks, and shoulders; more common in African-Americans, Asian-Americans, and Hispanics
Port-wine stain (nevus flammeus)	Flat, red, purple, or jet black lesions	Face and scalp
Strawberry hemangioma	Soft, red, raised	Anywhere
Transient neonatal pustular melanosis	Brown or black spots	Anywhere; usually in African-Americans
Vascular nevi Capillary hemangioma: stork bite or angel kiss	Pink, blanch easily	Eyelids, nose, nape of neck
Vernix caseosa	Cheesy white substance	Entire body

TABLE 18–5. COMMON HAIR ABNORMALITIES OF NEWBORNS	
Color or Texture	Indication
White streak	Waardenburg syndrome (check for deafness)
Coarse red patches	Kwashiorkor (protein deficiency)
Dry, gray	Malnutrition
No pigment	Albinism

HEAD

Hair

Note the quantity, color, distribution, and texture of the hair. The hair should be evenly distributed over the skull, not patchy or with abnormal whorls (cowlicks). The quantity can vary from fine fuzz to long strands. The color of the hair should be evenly pigmented. Remember that abnormal hair may indicate a congenital anomaly (Table 18–5). Assess the parents if unusual hair patterns or hairlines are exhibited in a newborn.

Skull

Note the overall contour, size, shape, and symmetry of the skull. Palpate the skull and suture lines. Overlapping of suture lines or splitting up to 1 cm of the suture lines is normal after birth; however, suture lines should not be palpable after age 5 to 6 months. Palpate the skull in the upright position for swelling, bulging in the fontanels, and softness of the skull. Bulging, pulsations, and tenseness of the fontanels usually indicate increased intracranial pressure. Softness may indicate rickets, syphilis, and hydrocephalus. An abnormally large head may indicate hydrocephalus or a chromosomal, congenital, or metabolic disorder.

Estimate the dimension of the anterior and posterior fontanels. Other palpable fontanels are the sphenoid and mastoid. The anterior fontanel may be small or absent at birth if significant overlapping of the suture lines has occurred. The anterior fontanel should be diamond shaped and measure 4 to 5 cm by 2 to 3 cm. The anterior fontanel should close by age 9 to 19 months.

The posterior fontanel may also be absent at birth. The average size of the posterior fontanel is 1 cm by 1 cm or about the size of your fingertip. This fontanel usually closes by age 1 to 2 months.

Abnormal size or shape of the fontanels may be an indication of hyper- or hypothyroidism. An unusually large or delay in closure of the fontanels may indicate a delay in bone growth.

Scalp

Check the scalp for normal and abnormal findings. Desquamation is normal, which indicates that the child was overdue. Molding of the skull is also normal. It is important to be able to differentiate between caput succedaneum and cephalohematoma.

250

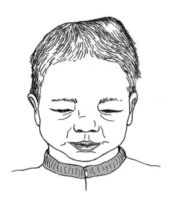

FIG. 18.1. Cephalohematoma.

Trauma causes caput succedaneum, resulting in edema of the scalp, which crosses the suture lines. The edema is usually over the presenting part. This is not a problem and will resolve in a few days. With cephalohematoma (Fig. 18–1), the edema is restricted to one side of the skull and does not cross suture lines. Cephalohematoma is caused by bleeding between the periosteum and the skull. A total of 25% of cephalohematoma are caused by a skull fracture. Complications of cephalohematoma include anemia, hypotension, hyperbilirubinemia, and infection. Cephalohematoma may take weeks to months to resolve.

Face

Inspect the infant's face for overall appearance, color, shape, and symmetry. Observe the facial expressions. Note that with facial nerve injuries, the affected side does not react. Check for bruising or birth injuries such as forceps marks.

Eyes

For the eyes, note the overall size, symmetry, shape, palpebral fissure, interpupillary distance, and absence of tearing (not usually present until age 2 to 3 months). Note bruises, edema of the eyelids, hemorrhages, and inflammation from medications. There may be mucoid discharge from a newborn's eyes, which is normal. Inspect the eye structures (e.g., pupils, iris, sclera) for pupillary light reflex (direct and consensual), iris color, color of sclera, and movement. Eye tests that must be done with newborns include red reflex (see Chapter 6), blink in response to light, fix and follow, and conjugate movements.

Ears

Inspect the ears for placement, appearance, size, shape, and patency of canal. Determine if the ears are low set, as seen in individuals with fetal alcohol syndrome and other congenital abnormalities. About 10% to 20% of the ear length should be above the crease of the eye. Abnormal shape or size may be a familial trait or may indicate deafness. The normal external ear is oval in shape. If a round-shaped external ear is noted, suspect Down syndrome. Inspect for ear tags, pits (may be familial or associated with anomalies), and firmness of recoil. Usually the canal is full of vernix and debris from the birth process, so an otoscope examination is not done. Newborns' hearing is usually tested by an audiologist before discharge using brainstem auditory evoked response (BAER) testing to screen for unilateral, bilateral, conductive, and sensorineural hearing loss.

Nose

Newborns are obligate nose breathers. Inspect the nose for size, shape, and placement. Also, check for patency of the nares to rule out choanal atresia, a blockage between the outside of the nose and the oral pharynx. This is easily done by having the child suck, blocking one nostril at a time, and observing for difficulty breathing and cyanosis. Marked nasal congestion is seen in those with congenital syphilis, and frequent sneezing is seen in newborns with narcotic addiction.

Lips

Observe the lips for symmetry, color, and malformations. Mild circumoral cyanosis may be present for the first 24 hours, especially if the infant has been crying. The lips should be pink. Cyanosis of the lips may indicate central cyanosis, and the child should be referred to a specialist immediately. Note the philtrum between the upper lip and the nose. Shortening or elongation of the philtrum is seen in infants with several congenital anomalies. The major malformation seen in newborns is cleft lip.

Mouth

Inspect the size and shape of the oral opening and interior structures. The gingivae may have Epstein's pearls, which are clusters of epithelial cells and are completely normal. However, Epstein's pearls must be differentiated from natal teeth, which should be removed because of the chance of aspiration. Inspect the uvula. A unifid and bifid uvula are normal as long as they raise midline.

Inspect the pharynx for any debris. Palpate the hard and soft palates with a gloved finger to locate any clefts, which could lead to speech difficulties if they are not corrected. A high-palate may be normal but is also present in individuals with several syndromes, including trisomy 18 and Noonan's syndrome.

Note the movement of the tongue. The tongue should move in all directions and lack sustained quivering or trembling. Check the size of the tongue. Macroglossia is a sign of congenital hypothyroidism (cretinism), Down syndrome, and others. There are two frenula in the mouth. Note the frenula under the tongue and between the upper lip and gum line. If either of the frenula is too tight (i.e., the infant cannot stick out his or her tongue or cannot extend the upper lip over the gum line), it may cause the child difficulties with feeding and speech.

Now is a good time to check the suck reflex and the rooting reflex. To test the suck reflex, insert a gloved finger in the newborn's mouth. The infant's suck should make a nice seal and exert firm pressure. To test the rooting reflex, stroke the skin just lateral to the side of the mouth toward the cheek. The infant's head should turn toward the side that has been stroked and he or she should begin to suck.

NECK

Hyperextend the neck to visualize placement of the trachea and webbing (seen in individuals with Turner syndrome). Observe for the thyroid gland, which usually is not visible in newborns unless it is enlarged. Turn the head in all directions to determine if the child has full range of motion. If there is a tilt toward either shoulder, suspect torticollis, which represents a shortening of one side of the sternocleidomastoid muscle. Torticollis may be present at birth but more commonly worsens during the first few weeks of life. This can be caused by trauma or can be congenital in nature. Note any masses, hematomas, or cysts. Determine if the trachea is midline.

UPPER EXTREMITIES

Inspect for symmetry, overall appearance, deformities, position, tremors, and symmetrical spontaneous movement. Inspect for birth trauma that is caused by overstretching. There are three common types: Erb's palsy, Klumpke's paralysis, and entire brachial plexus palsy (Table 18–6). Palpate both arms bilaterally, flexing and extending to note muscle strength, tone, and joint mobility. Also count the number of fingers and note the curvature, webbing, and taper of the fingers along with nail size and shape. Note the palmar creases. The simian line is found in 4% of the normal population and is seen also in children with Down syndrome. Check the color of the hands. Cyanosis of the fingers or hands is common. This is known as acrocyanosis and is usually a reflection of a newborn's normal peripheral vascular instability. Note the position of the hands, which should be with the fingers flexed in a fist with the thumbs under the fingers.

Elicit the palmar grasp reflex by placing your finger at the base of the newborn's fingers. The fingers should curve around your finger.

LUNGS

First inspect the pattern of breathing and count the respirations. The normal respiratory rate for newborns is 40 to 60 breaths per minute. Periodic breathing can be normal if the pauses are less than 10 seconds. Pauses that are

TABLE 18–6. BIRTH TRAUMA OF UPPER EXTREMITIES: THREE COMMON TYPES

Type	Presentation	Nerves Involved	Recovery
Erb's palsy	Cannot move the upper arm but still has palmar grasp	C5, C6	80%
Klumpke's paralysis	Hand and forearm are flaccid but upper arm moves; no palmar grasp	C7, C8, T1	< 50%
Entire brachial plexus palsy	No movement in entire arm and hand	C5–T1	Usually permanent

greater than 20 seconds are abnormal and should be monitored. Signs of distress are retractions, heaving, grunting, and increased rate. Note the appearance of the thorax, which should be round and symmetrical. Note that newborns are abdominal breathers.

Next auscultate the lung fields and compare sides. Fine crackles and transient hoarseness are normal in newborns; however, cough, stridor, and continued hoarseness are abnormal. Last, note the child's breathing patterns. Observe for any signs of respiratory distress such as nasal flaring, grunting, intercostal or substernal retractions, and irregular respiratory pattern.

Palpate the sternum, breast, all lung fields, and precordium. Palpate the clavicles for fractures. In newborns, the xyphoid may appear prominent. If the sternum bows inward, pectus excavatum is present. If the sternum bows outward, it is known as pectus carinatum (see Chapter 7). Palpate the breast tissue. The nipple nodules should be visible and palpable and approximately 1 cm in diameter. Mild erythema, swelling, and milky discharge may be present. Physiologic galactorrhea (i.e., milky discharge) results from maternal hormonal influence and usually resolves within a few weeks.

Note any accessory (supernumerary) nipples, which follow the milk line (curving from the axilla, through the nipples, and then vertical to curving toward midline just below the umbilicus). Accessory nipples are common in children of African-American descent.

CARDIOVASCULAR

Inspect the child's overall color, breathing pattern, and precordial activity (which should not be visibly bounding). Assess the skin, lips, nail beds, and earlobes for cyanosis. Note the behavior of the newborn. Is there any evidence of fatigue, vomiting, or sweating while the infant is at rest or feeding? Palpate all peripheral pulses bilaterally, compare the right brachial to the right femoral pulses to check for coarctation of the aorta (the femoral pulse will be decreased or absent), and note capillary refill time (normal is less

TABLE 18–7. PULSES*	
Value	Interpretation
0	Absent pulses
1+	Barely palpable pulses
2+	Normal pulses
3+	Full, increased pulses
4+	Strong, bounding pulses

* See Chapter 8 for the locations of all pulses.

than 3 seconds). Palpate the liver (if enlarged, consider congestive heart failure) and heart size using the scratch test (see Chapter 8).

Pulses

Auscultate the apical pulse. The average heart rate of the normal newborn is 120 to 160 beats per minute. When at rest, the heart rate can be as low as 80 and can be up to 200 when the infant is crying. Pulses should be palpated bilaterally. Compare the right brachial to right femoral pulses to check for coarctation of the aorta. With coarctation, the femoral pulse is decreased or absent. All pulses should be documented. Use Table 18–7 as a guide for documenting the presence or absence of pulses.

Heart

Auscultate all five areas of the heart with the bell and diaphragm of the stethoscope. Heart sounds in newborns are heard best and loudest over the left chest area. Note the rate, rhythm, intensity, and any unusual sounds. Murmurs are common in the first 24 to 48 hours until the circulatory system stabilizes. If a murmur is apparent, document where the murmur is best heard; whether it is systolic or diastolic; if it radiates; and its quality, pitch, timing, duration, and intensity (Table 18–8).

TABLE 18–8. GRADING OF MURMURS	
Grade	Description
I	Very faint; heard with concentration
II	Faint; heard immediately
III	Moderate intensity
IV	Loud; associated with a thrill (i.e., vibration on chest wall)
V	Loud; heard with stethoscope barely on chest
VI	Very loud; stethoscope off chest
Charting example	Grade 2/6 or II/VI

Innocent Murmurs

Closing of the Ductus Arteriosus This innocent murmur usually disappears within 2 days after birth. It is caused by the decrease in pulmonary vascular resistance. This murmur can be classified as grade 2/6 blowing, is systolic, and is best heard in the upper left sternal border (see Chapter 8).

Peripheral Pulmonic Stenosis or Peripheral Pulmonary Branch Artery Stenosis This innocent murmur is heard best over the peripheral pulmonary arteries. The murmur of peripheral pulmonic stenosis can be heard equally on the front of the chest, in the axilla, and on the back. This murmur is classified as a grade 2/6, and it is short, blowing, and midsystolic, and should disappear by age 3 months.

ABDOMEN

Inspect the overall contour, shape, and symmetry of the abdomen. Note distention, midline defects, or collapse. Note whether a diastasis recti is present. This is a separation of the medial rectus sheath and usually resolves in a couple of years. Diastasis recti is more visible when a newborn is crying or straining.

Check the umbilical stump, which should have two arteries and one vein visible at birth. Incidence of only one artery is associated with skeletal, gastrointestinal, and renal anomalies. After the cord is clamped and dye has been applied, the presence of arteries and veins cannot be visualized. Note any odor or discharge from or around the stump. Palpate the umbilical stump for laxity, which may represent an umbilical hernia. If a newborn has an umbilical hernia that protrudes, note the size and the ability to be reduced. An umbilical hernia usually closes spontaneously by age 3 to 5 years.

Auscultate bowel sounds and vascular bruits before palpation and percussion. Palpate all four quadrants, liver, spleen, and kidneys, noting tone and masses. The liver in a newborn is 1 to 2 cm below the anterior costal margin, right midclavicular line. The spleen is normally not palpable in newborns, but the lateral tip may be palpable. The kidneys are difficult to palpate but are the most common abdominal mass in this age group. The right kidney is easier to palpate because it is positioned lower. Many times newborns will cry during the abdominal examination. Try offering a pacifier. If this does not quiet the infant, palpate at the end of expiration (end of a cry).

INGUINAL AREA

Palpate the inguinal area for masses and enlarged lymph nodes. Also palpate the femoral arteries. Compare the right brachial and right femoral pulses. If the femoral pulse is absent or delayed, it usually indicates coarctation of the aorta.

GENITALIA

Girls

In a full-term infant, the labia majora cover the labia minora. The clitoris should be covered by the labia in the adducted position. There may be some erythema, swelling, blood, or white mucus draining from the vagina. This is normal for the first 3 to 7 days (sometimes up to 1 month) and is caused by maternal hormones. Note any swelling or bruising from birth trauma.

Retract the labia gently to visualize the genitalia. Inspect the clitoris, urethra, vagina, and anus. Note the patency of the vaginal opening and the anus. Patency of the anus is apparent with the passage of meconium and stool. Also check that there is adequate separation of the anus from the vagina. This should be approximately 2 to 4 cm.

Boys

Do *not* retract the foreskin. Foreskin is not fully retractable until age 3 years. Note the size, absence of curvature, and location of the urethra. Note whether the urethra is on the tip of the penis, the underside (hypospadias), or the top (epispadias). Look for chordee (i.e., bent penis), which is associated with hypospadias and epispadias. Check the length and size of the shaft. Check for bruising or edema from birth trauma. Note the color, appearance of rugae, and median raphe. The tip of the newborn's penis may be vascularly engorged and bluish. Check for patency of the urethra by observing the urinary stream.

Palpate the testes for size, masses, fluid, edema, and evidence that the testes are descended. The normal newborn teste is 1.5 to 2.0 cm. Differentiate between retractile testes and cryptorchidism (i.e., failure to descend) by placing the finger of one hand just above the scrotal sac on one side and pushing gently downward. With the other hand, palpate the sac to determine the teste is present. If you are unsure, transilluminate the scrotum for the testicular shadow. Note enlargement of scrotum caused by inguinal herniation or presence of a hydrocele (i.e., fluid remnant in the scrotum). Patency of the anus is apparent with the passage of meconium and stool.

HIPS

Inspect for inequality in size and length of the legs, resistance to abduction, placement of medial thigh creases, and degree of flexion of the hips and knees. Congenital hip dysplasia occurs in approximately 2.5 to 6.5 cases per 1000 newborns. Therefore, it is very important to know the indicators (Table 18–9).

Perform the Ortolani and Barlow maneuvers until the child is walking (see Chapter 12). Clicks usually are normal, but clunks usually are abnormal. If the hip is unstable (i.e., it dislocates), make sure the child is referred to an orthopedist as soon as possible.

TABLE 18–9. CONGENITAL HIP DYSPLASIA	
Inspect For	**Indications of Congenital Hip Dysplasia**
Size and length of legs	Inequality
Abduction	Crying in connection with abduction (often normal)
Medial thigh creases	One side has two; other side has three
Hips and knees	Degree of flexion not equal

LOWER EXTREMITIES

Inspect for symmetry, overall appearance, deformities, size, shape, symmetry of spontaneous movements, anterior medial thigh creases, and degree of flexion. Mild bowing of the tibia is normal because of uterine position. Flexion contractures of the hips and knees are also normal because of uterine position. Asymmetry of the thigh and gluteal folds is usually an indication of congenital hip dysplasia. Note the tone and strength of the muscles bilaterally by assessing with passive manipulation.

Feet

Count the toes and inspect for webbing, overlapping, and deformities. Inspect for edema (seen in children with Turner's syndrome), creases on the plantar surface, nails, and position. Note the alignment of the toes, metatarsals, and forefoot, both in the resting position and with spontaneous movement. Note any curvature of the ankles. If spontaneous movement corrects the curvature, then there is no problem. If spontaneous movement does not correct the curvature but accentuates the curvature, then surgical correction is usually necessary.

Two abnormalities that are commonly seen are metatarsus adductus and talipes equinovarus (i.e., clubfoot). Look at the plantar surface of the foot. The forefoot (i.e., the toes and metatarsals) should be in straight alignment with the hindfoot. With metatarsus adductus, the forefoot curves inward. Stabilize the heel with your index finger and thumb and try to straighten out the forefoot by pushing laterally against the curved edge. If the foot can be straightened with moderate pressure, this deformity may correct spontaneously or passive range of motion exercises may be needed. If the foot does not straighten or is rigid, serial casting may be necessary. Metatarsus adductus usually resolves within 2 months.

With talipes equinovarus, the foot is turned inward, and the lateral edge of the foot is more distal than the medial edge. Range of motion is limited or absent. Surgical correction is needed.

Check the plantar grasp reflex by placing one finger under the toes. The toes should curve over the fingers. Check the Babinski reflex by running a finger from the heel on the lateral aspect of the plantar surface and curving around under the toes. Until 18 age months, the toes should flare.

BACK

Look at the midline and then at parallel structures. Check the occiput for birthmarks (stork bite or angel kiss) and neck webbing (Turner's syndrome). Note symmetry of the scapula, iliac crests, posterior medial thigh creases, and buttock creases. Inspect for a pilonidal dimple or sinus tract. Check the lower back for Mongolian spots, hair tufts, dimples, and hemangiomas. Check the anus for sphincter tone by gently palpating with the tip of your little finger.

Palpate the entire back for curves and abnormalities of the spinal column. Palpate the scapula for crepitus. Auscultate the posterior lung fields.

NEONATAL REFLEXES

There are several primitive reflexes that should be elicited during the physical examination. They are outlined in Table 11–6.

 # ANTICIPATORY GUIDANCE

There are five main categories for anticipatory guidance for all children: safety, parenting, nutrition, dental issues, and immunizations and screening.

SAFETY

For newborns, a number of topics, including newborn care and safety measures, should be covered (Table 18–10).

PARENTING

No discipline is needed in this age group. Newborns need to have all of their needs met, bond with the caregiver, and get plenty of rest. Many parents are concerned about spoiling their newborn. Encourage the parent to meet the infant's needs. Let the parent know that it is important to cuddle and talk to the newborn. Encourage the parent to place the infant in the crib for sleeping.

NUTRITION
Bottle Feeding

Feed approximately 1 to 2 oz every 3 to 4 hours. Encourage the parent to feed the newborn held in a semi-sitting position and not to prop bottles. Burp the child about midway through and after each feeding. Always mix formula according to instructions. Iron-fortified formula is recommended. Wash bottles, nipples, and collars thoroughly in hot soapy water. Do not use a microwave to warm up formula.

TABLE 18–10. ANTICIPATORY GUIDANCE: NEWBORN CARE AND SAFETY

CIRCUMCISION

- If circumcised, clean the area with warm water only.
- A yellowish crust over the head of the penis is normal in the healing process.

CRADLE CAP

- Prevent by washing hair frequently, and stimulate scalp with a brush daily.
- If cradle cap occurs, wash the hair daily with a mild soap or baby shampoo.
- Shampoo such as Selsun Blue mixed one part shampoo to three parts water may also be used two to three times per week.
- Brush or comb the scalp to help remove loose crusts.

GENITAL CARE

- Girls: Wipe front to back and clean well between the labia.
- Boys : Wipe under the scrotum and the penis.

FEEDING

- Breast fed: Every 2 hours
- Bottle fed: Every 3–4 hours
- Water supplements: Not usually necessary

SKIN CARE

- Powder and oil: Not recommended
- Bathing: Not necessary daily; wash hands, face, and diaper area daily
- Umbilical cord care: Keep clean and dry; fold diaper under cord; clean with alcohol three times per day and as necessary; takes 1–2 weeks to drop off; if umbilicus becomes red and malodorous, or drainage occurs, consult your healthcare provider

STOOLS

- Varying consistencies
- Breast fed: Yellow and soft with curds
- Bottle fed: Dark yellowish brown, curds

THERMOMETER USE

- If baby feels feverish or cool or if you suspect an illness, take the axillary temperature; if elevated to greater than 100.4°F, call the healthcare provider; if the temperature is low, add covers and recheck in 30 minutes

SAFETY

- Always use a car seat in the backseat; must be facing backward until the infant is 20 lb and age 1 year
- Do not leave alone with siblings or pets
- Do not leave unattended on a surface from which the child can fall
- Never shake a baby; shaking can cause brain damage
- Always support the child's head
- The child should sleep on his or her back
- The child should not sleep in the same bed with the parents

WHEN TO CALL THE HEALTHCARE PROVIDER

- Fever (temperature greater than 100.4°F)
- Vomiting persistently
- Extremely frequent, runny stools
- Refuses to eat
- Unusually fussy
- Changes in color
- Does not look right
- Just not sure child is all right

Breastfeeding

Feed every 2 hours or on demand for 10 to 15 minutes on one breast. For the next feeding, alternate breasts. Make sure the child's body is in alignment. When feeding, the neck should be straight in alignment with the body rather than turned to the side. To be sure a newborn is getting enough breast milk, weigh the child daily. The normal weight gain for newborns is 1 oz/day, or 2.2 lb/month.

DENTAL ISSUES

Instruct the parents that the teeth will start appearing anywhere between age 6 and 15 months. Instruct the parents to begin cleaning the newborn's mouth and gums now by wiping his or her tongue and gums with a moist cloth.

IMMUNIZATIONS AND SCREENING

The child should receive the first hepatitis B immunization while in the hospital. If this was not done, the immunization should be given at the 2-week visit. Screening is an important way to protect children from life-threatening diseases. Although usually done in the hospital, phenylketonuria (PKU) newborn metabolic screening needs to be repeated at the 2-week well-child examination. This laboratory test is required by law. It is done to determine if the child is unable to metabolize PKU in food, which may result in mental retardation.

Different states have different metabolic screening requirements for tests such as PKU, galactosemia, hypothyroidism, sickle cell anemia, maple syrup urine disease, and so on. Early treatment makes a significant difference in outcome.

 # REFERRALS

Assess the parents' age, financial support, emotional support, and living conditions. If the parents are very young, have no financial support, have no emotional support system, or live in suboptimal living conditions, consider a referral to the public health nurse, the Women, Infants, and Children (WIC) program, the hospital sociologist, or support groups within your community.

TEST YOUR KNOWLEDGE OF CHAPTER 18

1. What are the components in the history for newborn children?
2. What are the components of screening for newborn children?
3. How are the OFC and chest circumference measurements determined?

4. What is the sequence of the physical examination for newborn children?
5. Describe the birthmarks commonly seen in newborns.
6. Describe the head assessment for newborn children.
7. Describe the complete cardiovascular and respiratory examination in newborns.
8. Discuss innocent murmurs commonly found in newborns.
9. Differentiate between Erb's palsy, Klumpke's paralysis, and entire brachial plexus palsy.
10. Describe the examination for congenital hip dysplasia.
11. What are common problems found with the feet of newborns? How can you differentiate between them?
12. What are the five areas of anticipatory guidance for newborns?
13. Discuss the safety information the parents of newborns should know.
14. Discuss care information the parents of newborns should know.

BIBLIOGRAPHY

Algranati, P. S. (1992). *The pediatric patient: An approach to history and physical examination*. Baltimore: Williams & Wilkins

Goldbloom, R. B. (1997). *Pediatric clinical skills*. Philadelphia: Churchill Livingstone.

Mountain States Genetics Network. (2001). *Newborn screening. 2001 practitioner's manual*. Utah Department of Health.

Schmidtt, B. D. (1999). *Instructions for pediatric patients*. Philadelphia: W. B. Saunders.

CHAPTER

19

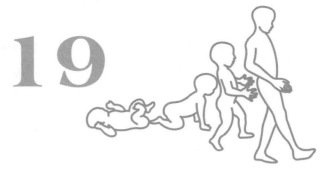

Infancy

The First 12 Months of Life

GILLIAN TUFTS

OBJECTIVES
- Establish a well-child basic examination for each of the age-specific well-child visits.
- Determine developmental milestones for the infant's age group.
- Ascertain specific anticipatory guidance needs for this age group.

The first 12 months of a child's life is a dynamic time. During this time, there are many firsts: first smile, first words, and first steps. The following guidelines may aid you in monitoring, in an integrated fashion, the physical, emotional, social, and cognitive development of infants. They also show what to include in the physical examination. For each age group, this chapter reviews the monitoring of cognitive, fine and gross motor, and verbal development. Review of emotional development, which is vitally important for the infant's well being, is also included. This chapter provides information in each of these developmental areas for the 2-month, 4-month, 6-month, and 9-month well-child visits (Fig. 19–1).

Anticipatory guidance for each visit is also reviewed. One of the most important benefits of regular well-child visits, anticipatory guidance provides the parents with accurate information on what to expect before the next well-child visit. Topics such as developmental changes, safety and accident prevention, dental issues, nutrition and feeding, sleep, discipline, and other parenting issues are covered. Anticipatory guidance should be tailored to the infant's age group and be specific to the individual family's situation.

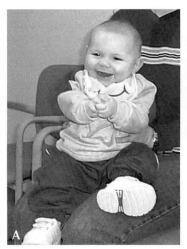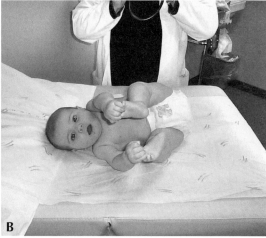

FIG. 19.1. (*A*) Four-month-old infant at well-child visit. (*B*) Six-month-old infant turning over.

The infant is an integral part of his or her environment. It is important to include an assessment of the family. Recent changes in living arrangements, jobs, finances, or marital status can produce stress in families. Increased stress experienced by the primary caregiver can directly affect the caregiver's ability to adequately meet the infant's needs. At each visit, review what birth control method is being used. During each visit, also include positive words for the parents.

Before moving into the specifics of each interval visit, there are some developmental generalities to keep in mind. The manner in which the infant responds to stimuli will evolve and mature. Over the first weeks to months the infant progresses from the generalized involuntary reflex to the purposeful voluntary action. Physical development matures in an organized manner: cephalic to caudal and proximal to distal. Last, over the first year, the infant progresses from a dependent newborn to a budding independent and autonomous toddler.

APPROACH

For all ages, approaching the visit in a calm, relaxed manner puts both the parents and the infant at ease. A relaxed, comfortable parent may decrease the anxiety and fear the child experiences. The approach to the examination of a 2-month-old infant differs from that of a 9-month old infant. The normal cognitive and social changes over this period often make the latter examination more difficult. Before the emergence of stranger and separation anxieties of a 6- to 9-month old infant, infants generally enjoy the social interaction of the medical history and physical examination. It may be best to leave the intrusive portion of the examination until the end, such as checking the tympanic membranes and pharynx or the evaluation of hip abduction. The physical examination may begin with the child sitting in the parent's lap. A younger infant can then be moved to the examination table to complete the examination and for the evaluation of the development milestones. To ease the infant during the examination, the provider can make repetitive soothing sounds, such as clicking the tongue, or make soothing motions, such as rocking or holding the infant's hand while listening to the heart or lungs. The provider may need to pause during the examination of a younger infant to allow for feeding, consoling, or changing of a diaper.

To allay the fear of an older infant, start the history while seated across the room, then gradually move closer while conversing with the parent. Allow the child to touch or play with the equipment. For example, handling a tongue blade or ear speculum before its use may decrease anxiety and increase cooperation. These actions can help distract the infant from the examiner and the examination. After the history has been taken, begin the physical examination of the infant on the parent's lap. Checking a reflex or listening to the heart and lungs can easily be performed while the infant is still comfortably next to the parent. Then, depending on the comfort level of the infant, he or she can be placed on the examination table, or the examination can be completed on the parent's lap. Talking softly and gently; moving slowly; and, depending on the infant's age, having the infant seated for some portion or possibly for all of the visit on the parent's lap help to make the visit more successful.

At each well-child visit, provide the parents time to express their concerns, needs, and expectations. Optimal growth and development for children can be accomplished only through an understanding of the family as a whole. A positive relationship between the parents and the provider is one that promotes child health and a willingness to work together on the problems that arise, thereby optimizing assessment and treatment of the child.

DEVELOPMENTAL MILESTONES

Developmental skills of the child are assessed at each visit. The developmental milestones provide a systematic manner by which you can observe neurologic growth of the infant. If delays or red flags are noted during a visit, early intervention can be made to promote optimal growth and development for that infant. The ultimate goals of development are the same for all infants.

For gross motor skills, gradual cephalocaudal development is expected. Head and trunk control is seen first with loss of head lag, the ability to sit independently, and development of locomotion (i.e., crawling and walking). Concurrently, there is a progressive loss of primitive reflex responses and emergence of postural responses as equilibrium balance develops, demonstrating integration of the motor and sensory systems within the brain.

Fine motor control of the infant improves over the first year of life from batting at objects to the ability to pick up small objects with the fingertips, the pincer grasp. During the second year of life, fine motor development continues as the infant learns to use these skills with self-care and in play. The skills of self-feeding and dressing eventually emerge from the development of fine motor control.

Language development is divided into two developing abilities: receptive and expressive. Receptive language development occurs first when the infant learns to understand language. Expressive language development occurs with the infant learning to make his or her thoughts, needs, and desires known. Cognitive skills over the first year of life include learning that the self is separate from the environment and, during the latter half of the first year, learning object permanence.

Social skills are those skills that the infant learns in order to form interpersonal and social relationships. Emotional development is the infant's ability to trust his or her environment and to learn how to express feelings, such as pain, anger, pleasure, displeasure, and fear.

 ## PERIODICITY

The timing of well-child visits is well established. In general, the goal of these visits is to provide health maintenance in a continuous and comprehensive manner. Specifically, goals are to:

- Establish an effective relationship with the parent
- Gain an understanding of the child's cultural background
- Assess for family stressors that identify at-risk families
- Gain early detection of disease processes
- Gain early detection of developmental and behavioral problems
- Provide health maintenance
- Provide anticipatory guidance

The current recommendation by the American Academy of Pediatrics (AAP) includes not only the timing of well-child visits but also what to address during each visit (Table 19–1). At any time, additional visits can be added, depending on the individual need of the infant and the family.

 ## THE 2-MONTH WELL-CHILD VISIT

By the end of the second month, the infant has adjusted to extrauterine life. The parents typically have more confidence at this visit than they had at the 2-week visit.

HISTORY

Begin with the interval history. Ask the parents what concerns and questions they have about caring for their child. Review the infant's feeding, elimina-

TABLE 19–1. PERIODICITY OF THE WELL-CHILD EXAMINATION

	AGE IN MONTHS			
	2	4	6	9
Interval history	X	X	X	X
MEASUREMENTS				
Length and weight	X	X	X	X
Head circumference	X	X	X	X
SENSORY SCREENING				
Vision	X	X	X	X
Hearing	X	X	X	X
DEVELOPMENTAL				
Behavior screening	X	X	X	X
PROCEDURES				
All infants				
Immunizations	X	X	X	X
High-risk infants				
Hct or Hgb				X
Lead screening				X
ANTICIPATORY GUIDANCE (INCLUDING BUT NOT LIMITED TO)				
Growth and development	X	X	X	X
Safety	X	X	X	X
Dental issues	X	X	X	X
Nutrition	X	X	X	X
Sleeping position	X	X	X	X
Parenting	X	X	X	X

tion, and sleeping patterns. Also obtain a review of systems. Along with the weight, the number and amount of feedings can be used to assess the infant's nutritional status. At age 2 months, the pattern of sleep may still be erratic. The stooling pattern is also likely to be irregular. An infant at this age may still have a loose stool after each feeding. Ask about the number of wet diapers and the color of urine. If the urine is dark yellow, the infant may need additional water after feeding or possibly the infant is underfed (assess along with the weight). Ask about any illness signs or symptoms or if there have been any illnesses or emergency room visits since the 2-week examination.

Ask about changes in the family situation. Changes in finances, jobs, or living arrangements can increase familial stress. Also ask about acceptance of the infant by the older siblings. Ask the parents if they getting enough rest. Have they returned to work, or are they planning to do so soon? What birth control method is being used? Table 19–2 summarizes the subjective information to obtain at the 2-month well-child visit.

267

TABLE 19–2. SUBJECTIVE INFORMATION: 2-MONTH WELL-CHILD VISIT			
Feeding	**Sleep**	**Review of Systems**	**Family Assessment**

• Breast, bottle, or both
• If formula-fed:
  ○ Type
  ○ Iron forti-fied
• Number of feedings over a 24-h period
• Amount per feeding; for breastfed infants, how long each breast
• Problems noted, such as spitting up
	• Number nighttime awakenings
	• Hours asleep dur-ing day
	• Position of sleep
	• Where infant sleeps
		• Fussy or colicky
		  ○ Tearing of eyes
		  ○ Nasal symptoms
		  ○ Cough
		  ○ Vomiting or spit-ting-up pattern
		  ○ Frequency and consistency of stools
		  ○ Number of wet diapers, color of urine
		  ○ Equal use of extremities?
		  ○ Skin rashes?
			• Changes in:
			  ○ Living arrange-ments
			  ○ Job situation
			  ○ Finances
			  ○ Marital status
			• For primary care-giver:
			  ○ Sufficient rest
			  ○ Support system
			  ○ Return to work
			• Birth control method

Observe the interaction between the parents and child. Note how the parents are holding the child, how they are talking to the child, and how the parents and the child respond to each other. Lack of interest of either party may be an indication of parental depression or a lack of bonding. Any of these are behaviors that may indicate a family at risk. Early intervention promotes overall well-being for the family. Ask the parents what strategies they are using to comfort the infant.

PHYSICAL ASSESSMENT

Begin the examination of the infant with general observation for brightness of the eyes, the skin color, and the amount of head control. Compare the weight, length, and head circumference with previous measurements. In general, infants at this age gain about 6 ounces per week. For a child with a head circumference greater than 95%, look at the curve from the previous visit, the developmental status, and the parental measurement. Approximately 50% of those with macrocephaly (i.e., head circumference that is greater than two standard deviations above the fiftieth percentile for the child's age) have familial macrocephaly, a benign condition. Review the findings on the growth chart with the parents. This can be a time for commenting to the parents on how well their infant is growing, which is a reflection of their care.

The physical examination is then done from head to toe. Special areas to note for 2-month-old infants are included in Table 19–3. The examination can be started on the parent's lap, but then the infant should be moved to the

TABLE 19–3. MEASUREMENTS AND PHYSICAL EXAMINATION: 2-MONTH WELL-CHILD VISIT

Measurements	Physical Examination
• Length	• HEENT: General shape of head
• Weight (unclothed, without diaper)	○ Fontanel, size
	○ Head control
• Head circumference	○ Red reflex, eye alignment
• Temperature, pulse, respirations	○ Eyes: Fix and follow
	○ Nose patent
	• Oral
	○ Condition of structures
	• Neck: Supple
	• Pulmonary
	○ Rate, adventitious sounds
	• Cardiovascular
	○ Heart murmur
	○ Brachial and femoral pulses equal?
	• Abdomen
	○ Contour, hernias, masses
	• Boys
	○ Testicles both present?
	○ Hydrocele present?
	○ Circumcised?
	• Girls
	○ Labial adhesions present?
	• Extremities
	○ Symmetric leg folds
	○ Hip abduction
	○ Feet: shape and flexibility
	• Skin
	○ Hemangiomas, rashes, burns/bruises (the latter are signs of physical abuse)
	• Neurologic
	○ Presence or absence of primitive reflexes

HEENT = head, eyes, ears, nose, and throat.

examination table to complete the physical and for evaluation of the developmental milestones. Check the red reflex and for strabismus. In most cases, the eyes should be aligned by the 2-month visit, but definitely by the 4-month examination. At age 2 months, visual acuity is 20/200, and there is an increased ability to follow objects vertically. Visualize the tympanic membranes and the oropharynx.

Auscultate the heart and lungs for rate, rhythm, and abnormal sounds. The murmur of a patent ductus arteriosus, occasionally heard at the 2-week visit, should now be gone. Palpate the abdomen for masses or hernias.

In boys, check for the presence of both testicles and palpate the scrotum for the presence of a hydrocele. Hydroceles do not change in size through-

TABLE 19–4. NORMAL RASHES OF 2- AND 4-MONTH-OLD CHILDREN

- Seborrheic dermatitis
- Atopic dermatitis
- Neonatal acne
- Hemangiomas
- Mongolian spots
- Cutis marmorata

out the day and transilluminate. For girls, check for adhesions of the labia minora.

Assess the musculoskeletal system. Determine if the neck is supple and without mass. Perform the Ortolani and Barlow maneuvers (see Chapter 12) to rule out congenital problems of the hip. Check the feet. Kidney bean–shaped feet that are flexible may indicate that metatarsus adductus is present. Inspect the skin for rashes, lesions, or signs of abuse. Table 19–4 lists the dermatological problems that can normally be found at this age.

Assessment of the infant's neurologic development begins as soon as you enter into the room. Note the infant's response to you and how the head is being held. Note how the infant responds to the parent. When the parent is speaking, does the infant regard the parent's face? Is the social smile or reciprocal smile present? Are the hands fisted? By age 2 months, the hands are fisted only about 50% of the time.

Assess the neurologic development, including both the gross and fine motor milestones. While performing the various maneuvers to assess development, ask the parents what they have noted regarding the infant's development. Check for the head lag. Place the infant in the prone position. At age 2 months, the head should lift off the table. By age 3 months, both the head and shoulders should typically lift when the infant is in the prone position. While performing the physical examination and assessing the development, you can take the opportunity to discuss and demonstrate the capabilities of 2-month-old infants. This aids in parental education of reasonable expectations of the child. Table 19–5 shows what can be expected of 2-month-old infants as well as areas of concern.

EGO DEVELOPMENT: TRUST VERSUS MISTRUST

Although not as obvious, assess the infant's emotional development. This is done by asking the parents how they handle meeting the infant's needs and through observing the interactions between the parents and the child, as mentioned earlier. According to Erikson's stages of ego development, infancy (birth to age 1 year) is the stage of trust versus mistrust. Erikson divided this first stage of life into two phases. Generally, during the first 6 months of life, the infant's most important social activity involves food. Newborns and young infants have little tolerance for delay of gratification.

TABLE 19–5. DEVELOPMENTAL MILESTONES OF 2-MONTH-OLD INFANTS	
Type of Skill	Red Flags
GROSS MOTOR	
Head bobs + Head lag + Moro reflex + Asymmetrical tonic neck reflex Head or chest up when prone	Rolling over before age 3 months may indicate hypertonia
FINE MOTOR	
Grasp reflex is waning Hands unfisted ~ 50% time May briefly hold object	Fisting after age 3 months is an early indi- cator of neuromotor dysfunction
LANGUAGE	
Reciprocally coos Regards speaker	
COGNITIVE	
Piaget: Sensorimotor Tracking objects > 180 degrees	
EMOTIONAL	
Erikson: Trust versus mistrust May express interest, distress (hunger), or enjoyment (smiling)	Irritability
SOCIAL	
Reciprocal social smile Bonding by the parent Eyes follow moving person	Delay in social smile may be sign of visual or cognitive impairment or maternal depression

The task of an infant is to form a sense of trust in the surrounding world. Infants also learn to love and be loved. Mistrust develops during this time when the basic needs of feeding, comfort, and stimulation are inconsistently or inadequately met. At this age, infants are capable of showing interest, distress, and pleasure. Infants enjoy and show pleasure in interaction with people.

COGNITIVE DEVELOPMENT: SENSORIMOTOR PHASE

Cognition development begins at birth. According to Piaget, the period from birth to age 24 months is termed the sensorimotor phase. During the first year of life, the infant passes through four stages. A 2-month-old infant has completed the first stage of neonatal reflex (i.e., behavior is reflexive only) and has passed into the primary circular reaction. In this stage, the infant begins to replace reflex behavior with voluntary action, such as bringing the thumb to the mouth for the purpose of sucking. The infant is also working on the concept of separation, which is learning separation of self from objects in the surrounding environment.

TABLE 19–6. IMMUNIZATIONS DUE AT THE 2-MONTH WELL-CHILD VISIT*
- DtaP
- Hepatitis B
- HIB
- IPV
- Pneumococcal polysaccharide vaccine

* Check *www.cdc.gov* for updates.
DtaP = Diphtheria, tetanus, acellular pertussis; HIB = *Haemophilus influenzae* type b; IPV = inactivated polio vaccine.

IMMUNIZATIONS

The first set of immunizations is due at this visit (Table 19–6). The first hepatitis B shot is typically given before discharge from the hospital. If available, give the infant a combination shot; for example, HIB (*Haemophilus influenzae* type b) with combinations of DtaP (diphtheria, tetanus, and acellular pertussis vaccine) or Hep B (hepatitis B vaccine). Review possible vaccine reactions with the parents and provide them with information regarding each type of vaccine.

ANTICIPATORY GUIDANCE

Anticipatory guidance can be divided into several topics. These issues are related. For example, the stage of growth and development of the infant will affect the safety recommendations made during the visit. Over the next 2 months, before the infant returns for the 4-month well-child visit, many changes will occur. Anticipatory guidance helps the parents be prepared for these normal developmental changes and enable them to better meet the infant's needs. For example, over the next 2 months, the infant will lose several of the primitive reflexes, which is a normal developmental change. These changes have implications for safety, which are important for the parents to anticipate to keep the environment safe for the infant. Social and cognitive changes, along with the developmental changes, lead to changes in the way the infant interacts with the environment. Anticipatory guidance is divided into five areas: growth and development, safety, nutrition, dental issues, and discipline and parenting. By the end of the office visit, always include a compliment for the infant's growth, care, or development. Parenting is a complex task, so a compliment from the provider gives reassurance to the parent.

Growth and Development

Infants at this age gain 1 oz/d and 0.5 to 1.0 in/mo. Physically, the infant responds less reflexively and is becoming more voluntary in his or her actions. The loss of the asymmetric tonic neck reflex allows the infant to roll, first, front to back and, later, back to front. Upper arm activity is less random and becomes more purposeful. By age 4 months, the infant will be able to grasp and hold objects and may begin to bat at toys. Soon it may be the time for the parents to offer the infant a toy that can be grasped, such as a rattle.

Bifocal vision is developing, and the infant can focus on faces and colors. This may be a good time for use of a mobile in the crib. Sound discrimination (i.e., the ability to recognize the caregiver's voice) improves. Mothers may notice the baby turning toward their direction in response to their voice. As the infant nears age 4 months, the parents may notice crying when the child is left alone, when the caregiver leaves the room, or when the infant is put to bed. Reassure the parents that this is part of normal development. Object permanence, which is seen in older infants, has not yet been established.

Sleep

Over the next 2 months, the sleeping, feeding, and elimination patterns of the infant will become more organized. Encourage the parents to establish a regular schedule of feeding and sleeping. By providing structure, the parents can further establish the organization of these newly formed patterns.

Sleeping is an important issue because it affects the whole family. It is important to review with the parents how sleeping patterns will change over the next 2 months. Remind the parents that positioning on the back (i.e., supine) or side is the recommended position for sleeping. The prone position has been found to be a major factor in the occurrence of sudden infant death syndrome (SIDS). At age 2 to 4 months, most infants continue to awaken at night to feed. Breastfed babies may have faster stomach emptying versus formula-fed infants. Early introduction of solid foods does not produce longer sleep periods.

Review hints to prevent sleep problems. The significance of nighttime awakening differs from family to family and culture to culture, so individual family assessment is needed. Recommend a consistent bedtime routine. This helps the infant learn what activities are associated with the time for sleep. With nighttime awakenings, keep the interaction to a minimum, with little talking, no lights, and no diaper changing. The parents may try delaying nighttime feeding slightly or giving slightly less in amount. Or if the infant is breastfed, they may feed for less time. These actions help the infant learn to go back to sleep by him- or herself and that nighttime is for sleeping, not playing or interacting.

You may discover during your assessment that the infant is sleeping with the parents. In many cultures around the world, this is common and considered normal. In general, in the United States, bed sharing or co-sleeping is not recommended and may be hazardous under some circumstances. Suggest to the parents that as an alternative, the infant's crib or bed be placed close to the parents' bed. The AAP recently recommended against bed sharing in its policy titled "Infant Sleep Positions and Sudden Infant Death Syndrome." If the family desires to continue bed sharing, recommend that:

- The infant remains in the nonprone position (supine or on side).
- Avoid placing the infant on soft surfaces, such as waterbeds or sofas.
- Avoid soft materials or loose covers, such as pillows, quilts, comforters, or sheepskins.
- Keep the bed away from walls or other furniture to prevent entrapment.
- Do not permit other adults or children to share the bed along with the infant.
- The parents should not smoke.
- The parents should not use alcohol or other substances that may impair arousal.

Stimulation

Stimulation of the infant in various manners further promotes growth and development. For gross motor control, the parent can exercise the infant's arms and legs while bathing and help the infant roll from front to back. To encourage fine motor development, the parents can provide objects of varying textures and objects to visualize, such as mobiles (but advise them to be cautious of the strings). Talking and singing to the infant aid language development. Music provides another form of stimulation. Holding and touching the infant regularly aid bonding by the parent and attachment by the infant.

Stimulation is important for development, but avoid overstimulation of the infant. The risk for overstimulation is individual. Encourage the parents to try to minimize prolonged social activities and learn the infant's cues to overstimulation. Prolonged crying when overstimulated should be avoided, but if it does occur, provide a quiet, soothing environment.

Safety

When bathing the infant, the parent should always check the water temperature with an elbow before placing the infant in the water. In general, the tap water temperature should be less than 120°F (49°C) to prevent accidental burns. An infant should never be left alone in the bath because drowning can occur in only 1 or 2 inches of water.

Always have infants restrained in a car seat, rear-facing, in the back seat. An infant should never be held in an adult's lap in the car.

Infants should not be left unattended because they are likely to roll over. Caution the parent to always have a hand on the child when the child is on the changing table, bed, or other furniture.

Keep small objects away from the child. The ability to grab objects improves in the following months, and the infant may be able to grasp and place objects in the mouth.

Always encourage parents to have a smoke alarm in the household. Encourage them to have a plan if a fire does occur and an escape plan that includes the infant.

Instruct the parents to not smoke while holding the infant, and if at all possible, have all smoking done outside the home (Table 19–7).

TABLE 19–7. SAFETY ISSUES FOR 2- TO 4-MONTH-OLD INFANTS

- Always test bath water before placing infant in the water.
- In general, have tap water, < 120°F (49°C).
- Never leave the infant alone in the bath.
- Always have the infant strapped in a rear-facing car seat when in the car.
- Never leave the infant alone when on furniture.
- Keep small objects away from the infant.
- Have smoke alarms in the home.
- Have a fire plan in place.
- Do not hold the infant while drinking hot liquids or smoking.
- Check the adequacy of nonparent caretakers.

Dental Issues

For 2-month-old infants, teething has not yet become an issue. Instruct parents not to prop the bottle while the infant is feeding. This helps prevent starting a habit that puts the infant at more risk for developing bottle caries after teeth are present. The American Academy of Pediatric Dentistry recommends that infants' gums be cleansed every day. With a soft washcloth wrapped around a finger, the gums should be gently massaged. Remind parents that feeding is a time of closeness and that much of the infant's early social interaction involves feeding. Typically, drooling begins around age 3 months. Drooling is not necessarily an indication of teething, only that the salivary glands have begun to function.

Nutrition

Breast milk, formula (iron fortified), or combination of both is sufficient for the infant until age 4 months and, possibly, until age 6 months. Energy requirements for 2- to 4-month-old infants is, on average, 98 to 108 kcal/kg. Both human milk and formula provide approximately 20 calories per ounce. A semi-sitting position is recommended for bottle-fed infants. Instruct the parents not to use honey for infants until the infant is 1 year old, to avoid infant botulism.

Encourage parents to delay the introduction of solid foods, such as cereal, until the next visit at age 4 months. Discourage the use of cereal in the bottle because the infant is unable to digest the cereal at this age, and it will not help the infant sleep through the night.

Iron requirements vary depending on the type of milk used. For breastfed infants, the baby's iron stores suffice until age 6 months. For formula-fed infants, recommend formulas fortified with iron (see Table 19–8).

Discipline and Parenting

Toward the end of the visit, review age-appropriate parenting skills. Discipline is not needed until the infant reaches at least age 6 months. Up to that point, the infant really only has needs, not wants. Remind parents that frequent holding or cuddling of 2- to 4-month-old infants does not result in

275

TABLE 19–8. NUTRITION IN 2-MONTH-OLD INFANTS

- Energy requirement is ~110 kcal/kg/d
- Milk (formula or breast) provides ~20 kcal/oz
- Use an iron-fortified formula
- Avoid bottle propping
- Avoid using honey

spoiling of the infant. Meeting the infant's needs, reducing frustration, and providing stimulation help to establish the infant's trust in his or her world. Last, encourage the primary caregiver to take some time for him- or herself. Also, encourage the caregiver and the partner to take time together—for example, occasional brief times away from the child.

Illness Care

Review with the parent the usual signs and symptoms of viral upper respiratory illness and viral gastroenteritis. Review home treatment and give instructions on when to call the healthcare provider's office or when to go to the emergency room. If the parent notices the following symptoms, the infant should be evaluated in the emergency room:

- Unusual irritability or lethargy
- Copious vomiting or diarrhea
- Signs of dehydration, such as poor oral intake along with reduced urine output, sunken fontanels, and no tearing

Remind the parents that when other family members are ill, good handwashing before handling the infant can help prevent spreading the illness to the infant. Encourage the parents to review illness and emergency care with the childcare provider if the infant is in daycare or in the care of other adults in addition to the parents.

THE 4-MONTH WELL-CHILD VISIT

This is a time of increasing interaction with the environment. The infant actively seeks social interaction. Often the schedule for feeding, elimination, and sleeping has become more organized. The more primitive reflex responses are disappearing, and voluntary, purposeful actions are increasing. The colic-type symptoms typically have eased as the gastrointestinal (GI) tract and neurologic system are maturing. Infrequently, colic in some infants may continue until 5 or 6 months of age.

HISTORY

Begin the visit with the interval history. First ask the parents about any concerns or questions they have. Then obtain history about feeding, elimination, and sleeping patterns. Ask about the number of feedings over a 24-hour period. If bottle feeding, ask about the amount given at each feeding. Ask about stooling pattern and consistency. Determine the number of wet diapers over a 24-hour period. Along with the weight, length, and head circumference, this information can be used to assess the infant's nutritional status. Review with the parents the infant's sleeping pattern. About 50% of infants sleep through the night at this age or at least have longer periods of sleep at night. If the infant is not sleeping through the night, assess how disruptive it is for the parents. Also ask what they do at night when the infant awakens.

Obtain a review of systems, including HEENT (head, eyes, ears, nose, and throat), cardiac, respiratory, GI, genitourinary, musculoskeletal, and skin. Ask the parents if there were any reactions to the immunizations given at the last well-child visit. Ask about any illnesses that have occurred since the last visit and if there have there been any emergency room visits.

It is important to assess the amount of stress experienced by the primary caregiver because it directly affects his or her ability to care for the infant. Ask about changes in the family situation since the last visit. Has the primary caregiver returned to work, or is he or she going to return soon? What childcare arrangements have been made? Have the parents had a chance to get out without the child? Ask about what birth control is being used (see Table 19–9).

DEVELOPMENTAL MILESTONES

Assessment of the developmental milestones begins when you enter the examination room. Note how the infant responds to you, how the head is being held, and how the infant is holding or using his or her hands. This is reviewed in more detail in the "Physical Assessment" section because it is often simpler and quicker to ask the parents what they have noticed while performing your own assessment.

Similarly, the social and emotional development can be assessed. Throughout the entire visit, be aware of how the parents and the child interact. Ask the parents how they spend their time with the infant. Do they talk or sing to the child? Are any toys being used? How do they comfort the infant? Also ask about periods of frustration and how the parents deal with it, assessing for the potential for abuse.

PHYSICAL ASSESSMENT

Compare the weight, length, and head circumference with previous measurements. The weight has generally doubled by the fourth to fifth month. Review the findings with the parents. This usually is a time for complimenting the parents on how well the infant is growing (Table 19–10).

The physical examination is then done from head to toe. The examination can be started on the parent's lap. The infant can then be moved to the examination table to complete the physical and for evaluation of the develop-

TABLE 19–9. SUBJECTIVE INFORMATION: 4-MONTH WELL-CHILD VISIT

FEEDING
- Type of milk: breast, bottle, or both
- Feedings over 24-hour period
- Amount per feeding
- Any solid foods yet
- Parental feeling on feedings and the expectation regarding starting solid foods

SLEEP
- Number of nighttime awakenings
- Hours sleeping during day
- Where infant sleeps

REVIEW OF SYSTEMS
- Temperament (e.g., calm or fussy)
- Persistent tearing of eyes
- Nasal symptoms
- Cough
- Vomiting or spitting-up pattern
- Frequency and consistency of stools
- Number of wet diapers; color of urine
- Using extremities equally
- Any skin rashes
- Any reaction to vaccines at last visit

FAMILY ASSESSMENT
- Changes in:
  - Living arrangements
  - Job situation
  - Finances
  - Marital status
- For primary caregiver:
  - Sufficient rest
  - Support system
  - Returning to work
  - Birth control method

---

mental milestones. While the infant is sitting in the parent's lap, check the red reflex and for strabismus. The eyes should be aligned by the 4-month examination. Visual acuity is now 20/100 or better. Check the tympanic membranes and the oropharynx. Palpate the fontanels and neck. The posterior fontanel should be closed by this point. The anterior fontanel remains palpable at approximately 2 cm in diameter. It should feel slightly depressed and pulsatile. The closure of the anterior fontanel occurs between age 9 and 18 months.

Auscultate the heart and lungs for rate, rhythm, and abnormal sounds. Move the infant to the examination table. Check the abdomen for masses or hernias.

TABLE 19–10. MEASUREMENTS AND PHYSICAL EXAMINATION: 4-MONTH WELL-CHILD VISIT

Measurements	Physical Examination
<ul><li>Length</li><li>Weight without clothes or diaper</li><li>Head circumference</li><li>Temperature (rectal)</li><li>Respirations and pulse</li></ul>	<ul><li>HEENT<ul><li>Fontanel size</li><li>Red reflex</li><li>Eye alignment</li><li>Tympanic membranes</li><li>Oropharynx</li><li>Neck supple?</li><li>Adenopathy?</li></ul></li><li>Cardiovascular<ul><li>Heart murmur</li></ul></li><li>Pulmonary<ul><li>Rate, adventitious sounds</li></ul></li><li>Abdomen<ul><li>Hernias, masses</li></ul></li><li>Boys<ul><li>Testicles both present?</li><li>Hydrocele present?</li><li>Circumcised?</li></ul></li><li>Girls<ul><li>Labial adhesions present?</li></ul></li><li>Musculoskeletal<ul><li>Leg fold symmetry, hip abduction, shape of feet</li></ul></li><li>Skin<ul><li>Rash</li><li>Lesions</li><li>Bruising or burns (which may be indications of physical abuse)</li></ul></li></ul>

HEENT = head, eyes, ears, nose, and throat.

In boys, assess for the presence of both testicles and palpate the scrotum for the presence of a hydrocele. In girls, check for the presence of adhesions of the labia minora.

Assess the musculoskeletal system. Perform the Ortolani and Barlow maneuvers to rule out congenital problems of the hip. Check the feet. Kidney bean–shaped feet that are flexible may indicate that metatarsus adductus is present. Note any rashes, lesions, or signs of abuse. The dermatologic problems seen in 2-month-old infants (see Table 19–4) are all also found at this age.

Assessment of neurologic system and social development can be included along with the physical assessment. While perform the various maneuvers to assess development, information regarding what the parents have noted can be obtained. Table 19–11 contains the various milestones of the 4-month-old infant. Ask the parents what they have noticed the infant doing at home. Note how the infant responds to the parents; when a parent is speaking, the infant should regard the parent's face. Is the social smile or reciprocal smile present? Are the hands fisted? By age 3 months, the hands should no longer be fisted. The hands can now be held in the midline. While the infant is still sitting in the parent's lap, place an object, such as a tongue blade, in the infant's hand. The infant should take and hold the object and may place it into his or her mouth. Regarding the object is normal at this age.

Assess the neurologic development, including the gross and fine motor milestones. This can be included with the physical examination when the infant is on the examination table. While performing the various maneuvers to assess development, ask the parents what they have noted regarding the infant's development. Check the head lag; there should be minimal to no head lag when the infant is pulled to sitting. Place the infant in the prone position. At age 4 months, the infant should hold the head erect and is likely to lift the body up onto the hands. The legs should be extended. The infant should be able to sit with support. The head is steady and no longer bobbing as it did at the 2-month visit. The first of the postural reactions are now present. The ability of the infant to keep his or her head vertical when the body is tilted is referred to as head righting. This reaction shows the beginning of integration between balance and equilibrium, a more complex neurologic response. When the infant is held standing, the legs are partially weight bearing, and the infant may push against the table or parent's lap. While performing the physical examination and assessing the development, you can take the opportunity to discuss and demonstrate the capabilities of 4-month-old infants with the parents.

Observe the interaction between the parents and the child. This is an excellent way to assess the infant's emotional development. Although reviewed as a separate topic, this assessment should be made throughout the entire visit. Note how the parents hold the child, how they talk to the child, and how the parents and the child respond to one another. Does the child look to the parent for reassurance? Lack of interest on either party may be an indication of depression in the parent, a lack of bonding, or a lack of attachment by the child. Any of these are red flags that point to a family at risk. Early intervention promotes overall well-being for the family.

EGO DEVELOPMENT: TRUST VERSUS MISTRUST

According to Erikson, the infant stage (birth to age 1 year) is the stage of trust versus mistrust. As with the 2-month-old infants, the task of the infant is to form a sense of trust in the surrounding world. The foundation of developing trust at this age is in terms of physical safety and comfort, and infants also learn to love and be loved during this stage. Mistrust develops when the basic needs of feeding, comfort, and stimulation are inconsistently or inadequately met.

TABLE 19–11. DEVELOPMENTAL MILESTONES OF 4-MONTH-OLD INFANTS

Normal Infants	Red Flags
GROSS MOTOR	
Moro reflex gone	Poor head control
Asymmetrical tonic neck reflex gone	
Up on hands when prone, head erect	
Rolling front to back	
Head lag gone	
FINE MOTOR	
Reaching for objects	Persistent fisting
Holds objects	
LANGUAGE	
Laughs out loud	Absence smile
Orients to voice	
Cry more distinctive to need	
Coos	
Listens to speaker	
COGNITIVE	
Piaget: Sensorimotor	Failure to reach for and grasp objects at
Hand regard	age 4–5 months
Regards objects when in hand	
Objects to mouth	
EMOTIONAL	
Erikson: Trust versus mistrust	
Expresses anger, joy, pleasure, and displeasure	
SOCIAL	
Recognizes the primary caregiver	
Attachment by the infant to the caregiver	
Smiles spontaneously	

COGNITIVE DEVELOPMENT

Attachment by the infant to the parent occurs during this time, according to Piaget. The infant now recognizes the primary caregiver and discriminates between familiar and unfamiliar faces. According to Piaget, the period from birth to age 24 months is termed the sensorimotor phase. During the first year of life, the infant passes through four stages. A 4-month-old child has passed through the first two stages of the sensorimotor phase. The infant no longer responds in a reflexive manner. His or her actions have become voluntary and based on cause and effect. The infant performs simple, repetitive actions and experiments with his or her environment, such as a mobile or a game with the parent. The infant is now beginning the third stage, moving into secondary circular reaction. Secondary refers to the infant interacting

TABLE 19–12. IMMUNIZATIONS DUE AT THE 4-MONTH WELL-CHILD VISIT*

- DtaP
- HIB
- IPV
- Pneumococcal polysaccharide vaccine
- Hepatitis B if not given already

* Check *www.cdc.gov* for updates.
DtaP = Diphtheria, tetanus, acellular pertussis; HIB = *Haemophilus influenzae* type b; IPV = inactivated polio vaccine.

with the environment rather than with the infant's own body. Memory is beginning. The action of experimenting with cause and effect furthers the infant's concept of separation, that is, learning to separate the self from objects in the surrounding environment.

IMMUNIZATIONS

The second set of immunizations are now due. The vaccines are similar to those given at the 2-month visit except that no hepatitis B is needed at this time. Remind parents that acetaminophen can be used for fever or fussiness. Remind parents that the next set of immunizations are due with the 6-month well-child visit (Table 19–12).

ANTICIPATORY GUIDANCE

The remaining time is spent reviewing what the parent may expect over the next 2 months before the next well-child visit. There are many growth and developmental changes, including physical, emotional, and social changes, that 4- to 6-month-old infants will experience. These normal changes determine what advice is given regarding growth and development, safety, dental issues, nutrition, discipline, and stimulation.

Growth and Development

The child should continue to gain 1 lb/d and 0.5 to 1.0 in/mo. Weight typically doubles by age 4 to 5 months. Before the next well-child visit, the infant will become increasingly physically active. The infant may sit with minimal support, may roll back to front (typically the infant has already rolled from front to back), and is weight bearing when held in a standing position. By age 6 months, the infant will be able to reach to grasp and place objects in his or her mouth.

Language development is in a pre-speech period that lasts up to about 10 months. During this period, the infant learns to localize sounds. Expressive language is beginning. Up to about age 3 months, the infant coos. Around age 4 months, the infant begins to "listen." The infant is silent as the parent or other adult speaks; after the speaker is quiet, the infant may mimic the

282

speaker and is then quiet as the speaker responds. Babbling is the addition of consonants; this occurs toward 6 months of age.

Safety

Safety is important. Simple measures can be taken to ensure the infant's safety. The following safety precautions should be reviewed with the parents for the 4- to 6-month-old infant:

- Falls occur with increased mobility, so never leave the infant alone on elevated surfaces.
- Possible aspiration or strangulation can occur, so keep small objects and cords out of the infant's reach.
- Have a smoke alarm in the home.
- Have a fire plan in place that includes the infant.
- Continue to use a rear-facing car seat.
- Never leave infant alone in the bath; an infant can drown in only 1 inch of water.
- Use tap water with a temperature less than 120°F (49°C); to prevent burns, always check bath water temperature with the elbow before placing the infant in the water.
- Do not drink hot beverages or smoke while holding the infant, and if at all possible, have all smoking done outside the home.

Before the next well-child visit at age 6 months, the parents may consider letting the infant use a walker. Discuss with the parents the potential dangers of using baby walkers and recommend against their use. Parent may think that walkers will aid in the child's learning to walk sooner, provide exercise for the infant, or provide a safe place for the infant to play. However, injuries can occur while children are in walkers. Rolling down the stairs is the most common means of injury, resulting in broken bones or head injuries. Infants in baby walkers can move faster than parents anticipate. An infant seated in a walker can reach higher, so the potential for burns by pulling objects down from the table or stove increases. Accidental poisoning may also occur if the infant reaches objects the parents thought were out of reach. Recommend that parents use a stationary walker or playpen instead.

Dental Issues

Many parents may have noted increased drooling, so they may have questions regarding teething. Drooling typically begins around age 3 months and is an indication of salivary gland function rather than teething. Also, infants do not automatically swallow the saliva before age 2 years. Typically, the first teeth erupt around age 6 months. Review these issues with the parents. Advise them to continue the daily cleansing of the gums with a soft washcloth. Also remind the parents not to prop the bottle while feeding. Not only are they missing a social opportunity with their child, but the habit of bottle propping, especially at night, promotes the development of dental caries.

TABLE 19–13. NUTRITION FOR 4- TO 6-MONTH-OLD INFANTS

- Either breast milk or formula is sufficient until age 6 months
- Caloric need remains ~110 kcal/kg/d
- Solid foods may be introduced when good head control is present
- Begin with iron-fortified cereal first
- Singly add fruits and vegetables next
- Avoid overfeeding

Nutrition

Nutrition is always an important issue for both parents and providers. Ensuring optimal growth and development requires adequate nutrition. Most infants are taking only milk at the 4-month examination. This may be breast milk, formula, or both. The caloric need of infants at this age is approximately 110 kcal/kg per day.

As the tongue thrust diminishes and head control improves, the infant will be ready for solid foods. The parent may consider introducing solid foods at any time before the 6-month visit, although breast milk or formula is enough for many infants until that time. Some infants may also show interest in table foods sooner than others, so when parents should begin to give the child solid foods should be individualized. Typically, rice cereal fortified with iron is recommended first, followed by fruits and vegetables. The cereal can be mixed with breast milk, formula, or juice. After they have been started, solid foods may be given once or twice a day, starting with 1 or 2 teaspoons and gradually working up to larger quantities. Introducing each new food one at a time to ensure there is no allergic or GI reaction is usually recommended.

Alert the parents to the possibility of overfeeding. Recommend that the parent not use feeding for quieting when the infant is fussy but not hungry. Encourage parents to be alert to the signs the infant gives them when he or she is satisfied and not to push to finish the last little bit of food. Nutritional issues are summarized in Table 19–13.

Discipline and Parenting

The topics of discipline, sleeping, stimulation, and illness care also should be covered. These are important issues for parents. Helping the parents understand their infant and what are reasonable expectations to have aid the parents in coping with an ever-changing infant and helps the parents meet the infant's needs.

As with 2-month-old infants, discipline is not needed with 4-month-old infants. Infants continue to need cuddling and holding. Remind the parents this will not result in spoiling. Meeting the infant's needs of comfort, feeding, stimulation, and nurturing continues to aid in establishing trust in the infant's world.

Review the usual signs and symptoms of viral upper respiratory illness and gastroenteritis. Review home treatment and give instructions of when to call the office or to go to the emergency room. Instructions regarding fever treatment and doses of commonly used over-the-counter medications, such as acetaminophen (not ibuprofen until age 6 months), may prove helpful to parents and save them a phone call or visit to the office. Review emergency room parameters. If the parent notices the following symptoms, the infant should be evaluated in the emergency room:

- Unusual irritability or lethargy
- Copious vomiting and diarrhea, which may result in dehydration
- Signs of dehydration, such as poor oral intake along with reduced urine output, sunken fontanels, and no tearing

Remind the parents that when other family members are ill, good hand-washing can help prevent spreading of the illness to the infant. Encourage the parents to review illness and emergency care with the childcare provider if the infant is in daycare or in the care of others besides the parents.

 # THE 6-MONTH WELL-CHILD VISIT

By this time, 6-month-old infants have become more involved with the world around them. They smile and babble with their parents. They enjoy reciprocal and face-to-face play and actively engage those around them in these activities. As you walk into the room, the infant is likely to be sitting on the parent's lap or on the examination table next to the parent with minimal support. Parents of 6-month-old infants are generally confident and comfortable. If uncertainty or anxiety is present, further probing into the family situation is warranted.

HISTORY

As with the previous visit, begin with the interval history. First ask the parents about their concerns or questions. Then review the infant's feeding, sleeping, and elimination patterns. Ask the parents if solid foods have been started, and if so, what type. Ask if there have been any problems with the introduction of solid foods.

Ask if the infant is sleeping through the night. Most 6-month-old infants can sleep for about an 8-hour period, and most still need one to two naps during the day. If night awakening is occurring, ask what the parent does during the awake periods and assess how disruptive this is for the parent. Some working parents may enjoy the uninterrupted nighttime interaction; others may be exhausted.

Perform a review of systems, including HEENT, cardiac, respiratory, GI, and skin. The stool is now more formed and less frequent. The parents may complain of changes in the pattern. Always check for an association between the introduction of solid foods or formula with the change in pattern the parents have noticed. Review of the musculoskeletal and neurologic systems can be done when assessing the gross and fine motor development. Ask

TABLE 19–14. SUBJECTIVE INFORMATION: 6-MONTH WELL-CHILD VISIT

Feeding	Sleeping	Review of Systems	Family Assessment

• Type of milk: breast, bottle, or both
• Feedings over 24-hour period
• Amount per feeding
• Any solid foods yet?
• Parental feeling on feedings and the expectation of starting solid foods
	• Number of nighttime awakenings
	• Hours sleeping during day
	• Where infant sleeps
		• Temperament (e.g., calm or fussy)
		• Persistent tearing of eyes
		• Nasal symptoms
		• Cough
		• Vomiting or spitting-up pattern
		• Frequency and consistency of stools
		• Number of wet diapers, color of urine
		• Using extremities equally?
		• Any skin rashes?
		• Any reaction to vaccines at last visit?
			• Changes in:
			  ○ Living arrangements
			  ○ Job situation
			  ○ Finances
			  ○ Marital status
			• For primary caregiver:
			  ○ Sufficient rest
			  ○ Support system
			  ○ Returning to work
			• Birth control method

about any illnesses that have occurred since the last visit or if there have been any emergency room visits. This may be an opportunity to review home care of the simple cold or viral gastroenteritis to save a future emergency room visit. Check if there were any reactions to the immunizations given at the last visit. Table 19–14 summarizes the information to gather at the 6-month visit.

Assess the family situation. Ask if there have been changes in the living arrangement or financial status since the last visit. Ask about the interaction between the siblings and the infant. Check if the primary caregiver is working and what childcare arrangements have been made. Have the parents had a chance to get out without the child? Review what type of birth control is being used.

Assessment of the infant's development begins as soon as you walk into the examination room. Note how the infant responds to you, the vocalizations of the infant, how the head is being held, how the infant is sitting, and how the infant is using his or her hands.

Similarly, assess the infant's social and emotional development. Throughout the entire visit, be aware of how the parents and child interact. Ask the parents how they spend their time with the infant. Do they talk or sing to the child? What toys are being used? How do they comfort the child? Also ask about how the parents deal with periods of frustration, assessing for the potential for abuse.

PHYSICAL ASSESSMENT

Compare the weight, length, and head circumference with previous measurements. Review the findings with the parents. This usually is a time to comment to the parents on how well the infant is doing.

The physical examination is then done from head to toe (see Table 19–15). Begin the examination on the parent's lap. Check the red reflex and the symmetry of the light reflex, a screen for strabismus. Check the tympanic membranes and oropharynx. Typically, the first tooth erupts around age 6 months. Palpate the fontanels and the neck. The anterior fontanel remains palpable, approximately 2 cm or less. It should feel slightly depressed and pulsatile.

Listen to the heart for rate, rhythm, and murmurs. Auscultate the lungs for respiratory rate and adventitious sounds. Then move the infant to the examination table. Palpate the abdomen for masses or hernias.

In boys, assess for the presence of both testicles and palpate the scrotum for the presence of a hydrocele. In girls, check for adhesions of the labia minora.

Assess the musculoskeletal system. Perform the Ortolani and Barlow maneuvers to rule out congenital problems of the hip. Check the feet for shape and flexibility. Check the skin and note any rashes, lesions, or signs of abuse.

While the infant is on the examination table, begin your assessment of the neurologic or developmental milestones. While performing the various maneuvers to assess development, information regarding what the parents have noted can be obtained. Table 19–16 contains the various milestones of the 6-month-old. Assess the fine motor development. While the infant is still sitting in the parent's lap, offer an object, such as a tongue blade, to the infant. Typically, at this age, the infant should take and hold the object. He or she may place it into the mouth and should transfer the object from hand to hand. You may note that the infant reaches and grabs for the stethoscope around your neck as you move closer to perform the examination. The movement is a smooth motion involving both arms and an open hand before clasping the tube of the stethoscope.

Assess the gross motor skills. With the infant still on the examination table, pull him or her from the supine to the sitting position. No head lag should be present. By age 6 months, the child often anticipates the maneuver and raises the head before the shoulders. While sitting, a 6-month-old child may still require support or may assume a tripod position (Fig. 19–2). In either case, the head is erect, and the spine is straight. By age 6 months, the protective equilibrium response has developed. When a sitting infant is pushed laterally, the trunk flexes towards the pushing force and the opposite arm extends to support the body. This motion maintains the infant's center of gravity. Lift the infant by the trunk and then gently lower the feet to the examination table. The infant should be partially to fully weight bearing. By age 7 months, the infant should be fully weight bearing and will often bounce when held in this position.

TABLE 19-15. MEASUREMENTS AND PHYSICAL EXAMINATION: 6-MONTH WELL-CHILD VISIT

Measurements	Physical Examination

• Length
• Weight without clothes or diaper
• Head circumference
• Temperature (rectal)
• Pulse and respirations
	• HEENT
	  ○ Fontanel size
	  ○ Red reflex
	  ○ Eye alignment
	  ○ Tympanic membranes
	  ○ Oropharynx
	  ○ Neck supple
	  ○ Adenopathy
	• Pulmonary
	  ○ Rate, adventitious sounds
	• Cardiovascular
	  ○ Heart murmur
	• Abdomen
	  ○ Hernias, masses
	• Boys
	  ○ Testicles both present?
	  ○ Hydrocele present?
	  ○ Circumcised?
	• Girls
	  ○ Labial adhesions present?
	• Musculoskeletal
	  ○ Leg fold symmetry, hip abduction, foot shape and flexibility
	• Skin
	  ○ Rash
	  ○ Lesions
	  ○ Bruising or burns (which may be indications of physical abuse)

HEENT = head, eyes, ears, nose, and throat.

EGO DEVELOPMENT: TRUST VERSUS MISTRUST

A 6-month-old child continues in the stage of trust versus mistrust in his or her surrounding environment. Consistent, loving care is essential to establishing basic trust and has lifelong effects. Trust results later in faith and optimism. Mistrust can develop not only through too much frustration, when needs are not met, but also in infants who experience too little frustration. It is important for the infant to learn about testing control over the surrounding environment rather than having the parent immediately meet every need. Erikson divided the first year into two stages. During the second half of the first year, infants learn interaction with their environment through advancing motor, visual, and verbal skills. It is the degree and quality of these interactions that promote trust.

288

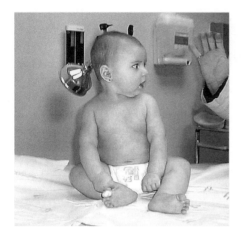

FIG. 19.2. Six-month-old infant in the tripod position.

COGNITIVE DEVELOPMENT: SENSORIMOTOR PHASE

Object permanence is the task of 6- to 8-month-old infants. Piaget places this age in the secondary circular reaction stage, in which the infant is now involved with activities separate from their bodies. Infants are learning that objects have permanence, which is that the object can exist even when it is no longer visible. For a 6-month-old infant, object permanence is developing. The infant is able to find partially hidden objects. In coming months, the child will enjoy peek-a-boo. Infants continue to experiment with cause and effect. They realize through experimenting that they are separate from their environment.

IMMUNIZATIONS

The third set of immunizations is now due (Table 19–17). The vaccines are similar to those given at the 4-month visit except that the last hepatitis B shot is included. Review problems with the previously received immunizations. Recommend that parents give the infant acetaminophen for fever or fussiness. Review with the parents that the next immunizations are due at the 12-month well-child visit.

ANTICIPATORY GUIDANCE

The topics of anticipatory guidance are many and are interrelated. As with the previous visits, the infant is developing rapidly. Many changes will occur before the 9-month visit. Reviewing the anticipated changes with the parents aids them in feeling better prepared to meet the needs of their growing infant. The infant will become more mobile over the following months, and safety is of concern. Eruption of the first teeth is likely to occur before the next well-child visit, if not already by this visit.

TABLE 19–16. EXPECTED DEVELOPMENTAL MILESTONES OF 6-MONTH-OLD INFANTS

Normal Infants	Red Flags
GROSS MOTOR	
No head lag present	W-sitting
With sitting, the head is erect and spine is straight	Bunny hopping
Sits with support, or propped on hands	Poor head control
Rolls over in both directions	
Equilibrium response	
Bears weight when standing	
Stands with support	
FINE MOTOR	
Grasping objects with both hands	Persistent fisting
Transfers objects from hand to hand	Hand dominance
Rakes small objects	Failure to reach for objects
Shakes, bangs, drops objects	
LANGUAGE	
Babbling, using consonants	Absence of babbling
Responds to name	
Using sound to get attention	
Respond to friendly versus angry tone	
Razzes (the raspberry sound)	
COGNITIVE	
Object permanence developing; looks after dropped object	
EMOTIONAL	
Fear	
Emerging self-identity	
SOCIAL	
Stranger awareness	Absence of stranger awareness
Person preference	
Differential facial expressions	

Growth and Development

Growth slows in the next few months. The child should gain approximately 1 lb or 0.5 kg per month and 0.5 in or 1.0 cm per month in length. The head and chest circumferences should equalize.

The infant is likely to become mobile by the next well-child visit. The infant will progress from sitting independently to getting on all fours to creeping and crawling. By age 9 months, the infant may be able to pull to stand. The fine motor control continues to develop, advancing from the immature rake of a small object at age 6 months to the radial-palmar grasp of a small toy by age 9 months. By the next visit at age 9 months, the infant may be able to reach for objects while on all fours. Hand dominance is not established until age 18 months if hand dominance appears earlier, it may be an indication of weakness in the contralateral hand or extremity.

Language at age 6 months of age is still in the pre-speech period. Before age 6 months, infants learn to localize sounds and participate in reciprocal vocalizations. Over the next few months, babbling begins, which may include a nondiscriminating "mama" or "dada" by 9 months. By age 9 months, infants may be able to follow verbal routines, such as waving bye-bye.

Stranger awareness may become evident. By age 6 to 8 months, infants typically protest when their caregiver leaves the room, or infants may exhibit fear of being touched or picked up by persons unfamiliar to them. Infants have been aware of the difference between parents and strangers since their earliest weeks and have shown preference for their parents' familiar faces over those of strangers. During the second half of infants' first year, they exhibit a more obvious recognition of strangers, often reacting overtly negatively. Infants may squirm or fuss to return to their parent, may cling to the parent, or may cry if being handed over to an unfamiliar person. This awareness has developed because the infant understands that the parent exists even when not present. The infant has not yet developed the cognitive capacity to know that the parent will return. Stranger awareness is a normal development event, but parents unaware of this may become concerned that something is wrong with their infant or that they are doing something wrong. Informing them of this normal developmental stage will help to allay their fears.

Sleep

By age 6 months, about 75% of infants can sleep for a 6- to 8-hour stretch at night. The following list includes hints for helping decrease the length and number of nighttime awakenings:

- Maintain a regular bedtime and bedtime routine.
- Encourage self-quieting by the infant. Place the infant in the crib while he or she is still awake but is drowsy. This may be the time to introduce a special blanket or stuffed animal for comfort.
- Leave the door to the room open after the infant has been placed in the crib.
- Avoid small frequent feedings during the day.

291

- Keep the lights off and the interaction to a bare minimum during nighttime awakenings.
- During nighttime awakenings, spend less than 1 minute soothing the infant, such as gentle touching or talking. Do not pick up the infant. Repeat the soothing action every 5 minutes, gradually lengthening the interaction to every 15 minutes.
- If the infant is still feeding, make the interaction brief and boring. Slowly decrease the amount of feedings given

These techniques can be used by parents to prevent sleep problems from developing or can be used after a problem has begun. The goal is to encourage the infant to self-quiet, self-comfort, and go to sleep comfortably without help from the parents. The action of repeated soothing of the infant during the night is used to help lessen fear or anxiety in the infant.

Stimulation

Interaction between the infant and the parents furthers the infant's development in all areas. For gross and fine motor development, infants need opportunities for play and experimentation. Encourage the parents to provide a safe area for the infant to explore and to provide age-appropriate toys, such as a mirror, rattles, or objects of various textures or colors. Talking, singing, and reading to the infant aid in language development and encourage the baby to vocalize more. Playing music provides another form of stimulation.

Safety

The world will become a wider place for the mobile infant. Many of the safety issues from previous visits remain the same, but now you need to expand your advice to parents. Encourage the parents to get down on the floor and look for possible safety hazards at the infant's level. The following is a list of the safety recommendations to review with the parents at the 6-month well-child visit:

- All cords or objects with small parts need to be removed from the baby's possible grasp.
- Place plastic plug covers over the electrical outlets.
- Install gates at the top and bottom of stairs.
- Install safety devices in drawers and cupboards.
- Lower crib mattress level.
- Do not leave the infant alone on elevated surfaces.
- Keep small objects and cords out of the infant's reach. Aspiration or strangulation may occur.
- Encourage parents to have a smoke alarm in the home.
- Encourage parents to have a fire plan that includes the infant.
- Use a rear-facing car seat.
- Do not leave an infant alone in the bath.

TABLE 19–18. FLUORIDE SUPPLEMENTATION RECOMMENDATION: AMOUNT OF FLUORIDE SUPPLEMENTATION BASED ON FLUORIDE CONCENTRATION OF THE WATER SUPPLY

Age of Child	Fluoride < 0.3 ppm	Fluoride 0.3–0.6 ppm	Fluoride > 0.6 ppm
Birth–6 months	0	0	0
6 months–3 years	0.25 mg	0	0
3–6 years	0.5 mg	0.25 mg	0
6–16 years	1 mg	0.5 mg	0

- Maintain tap water temperature less than 120°F (49°C) and always check bath water temperature with elbow before placing infant to prevent burns.
- Do not drink hot beverages while holding the infant.
- Do not smoke while holding the infant, and if at all possible, have all smoking done outside the home.
- Keep all chemicals in their original bottles and keep them elevated out of the infant's reach.
- Keep the poison control number by the telephone.

Dental Issues

Tooth eruption typically begins around age 6 months. The primary teeth eruption follows a typical pattern. See Chapter 5 for the schedule of teeth eruption of the primary teeth. For the discomfort of teething, suggest the infant be offered a cold, wet washcloth or a chilled pacifier on which to chew. Recommend that the parents begin cleaning the infant's teeth with a soft toothbrush after the teeth have emerged. Toothpaste is not needed at this age. As with the previous visits, discourage the practice of bottle propping when feeding or at bedtime.

Addressing fluoride supplementation is recommended at the 6-month visit. The time to begin fluoride supplementation depends on the age of the child and the fluoride content of the drinking water. See Table 19–18 to check when fluoride is needed and the amount recommended.

Nutrition

By the 6-month well-child visit, many infants have been introduced to solid foods. Instruct the parent to continue to breastfeed or to use iron-fortified formula for the first year. Although solid foods may have been and will be started, milk continues to be the major source of the infant's nutrition. If cereal is not already started, recommend iron-fortified cereals, mixed with breast milk, formula, or juice, as the first food. Then the parent should add fruits and vegetables one at a time to ensure there is no adverse reaction. After they have been started, solid foods may be given once or twice a day, starting with a teaspoon or two and gradually working up to larger quanti-

293

TABLE 19–19. FOODS TO AVOID IN 6-MONTH-OLD INFANTS

- Peanuts
- Popcorn
- Hotdogs and sausage
- Raw vegetable or fruit pieces: carrots, celery, apples
- Whole grapes, raisins
- Hard candy

ties. Finely chopped foods as well as pureed fruits or vegetables are best at this age. Remind parents to avoid foods that may cause aspiration or choking. Table 19–19 includes foods to avoid until an infant is approximately 2 years of age. Some references also suggest that the parents should avoid giving the infant whole eggs or strawberries until age 12 months.

Remind the parents about not overfeeding, to observe for the infant's cues when he or she is satiated, and to not use food for comforting the infant. Over the next few months, the infant may express interest in self-feeding. This is a messy but beneficial practice. Self-feeding promotes fine motor control. Instruct the parent to introduce the cup, offering the infant small amounts of water or juice, not more than 4 to 6 oz a day so as not to replace the calories received from milk.

Discipline and Parenting

As the infant becomes more mobile and aware of his or her environment, discipline may be needed for the infant's safety. At this age, discipline needs to be simple and consistent. For example, when an infant reaches for an electric cord or bites while breastfeeding, a simple, stern "no" followed by distraction or physical removal is all that is needed. Many strategies can be used:

- Structure a safe home environment.
- Distract the infant (e.g., with a toy).
- Physically remove the infant.
- Use a simple verbal disapproval such as a stern "no."
- Use "no" sparingly and only when appropriate.
- Use simple nonverbal disapproval such as eye contact with a stern look.

Remind parents of the infant's desire and need to explore the environment and encourage parents to structure their home such that little discipline is needed. Importantly, remind parents that the infant continues to need nurturing. Hugging and cuddling remain a very important part of infant care.

Ask the primary caregiver what he or she is doing to nurture himself or herself. Ask about the time the caregiver is taking to manage stress. Also ask if the primary caregiver and the partner have had a chance to get away, even briefly, without the infant. If the answer is no, encourage them to do so.

Review illness care. Ask what the parents should do if they suspect the infant is ill or has a fever. As with the previous visits, briefly review illness care for infants with viral upper respiratory infections or gastroenteritis.

294

Instructions regarding fever treatment and doses of commonly used over-the-counter medications, such as acetaminophen, may prove helpful to parents and save them a phone call or visit to the office. Ibuprofen may be used after age 6 months. Review emergency room parameters. If the parent notices the following symptoms, the infant should be evaluated in the emergency room:

- Unusual irritability or lethargy
- Copious vomiting and diarrhea to result in dehydration
- Signs of dehydration such as poor oral intake along with reduced urine output, sunken fontanels, and no tearing

Remind the parents that when other family members are ill, good hand-washing can help prevent spreading of the illness to the infant. Encourage the parents to review illness and emergency care with the childcare provider if the infant is in daycare or in the care of others besides the parents.

THE 9-MONTH WELL-CHILD VISIT

Nine-month-old infants are gaining independence energetically, are actively interested in the world, and have a desire to explore. The parent may note that these infants have less desire to be cuddled and held because their surroundings now hold their interest. At times, parents may view the growing independence with a sense of loss. The developmental milestones of a 9-month-old infant are more obvious. The day-to-day care of a 9-month-old infant may take more energy and thought from the parent than required before.

HISTORY

As with every well-child visit, begin the visit with the interval history. First provide time for the parents to express any concerns or ask questions. Then review how the infant spends his or her day. Ask about feeding, sleeping, and play patterns. Ask the parents about the types of food the infant is now eating and if there have been any problems. Ask about any periods of nighttime awakening. Some infants at this age who have been sleeping through the night may now be awakening. This may be caused by newfound physical skills (e.g., crawling or pulling to stand) or may result from anxieties left over from the day. If nighttime awakening is occurring, ask what the parent does during the awake periods. Check about any illness that has occurred since the last visit. Obtain a review of systems, including HEENT, cardiac, respiratory, GI, and skin. It is often simpler to review the musculoskeletal and neurologic systems when assessing the physical development. Ask how the infant is teething, the number of teeth present, and if there have been any problems. Check if there have any illnesses or emergency room visits since the last well-child visit. Table 19–20 summarizes the information to gather at the 9-month visit.

TABLE 19–20. SUBJECTIVE INFORMATION: 9-MONTH WELL-CHILD VISIT

Feeding	Sleeping	Review of Systems	Family Assessment

• Type of milk: breast, bottle, or both
• Amount per feeding
• Type of solid foods
• Problems with any foods
• Amount of juice or water
	• Number of nighttime awakenings
	• Hours sleeping during day
	• Where infant sleeps
		• Persistent tearing of eyes
		• Nasal symptoms
		• Cough
		• Teething
		• Frequency and consistency of stools
		• Using extremities equally?
		• Any skin rashes?
		• Any reaction to vaccines at last visit?
			• Changes in:
			  ○ Living arrangements
			  ○ Job situation
			  ○ Finances
			  ○ Marital status
			• For primary caregiver:
			  ○ Sufficient rest
			  ○ Support system
			  ○ Returning to work
			• Birth control method

Assess the family situation. Ask if there have been changes in the living arrangement or financial status since the last visit. Check if the primary caregiver is working and what childcare arrangements have been made. Ask if the parents have had a chance to get out without the child. Review what type of birth control is being used.

As with the previous visits, begin the developmental assessment as soon as you walk into the examination room, although it may be more difficult with infants of this age. Note the infant's responses to you; the infant may be wary of your presence, even though there was a smile at the last visit. Stranger awareness is in full swing at this age. It is best not to initially make direct eye contact with the infant. This is the time to sit across the room from the infant and gradually move closer, initiating eye contact only after conversing with the parents for a few minutes. The infant may not be comfortable vocalizing or playing in the strange examination room. Much of the developmental history may need to come from the parents.

Assess the infant's social and emotional development. Be aware of how the parent and the child interact throughout the entire visit. Does the infant turn to the parents for reassurance? If not, concern should be raised. Ask the parents how they spend their time with the infant and how they play with the infant. Do they talk or sing to the child? Are they reading to the infant? What toys are being used? How do they comfort the child? Also ask about how the parents deal with periods of frustration, assessing for the potential for abuse.

PHYSICAL ASSESSMENT

Compare the weight, length, and head circumference with previous measurements. Review the findings with the parents. If risk factors are present, screening for elevated lead levels or for anemia should be done at this visit. Each screening test is reviewed individually.

TABLE 19–21. MEASUREMENTS AND PHYSICAL EXAMINATION: 9-MONTH WELL-CHILD VISIT	
Measurements	**Physical Examination**
• Length	• HEENT
• Weight without clothes or	○ Fontanel size
diaper	○ Red reflex
• Head circumference	○ Eye alignment
• Temperature (rectal)	○ Tympanic membranes
• Pulse and respirations	○ Oropharynx
• If risk factors present:	○ Neck supple
Hct/Hgb and lead screening	○ Adenopathy
	• Pulmonary
	○ Rate, adventitious sounds
	• Cardiovascular
	○ Heart murmur
	• Abdomen
	○ Hernias, masses
	• Boys
	○ Testicles both present?
	○ Hydrocele present?
	○ Circumcised?
	• Girls
	○ Labial adhesions present?
	• Musculoskeletal
	○ Leg fold symmetry
	○ Hip abduction
	○ Feet shape and flexibility
	• Skin
	○ Rash
	○ Lesions
	○ Bruising or burns (which may indicators of physical abuse)

HEENT = head, eyes, ears, nose, and throat.

The physical examination is done from head to toe (Table 19–21). Begin the examination on the parent's lap. While reviewing the history with the parents, encourage the infant to touch and play with the otoscope or stethoscope. This may help ease the infant into the examination portion of the visit. Check the red reflex and the symmetry of the light reflex, a screen for strabismus. Check the tympanic membrane and oropharynx. Are there teeth present? Palpate the fontanel and the neck.

Auscultate the heart for rate, rhythm, and murmurs. Check the lungs for respiratory rate and adventitious sounds. Then try to move the infant to the examination table. Even if the infant is cooperative, it may be difficult to keep him or her lying on the table long enough to perform the examination. Some infants may object strongly, so the remainder of the examination can be completed on the parent's lap. To examine the abdomen, the infant may need to be laid across the parent's and your laps. Check the abdomen for masses or hernias.

In boys, check for the presence of both testicles and palpate the scrotum for the presence of a hydrocele. In girls, check for adhesions of the labia minora.

Assess the musculoskeletal system. Perform the Ortolani maneuver to rule out congenital problems of the hip. Check the symmetry of the posterior thigh creases. Check the feet for shape and flexibility. Limited flexion of the foot may indicate tight heel cords, a finding that requires further evaluation. Check the skin and note any rashes, lesions, or signs of abuse.

While the infant is on the examination table (or still on the parent's lap), begin the assessment of the developmental milestones. As mentioned earlier, infants of this age may not allow a complete neurologic check. Assuming the infant is on the examination table, note how well he or she is sitting. An infant at this age will be able to sit without assistance. The infant may move from the sitting position onto all fours and crawl forward or may try pulling to a stand. If there was difficulty keeping the infant still during examination of the abdomen, the assessment of gross motor control may already be complete.

The parachute response is now in place. This is a complex, integrated neurologic response to multiple sensory inputs. The parachute reaction occurs when the child is held horizontally by the waist, parallel to the floor, and is lowered rapidly to the floor. The arms and legs extend with hands open and fingers spread, as if to catch the infant's fall. The parachute response, along with the equilibrium response and head righting of earlier visits, demonstrates that balance and equilibrium are developing normally. Infants with central nervous system damage are slow to show these postural reactions. Hold the infant upright by the trunk. Any scissoring of the lower extremities requires further investigation.

Assess the infant's fine motor development. This can be done while still reviewing the history with the parent after the infant seems relatively comfortable in the situation. For example, while talking with the parent before the examination has been started, place an object in your hand and offer it to the infant. If the infant will not accept the object, ask the parent to try. At age 9 months, the inferior pincer grasp is present. The ability to grasp objects has developed from the reflexive palmar grasp of the neonatal period, to the hand regard and hand play of a 3- to 4-month-old infant, to the voluntary grasp and ability to transfer objects from hand to hand of a 6-month-old infant. Nine-month-old infants are learning to use their thumbs and fingers independently. The grasp now involves the extended thumb but flexed index finger. Table 19–22 contains the various milestones of 9-month-old infants.

EGO DEVELOPMENT: TRUST VERSUS MISTRUST

Nine-month-old infants continue in the stage of trust versus mistrust. Consistent, loving care is essential to establishing basic trust and has lifelong effects. Trust results in faith and optimism. During the second half of the first

TABLE 19–22. DEVELOPMENTAL MILESTONES OF 9-MONTH-OLD INFANTS

Normal Infants	Red Flags
GROSS MOTOR	
Sits independently	Persistent standing on tip-toes
Crawling or creeping on hands and knees	Scissors motion of lower
May pull to stand	extremities
Weight bearing with standing	Persistence of primitive reflexes
Parachute response	
FINE MOTOR	
Maturing grasp: the inferior pincer grasp; may use fingertips	Persistence of primitive reflexes
Able to point at and pick up small object	
May be able to isolate the index finger and poke	
Feeds self with fingers	
LANGUAGE	
Responds to own name	Inability to localize sound
May imitate sounds of others	
May say "mama" or "dada" but inappropriately	
Associating words with meanings	
May begin to integrate babble and intonation	
Looks where finger is pointing to, rather than looking at the pointer	
Responds to "no"	
COGNITIVE	
Bangs objects on surface	
Learns object permanence	
Plays peek-a-boo	
EMOTIONAL	
Avoidance reaction	
SOCIAL	
Stranger awareness	
Separation anxiety	
Sense of self	

year, infants learn interaction with their environment through advancing motor, visual, and verbal skills. It is the degree and quality of these interactions that promote trust. Encourage the parents to provide a safe area and to allow the infant time to test and use the newly developing skills.

COGNITIVE DEVELOPMENT: SENSORIMOTOR PHASE

Many 9-month-old infants can now locate objects that have been completely hidden. Although not yet completed, object permanence remains a task of this age. Infants often enjoy a game of peek-a-boo and may be comfortable

Age	Hematocrit (mean), %	Hemoglobin, g/dL
Full-term infants	51	13.5–16.5
2 weeks	53	13.4–16.6
2 months	35	9.4–11.2
6 months	31–36	11.1–12.6
2 years	33–36	10.5–12

crawling away from their parent because they can now remember where to return to find the parent. Piaget describes the 9-month-old infant as being in a stage of coordination of the secondary reactions. This is the fourth of six stages that infant and toddlers pass through during the first 2 years of life. The infant now is goal oriented. The desired action or object can be actively sought, and intention is developing. Previously, obstacles (hidden objects) would hinder the infant's effort, but 9-month-old infants are now capable of working to overcome barriers. These infants typically use the same strategies as before when confronted with new situations. The world is now beginning to make sense to these infants. They understand certain sequence of events, such as waving good-bye or understanding that a comb is used in the hair and can imitate the movement of combing the hair.

HEMATOCRIT

Infants are at risk for developing iron-deficiency anemia. At the 9-month visit, hematocrit or hemoglobin screening should be obtained if risk factors are present (Table 19–23). Evidence shows that those infants with iron-deficiency anemia can have behavioral or development problems. The risk categories include the following factors:

- Low socioeconomic status
- Birth weight < 1500 g
- Whole milk was given before age 6 months
- Low-iron formula was used
- Low intake of iron-rich foods

Iron-deficiency anemia is an easily identifiable and treatable condition. Most offices or clinics can perform screening using the fingerstick hematocrit. The results and treatment, if needed, can then be started before the family leaves the office. Exclusively breastfed infants are also at risk for developing iron-deficiency anemia because the infant's iron stores are depleted around age 6 months and breast milk is deficient in iron.

LEAD SCREENING

The AAP recommends that blood lead screening be performed as part of routine health supervision at about age 9 through 12 months and, if possible, again at about age 24 months. The rationale is for primary prevention to prevent lead poisoning and the sequelae of elevated blood lead levels, specifically, the resulting neurotoxicity of developing children. In areas where universal screening is not warranted, screening should be obtained in children who are at risk. Risk factors include:

- Living in dwellings built before 1977
- Visiting dwellings built before 1977 regularly, such as daycare
- Having a sibling or playmate with elevated blood lead levels
- Living with an adult whose job or hobby involves the use of lead
- Living near industry involved in lead

Exposure to lead may be through water, air, or the ingestion of lead-based paint. Lead-based paints were used before 1977, so an infant living in or visiting an older home may be at risk. If an infant is living in a home built before 1977, ask the parents about any peeling paint present or if there is any remodeling currently taking place. Ask about the pipes: do the parents know whether the plumbing includes lead pipes? Hobbies that potentially may involve lead include ceramics, furniture remodeling, and working with stained glass. When the blood lead level is checked at the office or clinic, care must be taken to prevent environmental contamination of the sample to reduce the problem of falsely elevated levels.

IMMUNIZATIONS

There are no specific immunizations due at the 9-month visit. Check to see if there are any immunizations missing from the first three visits. Any vaccines missing can be given at this time.

ANTICIPATORY GUIDANCE

By the time the infant returns to the office for the next well-child visit, he or she could very likely be walking and talking. The developing autonomy and independence will grow over the coming months, with implications for safety and discipline. As the infant grows into toddlerhood, the infant may begin to exert his or her own will. Anticipatory guidance will help the parents of 9- to 12-month-old infants be prepared for the coming changes. Whether it is providing a safe environment or having enough confidence to set limits, the coming months can be challenging for even the most experienced parents.

Growth and Development

The infant should continue to gain approximately 1 lb or 0.5 kg per month and 0.5 in or 1.0 cm per month in length. Mobility continues to progress. Over the next several months, the infant most likely will be cruising or walking alone. The infant will typically pull to stand first. Then the infant will begin cruising (i.e., walking while holding onto objects). Walking alone follows.

Fine motor development also progresses over the next 3 to 4 months. By age 1 year, the fine pincer grasp will be in place. This is the ability to grasp a small object between the fingertips. The infant may be able to make marks with a crayon by the next visit.

Toward the first birthday, the infant begins to realize that people and objects have names. For example, the random "mama" or "dada" that the infant was using before now begins to mean the mother or father. The receptive part of language development, the ability to understand language, is growing. The number of words the infant can understand by age 1 year is approximately 100. The expressive language skills are also developing. During the end of the first year until about the 18th month, the number of words an infant says can be used to assess the expressive language ability.

Sleep

The nighttime sleeping stretch has increased to 10 to 12 hours by age 9 months. The total sleeping time has decreased since the 6-month visit and will continue to decrease slowly as the first birthday approaches. If problems exist with nighttime awakening, review with the parent the techniques (see the section on the 6-month visit) to decrease the number of nighttime awakenings. Some infants may begin to awaken at night even though they used to sleep through the night. The infant's interest in the new motor skills or worry from separation anxiety may result in an increased number of awakenings at night. Reassure the parents that this is normal behavior. The use of repeated soothing techniques may help the parents in dealing with the changing sleep patterns. The goal is to encourage the infant to self-quiet or self-comfort and to go to sleep without help from the parents. The consistent use of a transitional object, such as a blanket or stuffed animal, may aid the infant in learning self-comforting measures. These objects can be used for bedtime or when the infant is exposed to new situations. The action of repeated soothing of the infant during the night is to help lessen fear or anxiety in the infant.

Stimulation

Parental interaction with the infant promotes development in all areas. Encourage the parents to play social games with the infant such as peek-a-boo or pat-a-cake. Encourage the parents to provide a safe area for the infant to explore and experiment. Age-appropriate toys, such as a mirror, rattles, or objects of various textures or colors, should be available to the infant. A cupboard in the kitchen with objects safe for the infant may serve as entertainment. Include such objects as plastic cups, bowls, or lids. Encourage the parent to continue talking or singing to the infant while feeding, dressing, or bathing. This aids in language development and encourages the baby to vocalize more. Reading to the infant not only promotes language growth but can also be used as a settling-down technique before sleep.

Safety

The world continues to open up to the mobile infant. As with the 6-month visit, many of the safety issues remain the same as for the previous visits. The advice to parents now needs to be expanded, however. Encourage the parent to get down on the floor and look for possible safely hazards at the infant's level. Also have the parents check for things at the eye level of the infant. This is the time when the infant can reach and pull things down (see the section on the 6-month visit).

Dental Issues

Tooth eruption typically has occurred by the 9-month visit. The primary teeth eruption follows a typical pattern (see Chapter 5). For the discomfort of teething, suggest the infant be offered a cold, wet washcloth or a chilled pacifier on which to chew. Recommend to the parents that they begin cleaning the infant's teeth with a soft toothbrush after the teeth have emerged. Toothpaste is not needed at this age. As with the previous visits, discourage the practice of propping the bottle when feeding or at bedtime. Assess the need for fluoride supplementation, which depends on the age of the child and the fluoride content of the drinking water. Review Table 19–18 in the 6-month old dental section to check when fluoride is needed and the amount recommended.

Nutrition

Many of the earlier interactions between the caregiver and the infant centered around eating. Control over the amount and type of foods the infant eats can become a problem in later months. Finger or table foods are appropriate at this age. Instruct the parents to allow the infant to feed himself or herself, giving the infant an opportunity to practice spoon- or finger-to-mouth coordination, promoting fine motor development. Finely chopped foods can be used. Remind the parents to avoid foods that may cause aspiration or choking (see Table 19–19). Instruct the parents to continue to breast-feed or to use iron-fortified formula for the remainder of the first year. Recommend waiting to begin whole cow's milk until after the first birthday. Remind parents about not overfeeding, to observe for the infant's cues when he or she is satiated, and to not use food for comforting the infant. Instruct the parent to introduce the cup, offering the infant small amounts of water or juice, not more than 4 to 6 oz a day so as not to replace the calories received from milk. Introduction of the cup will aid in weaning from the bottle over the next few months.

Discipline and Parenting

Over the following months, infants become more mobile and more curious about their environment. Setting limits and discipline is needed for infants at this age for their safety. Discipline needs to be simple and consistent. Encourage the parents to make the rules simple and few. It will then be easier for the parent to consistently carry out the rules. Often at this age, a simple stern "no" followed by distraction or physical removal is all that is needed (see the section on the 6-month visit for strategies). Remind the parents of the infant's desire and need to explore the environment and encourage the parents to structure their home such that little discipline is needed. Importantly, remind the parents that the infant continues to need nurturing. Hugging and cuddling remain a very important part of infant care.

Do not forget to ask what the primary caregiver is doing to nurture himself or herself. Ask about the time the caregiver is taking to reduce stress. Also ask if the primary caregiver and the partner have had a chance to get away, even briefly, without the infant. If the answer is no, encourage them to do so.

Review illness care. Ask what the parents should do if they suspect the infant is ill or has a fever. As with the previous visits, briefly review illness care during an upper respiratory infection or viral gastroenteritis. Instructions regarding fever treatment and doses of commonly used over-the-counter medications, such as acetaminophen and ibuprofen, may prove helpful to parents and save them a phone call or visit to the office. Review emergency room parameters. If the parent notices the following symptoms, the infant should be evaluated in the emergency room:

- Unusual irritability or lethargy
- Copious vomiting and diarrhea that may result in dehydration
- Signs of dehydration such as poor oral intake along with reduced urine output, sunken fontanels, and no tearing

Remind the parents that when other family members are ill, good handwashing can help prevent spreading of the illness to the infant. Encourage the parents to review illness and emergency care with the childcare provider if the infant is in daycare or in the care of others besides the parents.

TEST YOUR KNOWLEDGE OF CHAPTER 19

1. What are the components of a well-child visit?
2. Why is anticipatory guidance an important component of a well-child visit?
3. How should the examination of an infant be approached?
4. What are the developmental milestones of 2-month, 4-month, 6-month, and 9-month-old infants?
5. How does emotional development occur in infants?
6. How does cognitive development occur in infants?
7. What is the immunization schedule for infants?

8. What are the areas of anticipatory guidance necessary for the parent of an infant?
9. What is the progression of sleep pattern from a 2-month-old infant to a 9-month-old infant?
10. What safety tips should be stressed to the parents of infants?
11. What dental-care instructions should be given to the parents of infants?
12. How do nutrition requirements change as infants age?
13. What type of discipline should the parent of infants engage in?
14. What hints about illness care should be given to the parents of infants?

 BIBLIOGRAPHY

American Academy of Pediatrics, Committee on Environmental Health. (1998). Screening for elevated blood lead levels. *Pediatrics 101*(6), 1072–1078.

American Academy of Pediatrics, Committee on Injury and Poison Prevention. (2001). Injuries associated with infant walkers. *Pediatrics, 108*(3), 790–792.

American Academy of Pediatrics, Task Force on Infant Sleep Position and Sudden Infant Death Syndrome. (2000). Changing concepts of sudden infant death syndrome: Implications for infant sleeping environment and sleep position. *Pediatrics, 105*(3), 650–656.

Behrman, R. E., Kliegman, R. M., & Jenson, H. B. (Eds). (2000). *Nelson textbook of pediatrics*. Philadelphia: W. B. Saunders.

Dixon, S. D.. & Stein, J. T. (2001). *Encounters with children*. St. Louis: Mosby.

Green, M. (2000). *Bright futures. National Center of Education in Maternal and Child Health*. Arlington, Virginia.

Hall, R. T., & Carroll, R. E. (2000). Infant feeding. *Pediatrics in Review, 21*, 191–199.

Johnson, C. P., & Blasco, P. A. (1997). Infant growth and development. *Pediatrics in Review, 18*(7), 224–242.

Mills, M. D. (1999). The eye in childhood. *American Family Physician, 60*(3), 907–916.

Sanchez, O. M., & Childers, N. K. (2001). Anticipatory guidance in infant oral health: Rationale and recommendations. *American Family Physician, 61*(1), 115–120.

Zitelli, B. J., & Davis, H. D. (1997). *Atlas of pediatric physical diagnosis*. St. Louis: Mosby.

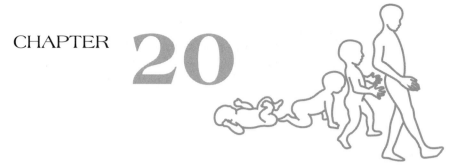

Toddlers

Ages 12 to 24 Months

GILLIAN TUFTS AND
JOANNE HAEFFELE

> **OBJECTIVES**
> - *Ascertain the developmental achievements of toddlers.*
> - *Develop an approach for physical examination appropriate for toddlers.*
> - *Develop physical examination skills used with toddlers.*
> - *Ascertain appropriate anticipatory guidance for parents of toddlers.*

Within the first year of life, children adapt remarkably to both their internal and external environments. The toddler period begins at age 12 months and continues to age 3 years, often beginning with the child's first steps. Typically by the end of the first year, children are able to sit, crawl, and cruise and are walking, or soon will be. A 12-month-old infant can remember and recognize family members. There is an attempt to socialize, communicate with purpose, and express themselves with specific emotional responses.

The family is still the center of the toddler's world as he or she acquires language, improves cognitive ability, expands physical coordination and skills, and achieves control over bladder and bowel function. All of these factors lead to self-awareness, familiarity with the environment, and a beginning concept of problem solving.

Toddlers appear proud, standing somewhat bowlegged, feet slightly apart, with their characteristic protruding belly. A complete assessment, including history, physical, testing, and anticipatory guidance, should be performed at each well-child visit (Table 20–1).

TABLE 20–1. PERIODICITY OF THE WELL-CHILD EXAMINATION FOR TODDLERS

Activity	Age, Months			
	12	15	18	24
Interval history	X	X	X	X
Measurements				
Height and weight	X	X	X	X
Head circumference	X	X	X	X
Sensory screening				
Vision	X	X	X	X
Hearing	X	X	X	X
Developmental/behavioral screening	X	X	X	X
Procedures				
Immunizations	X	X	X	
High-risk				
Hct or Hb	If risk factors are present			
Lead screening	If risk factors are present			
TB skin test	X			
Anticipatory guidance				
Growth and development	X	X	X	X
Safety	X	X	X	X
Dental	X	X	X	X
Nutrition	X	X	X	X
Sleep	X	X	X	X
Parenting	X	X	X	X

 # HISTORY

If this is the first time the child has been seen in the clinic, obtain information about the birth, prenatal period, and labor and delivery. Also, complete a medical history and surgical history, along with a list of medications (prescribed, over-the-counter, herbal) the child is taking, allergies (food, drugs, environment), and immunization status. If this child has been seen previously, begin the visit with the interval history. Check if there have been any illnesses, accidents, or emergency room visits since the last well-child visit.

Obtain a review of systems on all toddlers including head, eyes, ears, nose, and throat (HEENT); respiratory, cardiovascular, gastrointestinal, genitourinary, musculoskeletal, and neurologic systems; and the skin. The review of systems can be done while performing the examination to increase time efficiency. Ask about teething, the number of teeth present, and if there were any problems. Review the toddler's eating and sleeping patterns. Ask about the types of foods the child is now eating. Ask about milk intake, type (formula or cow's milk), and amount. Check to determine whether the transition from the bottle to the cup has been made or at least started.

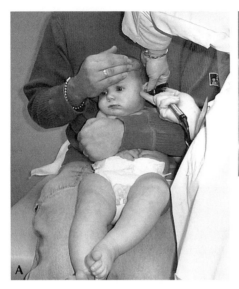
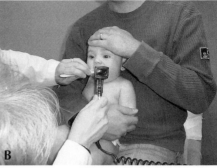

FIG. 20–1. (A) and (B) Restrain the child by holding the hands and head immobile.

Ask the parents if there have been any significant changes in the family situation. Ask about what method of birth control is being used or if another child is desired. Check if the child is in day care, and if so, ask the parents about their perception of how the child is coping. Ask about the use of a car seat and determine whether the seat is appropriate for the age and weight of the child. Throughout the toddler period, the child should be in a car seat when riding in the car.

🎾 APPROACH

You should approach the examination of toddlers in a calm, patient, and cheerful manner. Toddlers are most comfortable exploring the examination room while the healthcare provider is obtaining the health history from the parents. The physical examination should begin on the parent's lap, where the toddler will feel most secure and comfortable. The child can then be moved to the examination table with the parent helping to position the child. Allow the child to touch or play with the examining tools, such as the stethoscope, tongue blade, or otoscope.

Begin the physical examination with the least intrusive part of the examination, such as listening to the heart, lungs, or abdomen. Performing the examination first on the parent or the child's stuffed toy may help put the toddler at ease. Be sure to praise the child for cooperative behavior.

To improve cooperation during the examination, you can ask the toddler to help perform the examination. For example, before you begin the abdominal examination, you can ask the toddler to push on his or her abdomen, and then you can place your hands on top of the child's abdomen. At times, restraint is necessary. Have the parent assist by holding the child (Fig. 20–1) so the examination can quickly be completed.

TEMPERAMENT

During the latter half of the second year, toddlers may begin to exert their will. Ask the parent about the child's temperament. The temperament is how the child reacts to situations in general. Typically, words such as "easygoing," "difficult," or "slow to warm up" are used. Temperament becomes an issue when a toddler's temperament differs from that of the environment or family situation. Children who are difficult, described as highly active, are more irritable, or have irregular daily routines are vulnerable to developing behavior problems. Approximately 10% of children are considered "difficult." Also at risk are children who are slow to warm up, react negatively to new situations, react with moderate intensity, or may have somewhat irregular daily routines. These children also tend to be quieter. A total of 15% of children comprise the slow-to-warm-up group. Identifying these children early and helping parents develop strategies for dealing with the child may provide lifelong benefits. Ask the parents if they have any questions or concerns, and ask them how they deal with periods of frustration, assessing for the potential for abuse.

EGO DEVELOPMENT

Toddlers' ego development bipolar crisis is autonomy versus shame and doubt, according to Erikson. The positive developmental achievements of toddlers are autonomy and independent locomotion. Toddlers are always on the go, reaching for objects, and encountering barriers along the way. Toddlers begin to develop self-control and willpower. Parents must meet needs of toilet training, allow safe independence, and learn how to handle temper tantrums appropriately.

Usually at age 12 months, toddlers first begin to exert willpower. Challenges occur when toddlers struggle for autonomy and parents are not ready to let go and permit independence. Further resistance may occur when toddlers attempt self-feeding and refuse to go to bed without a struggle. Parents need to develop judgment and confidence to prioritize and set limits. Having patience while enjoying the toddler's independence may help to provide a stable environment.

COGNITIVE DEVELOPMENT

Until the age of 2 years, the child remains in the sensorimotor phase of cognitive development, according to Piaget. During the sensorimotor phase, the child learns about his or her world through watching, touching, and listening. Toward the end of the second year, the child begins the preoperational phase. During this time, generally between ages 18 and 24 months, the transition from the sensorimotor to preoperational phase occurs. Symbolic thought begins, and language and symbols are used in the thought processes. Memory and imitation are used in play. Object permanence is well established by this time. During the later months of the second year, toddlers are able to find an object that was hidden without watching the caregiver hide it.

As the child approaches the second birthday, he or she begins to move into the preoperational phase of cognitive development. This phase lasts until age 7 years. The thought process in the preoperational stage is concrete and tangible. The reasoning of a child in this stage is limited to the observable. These children are not yet able to generalize or make deductions. This is a time of egocentrism. Children in this stage of cognitive development see things in terms of how objects and events relate to them personally. This may appear as selfishness or self-centeredness, but actually, the child is not able to see someone else's point of view. The child's reasoning capability has not yet matured. The understanding of cause and effect is advancing. The child begins to think ahead about the effect that certain actions may have. By age 24 months, basic problem solving has begun and continues to be explored through trial and error during play.

DEVELOPMENTAL MILESTONES

Begin the assessment of the development milestones as you enter the examination room (Table 20–2). Some young toddlers may still be wary of strangers. It may be best to initiate interaction gradually. However, some children may remain wary, and much of the assessment of the gross and fine motor milestones, language, and social development must be obtained from parents rather than from direct observation.

Assess the toddler's social and emotional development. Be aware of how the parents and child interact throughout the entire visit. Does the child turn to the parents for reassurance? If not, concern should be raised. Ask the parents how they spend their time with the child. How do they play? Do they talk or sing to the child? Do they read to the child? What toys are being used? How do they comfort the child?

GROWTH AND DEVELOPMENT

The overall rate of growth slows during the second year. Usually by the child's first birthday, his or her weight has tripled. By the second birthday, the weight is generally four times that of the birth weight. Between ages 1 and 3 years, the toddler gains approximately 8 oz/month.

The height by the first birthday has increased by nearly 50% of the birth length. The toddler's length on average will increase by just less than 1 cm/month. The increase in length generally occurs in spurts rather than in a slow, steady pattern. It is not uncommon for the weight or height to remain the same for weeks before another growth spurt occurs. The height does not double until the child is 3 to 4 years of age.

The head circumference gains also slow during the second year. Head circumference by 1 year is nearly one third larger than the birth circumference. From ages 2 to 12 years, the head circumference changes very little, increasing by only approximately 1 inch/year.

The changes in growth and development are reviewed next, divided by age at examination: 12, 15, 18, and 24 months. The developmental skills can

TABLE 20–2. DEVELOPMENTAL MILESTONES BY AGE FOR TODDLERS

Age, Months	Social	Fine Motor	Gross Motor	Language
12	Plays ball; imitates activities Drinks from a cup	Waves "bye-bye" Puts block in cup Fine pincer grasp	Stands, cruises, and takes a few steps	Says two or three words Says "mama" or "dada" Follows simple commands
15	Helps in house Removes garments Uses spoon or fork	Scribbles Dumps raisin-sized objects Builds tower of two cubes Messy self-feeding	Walks well Stoops and recovers Walks backwards and sideways Climbs, bounces to music	Uses three to six words Naming Points
18	Little impulse control Temper tantrums start Feeds doll Undresses self Brushes teeth with help	Builds tower of four cubes Hand dominance Imitates vertical line Feeds self	Walks up steps holding on Runs Kicks ball forward	Uses six to 20 words Verbalizes wants Knows three body parts Receptive language developing Understands and follows commands Points to two pictures
24	Washes and dries hands Puts on clothing Protodeclarative behavior	Builds tower of six cubes Turns pages in book Imitates circle and horizontal line	Jumps up Throws ball overhand Walks up and down stairs with two feet per step	Combines words Names a picture Points to four pictures Knows six body parts 25% to 50% of speech understandable

be assessed through observing the child during the visit. Give the child a chance to get onto the floor to observe his or her gait. Offer the child an object to pick up to observe the fine motor skills. During the examination, the child can be asked to point out various body parts.

12-MONTH-OLD CHILD

At age 12 months, children are highly social and interested in exploring their environment. Their motor skills allow them locomotion, and their cognitive skills determine likes and dislikes. Difficulties arise as parents realize they are no longer completely in control, and the toddler does not always respond to the word "no."

Young toddlers should be able to stand and cruise, and begin to take a few steps alone. Most children are walking around their first birthday. The normal range for a child's first steps is 9 to 15 months. This is an exciting and important milestone for many families. The toddler's stance and walk are broad based, with the knees and hips flexed. The foot is placed flat-footed rather than the heel strike that develops during the third year of life. As the child matures, the walk becomes smoother and more narrowly based, with the arm and hand movements of the mature gait. At this age, the arms are held bent out from the body and move very little. The fully mature adult gait is seen at approximately age 5 years.

Fine motor skills continue to become more precise. Fine pincer grasp is present. The child can now grasp a small object between the thumb and fingertips. Accuracy of release of an object also has grown. The child can already or soon will be able to place a small object into a bottle. He or she may be able to build a tower of two blocks. The toddler should be able to wave "bye-bye."

Vocabulary at this age typically includes one to three words. "Mama" and "dada," which were previously said randomly, are now said with meaning. The child can follow simple commands, such as "give me the ball," with gestures. Over the next few months, these children are in the naming period of language development. They now realize that people and objects have names or labels. Jargoning, which is verbalization with normal speechlike intonation and rhythm but without using "real" words, occurs during the next months. The child will soon recognize and understand that his or her name means him or her. The child also understands the meaning of "no." A red flag for language development at this age is a lack of babbling or no response to music. Further evaluation is warranted if these language milestones have not been noted.

Social interactions are now becoming intentional. Typically, the concept of self has developed by this age, and these children have the capability to and are learning to form relationships with those around them. Because these children have learned that they are separate from their environment, sharing and empathy are beginning. Self-comforting measures can now be used, such as attachment to a special blanket or stuffed animal. Play at this age is usually solitary.

15-MONTH-OLD CHILDREN

At age 15 months, children are usually walking well independently. They are able to stoop and recover. They may be able to walk sideways and backwards now. Some toddlers may be able to run, but the run at this age is stiff legged. Climbing on the furniture is a newly found skill. Bouncing to music may be noted. The fine motor control continues to become more accomplished. The toddler can now place a small object into a bottle, may be able to stack a tower of three blocks, or scribble. A 15-month-old enjoys self-feeding with a spoon or with the fingers, although this can be messy. Children who are noted to be consistently behind in gross or fine motor skills need close evaluation. Cerebral palsy or another neuromuscular disorder should be considered.

At age 15 months, toddlers have a vocabulary of three to six words and often know one or two body parts when asked. They often can name a familiar object, such as a bottle. However, many wants or needs may still be communicated through nonverbal means, such as pointing at the desired object. They are able to follow one-step commands without gesture. At this age, toddlers enjoy listening to stories. A red flag for language development is a lack of understanding of familiar words or simple commands. Lack of consonant use may indicate a mild hearing loss.

At this age, children reach out socially. They may kiss, touching with their lips, and hug their parents. These children use their parents as a safe base from which to leave to explore and then return when reassurance is needed. A red flag in social development is a toddler who does not turn to his or her parent for reassurance but instead turns to a stranger. These children who do not have a secure attachment to their parents may show later behavioral problems.

18-MONTH-OLD CHILDREN

At age 18 months, children can walk upstairs, usually holding the rail or a parent's hand. These children can walk faster at this age, with little falling. At age 18 months, toddlers can seat themselves in a small chair. They are able to throw a ball and push or pull a large object. They may be able to undress themselves. Although delighted with these accomplishments, they often behave negatively because of a low frustration threshold. Often their low frustration tolerance leads to a flare in temper, or the classic "temper tantrum."

Fine motor control continues to blossom. Refining of previous skills such as grasping or the manipulation of objects occurs. Toddlers can now stack a tower of four blocks, dump an object from a bottle, imitate a vertical line, and scribble spontaneously. Scribbling is done by grasping the crayon with the entire hand. By age 3 years, hand control has developed so that drawing is accomplished by holding the crayon with the thumb and finger. At this age, children can feed themselves with a spoon and cup. Hand dominance appears around age 18 months. Before this point, children generally use both hands equally. Dominance that appears before this age may indicate weakness of the opposite arm or hand.

Most children of this age group can verbalize two or three things that they want and can speak more than 20 words. Toddlers can identify three body parts by pointing to them and can point to themselves. At this age, toddlers can typically name common objects shown on a card. Children's receptive language skills are further developed than expressive skills. These children can understand and follow two-step commands. They may spend short periods of time looking at books.

These children may now initiate social interaction with an adult by calling to them. They can now pucker their lips to give a kiss. Their play may include caring for or hugging a doll. An 18-month-old child's actions may be confusing to parents and to providers. One minute the toddler demands to do things for himself or herself, and the next minute the child is clinging to the parents. These toddlers are learning about their identity and who they are. The desire for autonomy and independence begins to emerge. During the first year of life, the emotional goal for the infant was attachment to the parents. During the toddler period, however—and possibly for the rest of childhood—independence is desired. At age 18 months, children are aware of what they want and that they have control over the choices that they desire. At this age, however, children are not capable of putting off gratification or expressing their frustration when they cannot have what they want. Anger and aggression may follow. The temper tantrum is the ultimate sign of this struggle. A temper tantrum may include crying, hitting, or having the child throw himself or herself to the ground. There is little impulse control at this age.

24-MONTH-OLD CHILDREN

By age 2 years, the stiff, wide-based gait of the young toddler has progressed to a more fluid, even gait, becoming more like the gait of an adult. These children can walk alone up and down the stairs with two feet per step. At age 2 years, toddlers can run well with little falling and are able to kick large balls. By age 2.5 years, children are able to jump in place.

The ability to stack a tower of cubes has now increased to allow stacking of six or seven blocks. These children may be able to make or imitate a circle or horizontal line. By this age, toddlers' language development is well established, and they can use two- to three-word phrases, such as "thank you" or "daddy up." They have a vocabulary of more than 50 different words. A 2-year-old child's sentences may now include a subject, verb, and object. A total of 25% to 50% of toddlers' speech is intelligible by age 24 months. Jargoning speech is no longer present. These children can point to six body parts. Listening to stories or sitting and looking through books is an enjoyable activity for these toddlers. They now have the capability of turning the pages singly. They are beginning to distinguish "you" from "me" and are able to use these pronouns. If the speech contains repeated, rote phases over and over that the child has heard, awareness should be raised. This is

TABLE 20–3. ANEMIA SCREENING: RISK FACTORS FOR ANEMIA

- Birth weight < 1500 g
- Low-iron formula fed during infancy
- Poor intake of iron-rich foods
- Whole milk started before age 6 months
- Low socioeconomic status

echolalia, and further evaluation is needed. Echolalia can be associated with autism.

At around age 2 years, children begin to involve an adult in their observations. This is referred to as "protodeclarative behavior," in which the child points to an object he or she considers interesting enough to share with an adult. This is a social activity. Earlier, the child may have only pointed to an object as a means of expressing that the object was wanted. Children with autism are able to point to objects they desire, such as food or drinks, but they rarely point to something they find interesting to share with another. This is a hallmark of autism, a lack of social ability. Play at this age remains parallel. The play of 2-year-old children engages simple imaginary play. By age 2 years, children have moved into the preoperational phase of cognitive development. These toddlers are learning to express ideas and solve problems through the use of symbols rather than direct motor manipulation or touching of an object as they have before.

SCREENING

ANEMIA

Anemia is defined as having a hematocrit level lower than normal for the child's age. Clinically, anemia means not having enough oxygen-carrying capacity in the blood. Screening for anemia is important when risk factors (Table 20–3) are present. It is acceptable to order either hemoglobin or hematocrit level, depending on the availability of the test within the office setting.

Toddlers with anemia are often iron deficient and present with pallor. On physical examination, they are often tachycardic with loud systolic murmurs. The usual cause is milk intake greater than 24 oz/d. The remainder of the physical examination is often normal.

LEAD

Lead screening should be assessed for populations at risk. Toddlers usually develop lead poisoning by ingesting a lead-containing substance. Older homes have been found to commonly use lead-based paint. Toddlers may ingest the lead if the paint flakes or peels, or they may inhale it as small dust particles. Important history questions to determine risk are as follows:

- Does the child live in a home built before 1978 (APA recommendations)?
- Is there evidence of pica?

TABLE 20–4. SYMPTOMS OF LEAD POISONING

GASTROINTESTINAL
- Vomiting
  ABDOMINAL PAIN
- Constipation
- Anorexia
  CENTRAL NERVOUS SYSTEM
- Lethargy
- Irritability
- Lack of attention span
- Projectile vomiting
- Failure to progress developmentally
  PERIPHERAL NEUROPATHY
- Hypoesthesias
- Paresthesias

- Does a sibling or close playmate have evidence of lead exposure?
- Is either parent working in an industry with exposure to lead?

Toddlers with lead poisoning may have few or no overt symptoms. Common symptoms are summarized in Table 20–4. Whole blood lead level is the desired screening test to best determine the child's risk for lead poisoning.

DENTAL ISSUES

Assessment of a toddler's dental health is important for recognition of problems as well as preventive issues. Current recommendations by the American Academy of Pediatric Dentistry are that all toddlers be examined within 6 months of the eruption of their first primary teeth. For most toddlers, this puts their first visit around age 1 year. All 20 primary teeth will have erupted by age 3 years. The goal is to screen all children for dental caries and initiate primary prevention. Toddlers who receive primary prevention may delay their first visit to age 2 years, when the child is more manageable. The American Academy of Pediatrics (APA) recommends the first dental visit be scheduled when the child reaches age 3. Dental abnormalities found on clinical examination include:

- Delayed eruption of teeth
- Spacing between the maxillary central incisors
- Malpositioning or rotation of an incisor
- Bulging of the alveolar ridge

VISION

Vision screening for toddlers is easily done through history questions and a modified physical examination. Ask the parents if they have observed their toddler pick up small objects and if the child can focus on and follow an

TABLE 20-5. VISION SCREENING

- Pupillary size, shape, and reaction to light
- Ability to follow the light
- Position of light reflection on the cornea
- Extraocular movements
- Strabismus; use cover/uncover test

object. Toddlers should be able to reach for small objects. If there is a family history of congenital cataracts or strabismus, an evaluation at age 12 months is indicated. A modified physical examination should be performed, in which all of the points listed in Table 20–5 are assessed. Documentation of normal results indicates appropriate assessment for this age group.

IMMUNIZATIONS

The immunizations indicated at the 12-month visit are listed in Table 20–6. Immunizations should not be delayed for mild illness, low-grade fever, or respiratory illness. If the last DtaP (diphtheria, tetanus, and acellular pertussis) vaccine was given less than 6 months before the 12-month well-child visit, it can be given at the 15-month visit. The varicella vaccine can be given at age 12 to 18 months. Inactivated poliovirus (IPV) vaccine can be given between ages 6 and 18 months. Thus, the IPV could be given before the 12-month visit to reduce the number of shots being given. Although the third hepatitis B vaccine should have been given at the 6-month well-child visit, always check to make sure it has been given. Check *www.cdc.gov* for updates on vaccination recommendations by state.

PHYSICAL EXAMINATION

The physical examination should be complete and include appropriate measurements from the periodicity table. A developmental assessment should also be performed, focusing on gross and fine motor control, language, and emotional and social growth. Height and weight measurements

TABLE 20-6. IMMUNIZATIONS FOR 12-MONTH-OLD TODDLERS

- DtaP #4
- HIB #4
- IPV #3 (can be given between ages 6 and 18 months)
- Prevnar #4
- MMR #1
- Varicella vaccine #1 (can be given between ages 12 and 18 months)

DtaP = diphtheria, tetanus, and acellular pertussis vaccine; HIB = *Haemophilus influenzae* type b; IPV = inactivated poliovirus vaccine; MMR = measles, mumps, and rubella.

should be plotted on a standard graph, noting normal progression. Share the information with the parents during the visit.

During the entire examination, observe the interaction between the parents and child. Look for interest and responsiveness through smiling facial expressions and vocalizations. Parents should respond with comfort to the toddler's calls of distress. Encourage parents to speak positively to their toddler. The healthcare provider can set an example by complimenting the child's behavior, growth, or development during the examination. Remember to include a compliment for parents. Comments made to parents during the visit on the well-being of their child and the good job that parents is doing can go a long way.

A head-to-toe examination is then performed. Specific areas that need examination and documentation are included in Table 20–7. Begin the examination with the child on the parent's lap. While reviewing the history with the parent, allow the infant to touch and play with the otoscope or stethoscope. This may help ease the toddler into the examination portion of the visit.

HEAD

Palpate for the presence or absence of the anterior fontanel. The anterior fontanel generally closes between ages 12 and 18 months. Inspect the hair for the presence of seborrhea or nits. Palpate the neck for adenopathy and thyromegaly.

EYES

Check the red reflex and the symmetry of the light reflex, a screen for strabismus. In older toddlers, the cover/uncover test can be performed. This test requires that the child be capable of longer fixation.

EARS

Check the external ears for placement and lesions. Perform an otoscope examination, noting the condition of the canals and tympanic membranes.

NOSE

Observe the nares for symmetry and drainage. Unilateral nasal drainage usually indicates a foreign body in the nasal canal. If the child is cooperative, an internal nasal examination may be done. If there is no suspicion of abnormality, defer this portion of the examination.

MOUTH

Note which teeth are present and the condition of the teeth. Visualize all the structures of the oropharynx to check for erythema and edema.

TABLE 20–7. PHYSICAL EXAMINATIONS FOR TODDLERS

Age, Months	12	15	18	24
Complete physical examination	X	X	X	X
Head				
Fontanels	X	X	X	X
Scalp	X	X	X	X
Neck	X	X	X	X
Eyes				
Red reflex	X	X	X	X
Strabismus	X	X	X	X
Ears	X	X	X	X
Nose and mouth				
Tooth eruption	X	X	X	X
Dental injuries	X	X	X	X
Tooth decay	X	X	X	X
Cardiac				
Murmurs, pulses, capillary refill	X	X	X	X
Abdomen	X	X	X	X
Genitalia	X	X	X	X
Musculoskeletal				
Upper extremities	X	X	X	X
Joints, muscles, strength	X	X	X	X
Hips*	X			
Lower extremities				
Varus, valgus, tibial torsion	X	X	X	X
Gait	X	X	X	X
Intoeing or out-toeing, stance	X	X	X	X
Feet	X	X	X	X
Neurologic				
DTRs	X	X	X	X
Cranial nerves	X	X	X	X
Babinski's reflex	X	X	X	X
Integument				
Birthmarks	X	X	X	X
Nevi				
Café-au-lait spots	X	X	X	X
Developmental milestones	X	X	X	X
Evidence of abuse or neglect	X	X	X	X

*When child is walking, can discontinue hip examination.
DTR = deep tendon reflex.

LUNGS

Auscultate the lungs for abnormal lung sounds (see Chapter 7). Monitor the respiratory rate and rhythm.

CARDIOVASCULAR

Auscultate the heart for abnormal heart sounds (see Chapter 8). If placement or size of the heart is in question, perform a scratch test. Palpate all pulses and check capillary refill.

ABDOMEN

Move the child to the examination table. Some toddlers may object strongly, and the remainder of the examination will need to be completed on the parent's lap. To examine the abdomen, lay the infant across the parent's and your laps. Auscultate all four quadrants for bowel sounds. Palpate the abdomen for masses or hernias.

GENITALIA

Boys

Palpate the scrotum for the presence of both testicles in the boys.

Girls

Observe the perineum and external genitalia. Gently spread the labia and observe the vaginal vault.

MUSCULOSKELETAL

Observe the symmetry of movement of the upper and lower extremities. Assess flexibility of the hands and feet. Observe the anterior and posterior thigh folds, and check for uneven knee levels, looking for developmental dysplasia of the hip that may have been missed earlier. When the child has started to walk, the Ortolani and Barlow maneuvers are no longer present. Parents may ask whether the child has flat feet or not, a common finding at this age. The arch of the foot may not be present until 3 to 4 years and appears flat at this age because of the presence of a fat pad.

Place the child on the floor and observe gait. While observing the toddler's gait, you can reassure and educate the parents. During the first months of walking, the child will have a wide-based stance. Out-toeing (i.e., walking with the toes pointed outward) is common during the first months of walking. After the gait is well established, intoeing (i.e., walking with the toes pointed inward) becomes a more common phenomenon. Thirty degrees or less intoeing or out-toeing is considered normal in the toddler age group. Transient toe walking is also considered normal. If toe walking persists, pathology should be considered. A stance that is mildly bowlegged is normal in 1- to 2-year-old children.

NEUROLOGIC

Assess the cranial nerves during the head examination. Attempt to elicit deep tendon reflexes. This is often difficult because the child must be relaxed to elicit the reflexes. Check for the disappearance of the Babinski reflex around age 18 months.

SKIN

Check the skin, noting any rashes, birthmarks, lesions, or signs of abuse.

ANTICIPATORY GUIDANCE

Anticipatory guidance is composed of age-specific guidelines for the promotion of healthy habits. Anticipatory guidance also can provide parents with ideas for stimulating and promoting motor control and social and language development. These guidelines should be discussed at the end of the visit and supplemented with written information for reinforcement. The areas covered should include growth and development, safety, dental issues, nutrition, and discipline and parenting.

12-MONTH-OLD CHILD

Growth and Development

At ages 12 to 14 months, and in some cases up to age 17 months, children have generally tripled their birth weight. The yearly weight gain for toddlers is on average 6 to 7 lb or 3 kg. The height of the toddler will increase by 2 to 3 inches over the next year. It is common for parents to notice a slowing in the toddler's appetite. Reviewing the slow-down in growth with parents is often the only reassurance that is needed.

Reassure parents that the range for taking the first steps is 9 to 15 months. If a child has not begun walking by the 12-month well visit, he or she most likely will be by the following visit. Because the child will become more mobile and curious over the coming months, remind the parents that the toddler must always be supervised.

The fine motor control continues to improve. Encourage parents to allow the toddler to feed himself or herself, either finger foods or with a spoon. Some parents have trouble with this because of the mess the toddler can produce. Remind parents that self-feeding not only promotes fine motor development (the pincer grasp) but also provides the child with an autonomous activity, which children of this age enjoy and need. Encourage parents to provide colorful toys that are stackable or toys that can be placed inside one another.

The vocabulary at this age typically includes one to three words. "Mama" and "dada" have now taken on meaning. Encourage parents to read, sing, and talk to their toddler on a regular basis. By doing so, language development and understanding are promoted. Reading books can be a close, enjoyable time for a toddler and parent. Encourage hand games such as peek-a-boo, patty-cake, and so-big. Teach the toddler to wave "bye-bye" if he or she is not doing so already.

Safety

Before the next well-child visit at age 15 months, the child will continue to become increasingly more mobile. If the child is not walking at this visit, he or she most likely will do so by the next examination. Encourage parents to get down on the floor and observe potential hazards at the child's height.

TABLE 20–8. SAFETY CHECKLIST FOR 12-MONTH-OLD CHILDREN

- Electrical outlets should be covered with guards.
- Keep all electrical cords out of the toddler's reach.
- Keep any container that is heavy or contains hot liquid away from the edges of shelves or tables, where the toddler could reach and pull it down.
- Keep the handles of pots toward the back of the stove.
- Place all poisonous or potentially harmful chemicals out of the reach of the toddler.
- Use a weight-appropriate car seat that is placed in the center of the back seat. When the child reaches 20 lb, the seat may face forward.
- Check the temperature of the water from the hot water faucet. It should be lower than 120°F.
- Never leave a toddler alone near a pool of water or in a bathtub.
- Avoid exposure to tobacco smoke.
- Remind parents about the use of sunscreen, SPF 15 or higher, when the child is playing outside.

They should be reminded to check for potential hazards within the child's reach. If there are stairs in the home, ask if a gate has been put up to block the child from climbing on them unattended. A child usually is not able to use the stairs without help until approximately age 2 years. Table 20–8 provides a list of other safety concerns about which to remind parents.

Dental Issues

Encourage parents to establish a daily routine for care of the child's teeth (Table 20–9). They should begin brushing the toddler's teeth daily using a soft child toothbrush. Toothpaste is not needed at this age. Remind parents not to put the toddler to bed with a bottle. The usual recommendation is to change from the bottle to the cup at age 12 months. Review the consequences of bottle mouth caries. If the child is still using a bottle at night or naptime, discuss strategies parents can use to gradually stop the use of the bottle. Such strategies include gradually switching from milk to water or substituting a transitional object (e.g., a new stuffed toy or blanket) for the bottle.

Recommend that parents give the toddler supplemental fluoride. The amount of fluoride given is based on the level of fluoride in the local drinking water and the child's age. Supplemental fluoride is effective for the prevention of dental caries. Review Table 20–9 to check when fluoride is needed and the amount recommended.

Thumb sucking is common during the toddler years. Conflicting theories exist explaining thumb sucking and the recommendation for discouraging the habit. More than 50% of all children have had the thumb sucking habit at some point. Often it is used as a comfort measure, and most toddlers do not suffer negative effects to their dentition. Thumb sucking can result in protrusion of the maxillary incisors and an anterior open bite, but there is controversy over what the long-term effect may be. The long-term prognosis may depend on whether the child has an acceptable occlusion. Trying to

TABLE 20–9. FLUORIDE SUPPLEMENTATION RECOMMENDATIONS: AMOUNT OF FLUORIDE SUPPLEMENTATION BASED ON FLUORIDE CONCENTRATION OF THE WATER SUPPLY

Age of Child	Fluoride < 0.3 ppm	Fluoride 0.3–0.6 ppm	Fluoride > 0.6 ppm
Birth to 6 months	0	0	0
6 months–3 years	0.25 mg	0	0
3–6 years	0.5 mg	0.25 mg	0
6–16 years	1 mg	0.5 mg	0

reduce the habit is impractical because of the immaturity of the toddler. Most children will stop the habit alone by age 4 years. The prognosis for long-term dental effects seems to worsen in those who continue the habit after age 6 years.

Nutrition

The growth of children during the second year has slowed compared with the growth during the first year of life. Along with the reduced growth rate, the appetite has also lessened. Parents may have noticed this and may appreciate reassurance that this is normal. The typical weight gain during the second year is 6 to 8 oz/mo. Encourage parents to feed their toddler at regular mealtimes and include two to three nutritious snacks per day. Encourage self-feeding. Toddlers enjoy experimenting and learn to like foods by touching and tasting them repeatedly. Encourage parents to offer nutritious fruits and vegetables, which give toddlers the necessary nutrients. Avoid foods high in sugar. Avoid foods small in size that may cause choking or aspiration. Foods to avoid include peanuts, popcorn, hot dogs, grapes, carrots, celery, raisins, corn, beans, candy, raw vegetables, and meat. Portion size for this age group is 1 teaspoon of each food per year of age. The recommended daily allowance for children between ages 1 and 3 years is 100 kcal/kg per day.

Encourage parents to make mealtimes into pleasant, social experiences. Encourage conversation during meals. Remind parents that the child may eat a small amount at one meal and then a large amount at the next. Let the child decide on the amount for each meal, but only have food available at certain times to avoid a snacking eating pattern. Remind parents that it may be difficult for children of this age to sit still long enough for a large meal.

If the mother is breast-feeding, discuss when weaning is desired. If the parents are bottle feeding, discuss changing from formula to whole milk and review the strategies for weaning from the bottle. The total amount of milk necessary daily is 16 to 24 oz. Greater than 24 oz of milk per day may cause anemia because of micro bleeding in the gut.

Discipline and Parenting

Encourage parents to praise their toddler for good behavior. Instruct parents to limit the number of rules to those that can be reasonably carried out and to consistently enforce them. To discipline a toddler, use restraint, distraction, or removal of the toddler from the trigger. Encourage parents to learn what situations may cause conflict and to avoid those situations, if possible. Discipline is used as a means of protecting the toddler and teaching basic behavior lessons. Discipline the toddler for aggressive behaviors such as hitting or biting. A very short time-out is acceptable at this age.

Allow the toddler to play alone as well as with playmates. At this age, play is generally done in parallel with other children—the children are playing side by side but not together. The young toddler relies more on motor skills for play, rather than imaginative play, as seen in older toddlers.

Encourage good sleep hygiene. Ensure that the parents establish a bedtime and regular routine before bed. This helps toddlers prepare for sleep. Toddlers should sleep in their own bed.

15-MONTH-OLD CHILD

At age 15 months, children are very mobile. They require constant attention from their caregivers. Although they have mastered such motor skills as walking, there is little internal guidance and control. With the toddler's increased mobility and curiosity, safety is of concern. They lack a sense of danger. For parents, this can be a difficult time, learning to allow the child more freedom to explore their world while maintaining safety.

Growth and Development

As with 12-month-old children, the height and weight gain is much less when compared with the first year of life. Along with this is a slow-down in the appetite. The typical annual weight gain is 6 to 7 lb. The typical gain in height is under 0.5 inches/month.

At this age, toddlers are generally walking well, are able to stoop to pick up an object, and can climb stairs while holding a hand or rail. Encourage parents to still take caution with stairs. By the toddler's next visit, the child should be able to push and pull large toys or be able to throw a ball. Encourage parents to have such toys available, if possible, and to spend some time playing with the child. Also encourage parents to provide space and time for the child to play freely but safely. With the onset of walking, parents may ask about shoes. It is best to recommend soft, supportive shoes, not rigid ones, to promote flexibility and permit movement. For children at this age, shoes are used more for protection of the foot than development of the arch, which occurs at a later time.

Children use their fine motor skills in play at this age. Encourage parents to provide toys that can be manipulated, such as stackable toys or toys that can be placed inside one another. A cupboard in the kitchen with plastic ware or pots and pans can provide the child with objects to manipulate and play with at little cost. Provide the child with a place for scribbling. Continue to encourage parents to allow their toddler to feed himself or herself with finger foods or with a spoon. Remind parents that self-feeding promotes fine

TABLE 20–10. SAFETY REMINDERS AT THE 15-, 18-, AND 24-MONTH WELL-CHILD EXAMINATIONS

- Use a weight-appropriate car seat that is placed in the center of the back seat. When the child reaches 20 lb, the seat may face forward.
- Check the bath water temperature and never leave the children unattended around water, whether it is the bath or the swimming pool.
- Keep all electrical cords and drapery cords out of the toddler's reach.
- Maintain a smoke-free environment.
- Place pots at back of stove and keep the handles of pots pointed toward back of stove.
- Keep all cleaning chemicals and medications up and out of reach of the toddler. Have the number for the poison control center near the telephone.
- Lower the toddler's crib mattress to the lowest rung because some children may climb out of the crib.
- Keep small objects, plastic bags, and balloons away from the toddler.
- Begin to teach the toddler caution when approaching a dog or cat.
- Continue to have gates at either end of the stairs.
- Keep the toddler away from lawn mowers, garage doors, and other moving machinery; streets; and driveways.
- Maintain enclosed outdoor play area.
- Use sunscreen that is at least SPF 15 to protect the skin from the sun.
- Choose caregivers carefully. Select one with a similar discipline philosophy.

motor development and provides the child with an autonomous activity, which is important to children at this age.

The vocabulary at this age typically includes one to three words. Encourage parents to read, sing, and talk to their toddler on a regular basis. By doing so, language development and understanding are stimulated. Reading books can be a close, enjoyable time for a toddler and parent. At this age, toddlers are able to turn the pages of book singly. Encourage parents to have age-appropriate books available for the toddler. Also encourage hand games such as peek-a-boo or patty-cake or making a game of naming the body parts.

Safety

This is an important issue for toddlers who have increased mobility but have not yet developed the judgment to recognize unsafe situations (Table 20–10). More highly active and mobile toddlers need additional monitoring. Recommend having dangerous objects or chemicals out of sight and reach rather than trying to teach the young toddler not to touch or handle them. Remind parents that the toddler can now walk, climb, reach, and grab for things. Keep dangling cords, chemicals, medicines, cigarettes, lighters, pots, curling irons, and other such objects out of reach. Also, remind parents briefly of some of the issues from previous visits, such as water safety; smoking in the household; and keeping small, mouthable objects out of reach. Encourage parents to consider the philosophy of their child's day-care provider, including his or her views on nutrition, play, and discipline.

TABLE 20–11. FOODS TO AVOID IN THE YOUNG TODDLER

- Peanuts
- Popcorn
- Hot dogs
- Carrot sticks
- Whole grapes
- Raisins
- Hard candy
- Large pieces of raw fruit or tough meat

Dental Issues

Instruct parents to clean the toddler's teeth once daily using a soft tooth-brush. Parents should be primarily responsible for brushing, but the toddler should help. Toothpaste is not necessary at this age. Instruct parents to con-tinue giving supplemental fluoride if the water supply is lacking fluoride. To prevent caries, remind parents not to put the toddler to bed with a bottle. Avoid frequent snacks or foods high in sugar. Recommend the first dental visit if this has not already been done.

Nutrition

Nutrition continues to be important for adequate growth and development, and mealtimes remain an important social time for the family. Encourage parents to include the toddler at the table, with a booster seat or high chair. Encourage conversation. Remind parents that although letting the toddler feed himself or herself can be messy, this is an opportunity to promote autonomy and manual dexterity. Review the child's diet and offer advice on the importance of basic food groups and avoiding commercially prepared, high-sugar foods. Continue to avoid foods that could lodge in the respirato-ry tract and cause choking. These are summarized in Table 20–11.

If the child is breast-feeding, discuss plans for weaning when the mother and the child are ready. If the child is still bottle feeding, discuss weaning from the bottle to the cup. This is an especially important issue if the bottle is being using at night. Discourage parents from using food for emotional comfort or reward.

Discipline and Parenting

Encourage parents to praise their toddler for good behavior and accom-plishments. Encourage the use of discipline rather than punishment as a means of teaching acceptable behavior. Continue the use of distraction, redi-rection, gentle restraint on a parent's lap, or removal from the item or situa-tion rather than corporal punishment. "Time-out" (i.e., separation of the child from the problem), whether it is an object or situation, is a popular means of discipline. This is a type of redirection and removal from the issue at hand, and it may be done on the parent's lap or by removing the toddler from the area of concern, such as to another room. One rule of thumb is to recommend 1 minute of time-out per year of age.

Between the ages of 15 and 18 months, the emotions of shame and guilt are developing. Encourage the use of discipline, focusing on the behavior of the child rather than on the child himself or herself (i.e., the behavior is bad, not the child). This approach helps to maintain a more positive self-image and, thus, promotes healthy self-esteem.

Continue to promote good sleep hygiene. Ask parents about their bedtime routine. Recommend a regular bedtime. Encourage parents to set routine activities before the child goes to bed. The toddler will learn to expect these activities as a signal for bedtime. Such activities may include bathing, reading, praying, or gentle playing. Suggest also including teeth brushing.

18-MONTH-OLD CHILD

Eighteen-month-old children can cause confusion for parents. At this age, toddlers can be happy and easygoing one minute and on the floor in a crying heap the next. The independent, exploring child can become clingy and fussy when challenged by an uncomfortable situation. At this age, children have a combination of a need for exerting will and a desire for closeness to the parents. Parents need extra patience during this time. Anticipatory guidance and education about what is normal behavior for this age group may provide parents with the reassurance they need.

Growth and Development

The rate of growth is much the same as for the previous two visits at 12 and 15 months. The child will gain approximately 3 lb before the next birthday. The height is increasing by about 0.5 inch/month. The growth may continue in an irregular pattern, in which periods of growth are interspersed with periods of little to no growth.

The gross motor capabilities continue to advance. Toddlers continue to need monitoring with walking up and down stairs. The continued use of gates may still be necessary. The child may now be running. Remind parents that constant supervision is needed. Children of this age enjoy throwing or rolling a ball and pulling a toy along the ground. Encourage parents to allow the child a safe place for play. Sand or water play with various tools, such as spoons, plastic cups and bowls, or funnels can be very enjoyable activities for 18-month-old children.

Fine motor control is promoted by having available blocks or other objects for stacking, sorting, and manipulating. Filling and dumping out toys aid in the development of coordination. Items such as plastic bottles or small cans, along with buttons, bottle caps, or wooden spools, can be used for sorting. The toddler may enjoy scribbling with a large crayon or pencil but should be supervised because the toddler does not yet have the sense of where and where not to use the crayon.

Between 18 and 24 months, when the next well-child visit is scheduled, the child's language will bloom. The toddler will begin to use pronouns as he or she approaches the second birthday. The vocabulary will swell to 50 or more words used in two- to three-word phrases. Let parents know that the toddler has a receptive vocabulary of 10 times the toddler's expressive vocabulary. This may help encourage parents to talk with their child more. Encourage parents to not only talk with their toddler but also read or sing as a means of stimulating language development. Teach the child simple songs such as "Row Your Boat" or "Ring Around the Rosy." The availability of books for the child is important. Encourage parents to start using the local library. Parents may note stuttering at this age. This problem is self-limited and not of any consequence.

The progression of sensorimotor to symbolic thought will occur during the months before the second birthday. Imaginative play emerges. The child will use one object to represent another during play, such as a block or cup being driven as a car. Feeding a doll with a make-believe bottle is common. In play, the child may imitate activities he or she observes taking place in the home, such as washing dishes, ironing, or performing yard work. Encourage parents to allow their child a place and time for play, where the child can safely play and spend time experimenting with little monitoring.

At this age, children have begun the state of development called "problem solving." With proper stimulation, these toddlers can rapidly advance intellectually. At this age, children solve problems through trial and error and need the time and space to practice their newly found skills. Encourage parents not to "interfere" with the trial-and-error process. Children need to explore problem solving on their own. Although parents of toddlers of this age group often get their children together in a social situation, the children are unlikely to share and often play side by side rather than in an interactive manner.

Safety

The issues of safety for 18-month-old toddlers are similar to those of 12- and 15-month old children. Remind parents that although the child appears to be maturing and rapidly acquiring new motor capabilities, the child's judgment, when it comes to safety, is lacking. Children ages 18 to 24 months need constant supervision. Parents need to be vigilant in their inspection of the child's play area, both inside and outside the home, to maintain safety. The car seat should continue to be used; water safety should continue to be monitored; and all objects such as chemicals, medications, lighters, alcohol, and firearms must be kept out of the reach of the toddler. Continue to keep plastic plugs in electrical sockets. Keeping a smoke-free environment is important for overall health. Instruct parents that 18- to 24-month-old children should never be left alone at home or in a car. If the child is riding on a bicycle, encourage the use of a bike helmet. Also encourage parents to use a helmet themselves. Ask parents about the day-care situation, if applicable.

Encourage parents to review eating and sleeping habits and the philosophy of discipline with the day-care provider.

Dental Issues

Instruct parents to clean the toddler's teeth once daily using a soft toothbrush. Parents should be primarily responsible for the brushing, but the toddler should help. Toothpaste is not necessary at this age. Instruct parents to continue giving supplemental fluoride if the water supply is lacking fluoride. Remind parents not to put the toddler to bed with a bottle to prevent caries. Avoid frequent snacks or foods high in sugar.

Nutrition

Nutrition is important for adequate growth and development, and meals are an important social time for the family. Encourage parents to include the toddler at the table, with a booster seat or high chair. Encourage pleasant conversation during mealtimes. Review diet and offer advice on the importance of basic food groups and avoiding commercially prepared, high-sugar foods. Recommend three meals a day with nutritious snacks in between. Continue to avoid foods that could lodge in the respiratory tract and cause choking. Avoid such foods as peanuts, popcorn, hot dog pieces, large pieces of raw vegetables or fruit, tough meat, and hard candy until the child has reached roughly 24 months of age. Instruct parents to continue the use of whole milk until the child reaches age 2 years; about 16 oz/day is recommended at this age.

Encourage parents not to allow mealtime to become a time for power struggles. Remind parents of the irregularity in the amount that the toddler may eat at each meal and that food jags, in which one food is desired over others, are common at this age. Instruct parents to look at the entire day or the 2-day food intake for a balanced intake and that not every meal needs to be balanced. Encourage parents to keep mealtimes and snack times as times for eating so that the child learns to eat only at those times. Discourage the use of food for comfort or reward.

Discipline and Parenting

There are many issues for 18-month-old children. This is the time to review the subjects of temper tantrums, toilet training, and rapprochement with parents. Parenting an 18- to 24-month-old child can be trying. The visits with the healthcare provider may be some of the few times parents get to express their frustrations and concerns. Take the time to listen to, educate, and support parents. It is important to identify situations in which parents may need more advice or support or situations in which there may be potential for abuse, either physical or emotional. Parents who have been abused themselves, with temperaments different from the child's, or with a rigid personality with little tolerance for conflict may need more guidance and support.

TABLE 20–12. TEMPER TANTRUMS: STRATEGIES AND RED FLAGS

STRATEGIES
- Focus on the behavior, not the child
- Pick the more important battles; don't expect 100% compliance from the child
- Removal, distraction, or redirection of the child's attention
- Use time-outs
- Verbalize what the child may be feeling
- Hold the child
- Learn what triggers a tantrum and avoid the situation
- If avoidance is not possible, develop strategies to circumvent the trigger

RED FLAGS
- Parents who have been abused themselves
- Differing temperament between the child and the parent
- A parent with a rigid personality who expresses little tolerance for conflict

More frequent visits for this type of family may be beneficial; more than one visit should be conducted every 6 to 12 months. Outside referral for the family or parent may be considered. Table 20–12 summarizes the actions parents can take when a temper tantrum occurs and red flags of which you should be aware.

For parents, the behavior of 18-month-old children can be demanding and confusing. These children may be cooperative and easygoing one minute and crying and stomping their feet the next. Temper tantrums may be mild to excessive. Remind parents that temper tantrums stem from acute frustration experienced by the toddler. Toddlers are learning that they cannot always have desired objects or that they must delay gratification. At times, the tantrum may occur in a public place, such as the grocery store or a large family gathering. A toddler may be experiencing sensory overload because there is too much visual, auditory, or tactile stimulation to handle. Tantrums may also occur at busy times of the day, such as while getting ready to leave in the morning or while a parent is preparing dinner.

Ask parents to be aware of the timing of the tantrums to possibly anticipate and prevent the situations from occurring. If the situation is unavoidable, consider distractions or other activities for the toddler. For example, perhaps the other parent or another sibling can help entertain or divert the toddler's attention. Ask parents what they do when a tantrum occurs. Provide advice for parents who are unsure of how to handle the child. First remind parents to focus on the behavior, not the child (i.e., the behavior is bad, not the child). Recommendations include removal, distraction, or redirection of the child's attention. Encourage the use of time-outs, which may provide the child and the parent time to regroup. Have parents verbalize what the child may be feeling, such as: "You're really mad" or "It's really bad when you can't have something that you want." If the child seems unable to calm himself or herself, have parents remove the child from the situation and hold the child. Bodily contact is important for toddlers who are feeling out of control. Temper tantrums are considered normal.

TABLE 20–13. TOILETING READINESS: CUES, STRATEGIES, AND HINTS

READINESS CUES

- Ability to undress self
- Shows interest in the toilet or in parents or sibling using the toilet
- Imitates toileting behaviors
- Aware of having a wet diaper or a diaper with a bowel movement present
- Increasing periods of dryness during the day or at night

STRATEGIES

- Use lots of positive reinforcement for use of the potty
- Do not use punishment or negatively reprimand for toilet training
- Toilet training may take weeks to months
- If the child does not seem ready yet, restart training at a later date

HINTS

- Stress may cause setbacks in training
- Boys may start later and take longer

Toileting issues may come up at this 18-month visit, or parents may have questions for the following months. At this age, children may begin to express interest in toileting. Generally, children are not toilet trained until the middle of the third year, around age 2.5 years. In some children, it may occur soon after their second birthday; for others, especially for many boys, it may not occur until after age 3 years. At this visit, however, the provider can review the signs of toilet training readiness (Table 20–13), but remind parents not to expect this event to occur until after the second birthday and, for many, closer to the third birthday. The process of toilet training for most families takes a few months. Encourage parents not to apply pressure or react negatively to toileting. There are several physical and neurologic processes that must be in place before the toddler is capable of this multistaged task. First, the child must have the neurologic development to have control over the anal and urethral sphincters. Next, the child must be able to sit still long enough to urinate or to have a bowel movement. Lastly, the child must have an understanding of the steps it takes to perform the task of toileting. This issue should also be readdressed at the next well-child visit.

Although parents may be uncomfortable to mention it, they may have noticed that the toddler touches his or her genitals. Review with parents that this is normal exploring behavior and encourage parents to focus on when the behavior is acceptable and when it is not. For example, if the behavior occurs at the grocery store, the parent could say, "It is not appropriate to touch yourself when we are here."

"Rapprochement" is not a term that parents may know or use, but they may have noticed or will notice the behavior. Between the ages of 18 and 24 months, the toddler may go through a transient period of increased clinging and need for parents. Parents may state that they cannot go anywhere without the child. This seeming regression in emotional and social behavior is normal. It is as if the child takes a step backward to take two or three steps forward in a few weeks to months. The child is reacting to the possibility of separation from parents, something that was seen during the latter half of

TABLE 20–14. DISCIPLINE FOR 18- TO 24-MONTH-OLD CHILDREN

- Daily praise for the toddler's activities or accomplishments
- Use time-outs, redirection, distraction, or removal
- Provide consistent limits
- Have rules, but not too many
- Have rules that are fair and age appropriate
- Offer the toddler choices—only two

the first year. Bedtime separation may again become an issue. Transitional objects may be helpful, such as a special blanket or stuffed animal. Having parents behave consistently with love and support so the child learns that they will always return may aid in decreasing fears.

Other issues of discipline and general approach are summarized in Table 20–14. These issues can be reviewed with parents as an overall approach to dealing with the difficult, challenging, and ever-changing 18- to 24-month-old child. Encourage parents to be consistent in their approach. Remind parents that 100% compliance from toddlers is not a reasonable expectation. Encourage parents to talk about their feelings and philosophies with each other so the approach is consistent between parents.

24-MONTH-OLD CHILD

At age 2 years, children continue to be a challenge for the family. These children have an increased verbal capability and are able to express, both positively and negatively, their wishes, needs, and opinions. The negative behavior starts to decrease at this time; however, the child still has an equal amount of good and bad days. You can aid parents significantly in pointing out that much of the toddler's behavior is normal. Remind parents that it is the job of 2-year-old children to explore, experiment, and test their environment and boundaries. Reassurance is what many parents need. Some parents may need more advice in dealing with some situations or issues, and a few families, who are having greater difficulty, may need outside referral or resources.

Growth and Development

The toddler's weight and height gain may slow even a little more over this next year. The toddler may only gain 5 lb or so before his or her next well-child visit at age 3 years. By approximately age 2.5 years, the weight of the child is 4 times the birthweight. The height may increase by only approximately 2 inches (or 5 cm) annually over the next several years. Typically, between the ages of 2 and 2.5 years, the child will reach 50% of his or her adult height. The head circumference increases only about 1 inches/year from this visit to approximately age 12 years. The body shape of the toddler will also change over the coming year. The body stance has less lordosis and protuberance of the abdomen. The legs, which may be bowed, will straighten out. The overall percent of body fat decreases, and toddlers emerge as leaner, more muscular preschoolers by their third birthday.

Two-year-old children can run well, jump, climb, and can walk up and down the stairs without help, although they still walk on steps with both feet per step. These children enjoy practicing these skills and continue to learn others. By their next birthday, toddlers will be able to walk up and down stairs with one foot per stair and walk on their toes, and they should be able to pedal a bicycle and hop on one foot. Encourage parents to play with the child outside, such as during trips to the park, to promote further gross motor skill development. As with 18-month-old infants, safety remains an issue. These children's judgment in identifying unsafe practices has not formed as well as their motor skills, so parents must be on their guard to prevent injury. Toddlers should not be left alone.

Fine motor development refinement continues. At age 2 years, the stack of cubes has grown to eight. These children may be able to draw a circle and construct a train consisting of several cubes. Encourage parents to allow the child the time and place for play. Children's dexterity will continue to grow as they have time to experiment and manipulate objects. Having toys such as blocks, stackable cups, or rings provides the child with the tools to experiment. Two-year-old children may enjoy doing simple puzzles. By age 3 years, children may be able to draw a stick figure, and their control has increased in ability so that they can stack a tower of 10 blocks or higher and draw a circle. By age 3 years, children are able to undress themselves and dress with help.

The language capability explodes during the next year. By age 3 years, the vocabulary will increase to 500 words. Parents can assist the vocabulary of the child through having frequent conversations and by reading or telling stories to the child daily. Encourage parents to point out things during the daily routine and talk to the toddler about them. By age 3 years, toddlers can tell stories about recent events. Approximately 75% of what the toddler says is understandable to a stranger. These children are able to say their full name and identify their gender. Bilingual children may appear behind and may mix the two languages.

Parents can foster the child's language skills through reading and communicating with the child. Parents may note stuttering at this age, which is self-limited and not of any consequence. This is an indication that the mind is working faster than the tongue. Encourage parents not to call attention to the stuttering. If stuttering continues beyond age 4 years, concern is warranted.

If delayed speech is noted at this age, suspect neglect, hearing loss, or mental retardation. Further investigation and screening are needed. The red flags of speech delay are often subtle. Many times, the assessment must come from parents because the child may be too shy or uncomfortable to speak at the office visit. If parents describe their toddler as capable of speaking well for his or her age but lacking the ability to understand simple instructions, using only a few words, or communicating largely through gestures, further evaluation should be done. Rather than waiting a year for the next well-child visit, have that child return within 2 to 3 months for evaluation of progress.

Over the next year, children's social skills grow considerably. Children are able to show concern for others, to play cooperatively with other children in small groups, and to develop friendships. Imaginative play blossoms over the next year. For 2-year-old children, pretend play may include copying events of the day. As children mature, play may become more complex to include scenarios that are outside the home. A child who is 2 or 3 years old may be ready for simple chores to do around the house. Give toddlers easy tasks to perform such as setting or clearing tables and picking up toys.

Safety

Safety continues to be of concern (see Table 20–10). The issues for this age group are similar to those of 15- and 18-month-old children. Remind parents that although the child appears to be maturing and rapidly acquiring new motor capabilities, good judgment, when it comes to safety, is lacking. At age 24 months, children need constant supervision. Parents need to be vigilant in their inspection of the child's play area, both inside and outside the home, to maintain safety. Young siblings cannot supervise the child. The car seat should continue to be used; water safety should continue to be monitored; and all objects such as chemicals, medications, lighters, alcohol, and firearms need to be kept out of the reach of the toddler. Have the poison control center number next to the phone. Keeping a smoke-free environment is important for overall health. Instruct parents that 24-month-old children should never be left alone at home or in the car. If the child is riding a bicycle, encourage the use of a bike helmet. Also encourage parents to use helmets themselves. Ask parents about the day-care situation, if applicable. Parents should review eating and sleeping habits and the philosophy of discipline with the day-care provider.

Dental Issues

By age 3 years, all 20 primary teeth should have erupted. Instruct parents to clean the toddler's teeth once daily using a soft toothbrush. Parents should continue to have the primary responsibility for brushing the teeth but should have the toddler's help. Toothpaste is now used. Instruct parents to use only a pea-sized amount each day. Parents should continue to give supplemental fluoride if the water supply is lacking fluoride. Ask about continued bottle use. If this is still present, develop strategies to stop the use of bottles. Remind parents to avoid frequent snacks or foods high in sugar to promote good nutritional habits and to reduce the likelihood of dental caries. Children should have dental examinations every 6 months.

Nutrition

Nutrition and a healthy diet are important for adequate growth and development. Eating is also an important social time for the family. Encourage parents to include the toddler at the table, with a booster seat or high chair. Encourage pleasant conversation during mealtimes. Review diet and offer advice on the importance of basic food groups and avoiding commercially prepared, high-sugar foods. Recommend three meals a day with nutritious snacks in between meals. Instruct parents to begin using low-fat milk, such as 2% milk, and dairy products.

Encourage parents to avoid mealtime power struggles. Remind parents of the irregularity in the amount that the toddler may eat at each meal and that food jags, in which one food is desired over others, are common at this age. However, parents should remain in control of what food is served, not the toddler. Remind parents that the growth has slowed and that their toddler's appetite may seem less than before. Reassure parents that this is normal. If parents express concern about the amount or type of foods eaten, remind them to consider the entire day or 2-day food intake rather than each meal alone. A balanced diet may be eaten over a period of 1 to 2 days in a 2-year-old. Encourage parents to keep mealtime and snack time as times for eating so that the child learns to eat only at those times. Discourage the use of food for comfort or reward.

Discipline and Parenting

Parenting 24-month-old children is trying. Autonomy and control remain important issues for children at this age. Review with parents the subjects of temper tantrums and toilet training. The visits with you may be some of the few times parents get to express their frustrations and concerns. Take the time to listen to, educate, and support parents.

Ask parents about their discipline techniques. Review discipline strategies with parents, and if there are discipline conflicts, encourage the parents to talk about ways they can work out a unified strategy. Toddlers will pick up differences in parental approach very soon. Remind parents to use distraction, removal, or time-outs for unacceptable behavior. The recommended rule for time-out is 1 minute of time-out per year of age. Time-outs can be done on the parent's lap or in a specific chair or location in the home. Encourage parents to avoid telling toddlers they are bad; rather, it is their behavior that is undesirable. Remind parents that impulse control is in the process of developing. By age 3 years, toddlers have mastered some degree of internal self-control, which is often shown by the toddler's ability to delay gratification.

Review toilet training. Go over the toilet readiness signs. Remind parents that current events can set back a child who appears ready or has started using the potty. Such events may include the introduction of a new sibling, illness, prolonged absence of a parent, or a family vacation. Reassure parents that this is normal. Instruct parents to use lots of positive reinforcement for use of the potty but not to punish or negatively reprimand the child for eliminating in his or her underwear or diaper. The potty training process may take weeks to months. If a 2-year-old child does not seem ready, encourage parents to wait a few months and reassess the situation. Remind parents that boys may take longer and may not show interest or readiness until after their third birthday.

Encourage parents to maintain regular routines and good health habits. Parents need to be good role models because at this age, children are notorious for imitating behavior. Good behavior should be reinforced because attitudes and habits are beginning to develop. Bedtime should be consistent, and a regular routine should now be established. Bedtime can be preceded by a warm bath, dental care, story reading or storytelling, a gentle discussion of the day's events, prayers, hugs, and kisses. By adhering to this routine, the toddler knows what to expect and understands that it is bedtime. Review with parents the amount of television watched and whether it is at bedtime. Recommend not more than 1 hour of television per day and discourage the use of television just before bed. Also discourage the practice of falling asleep by the television because this practice produces poor sleep habits.

TEST YOUR KNOWLEDGE OF CHAPTER 20

1. What are the components of the history and review of systems for toddlers?
2. Describe the approach to the examination of toddlers.
3. Discuss the temperament of toddlers and strategies for the parent to use.
4. What are the expectations of ego and cognitive development of toddlers?
5. Describe the expected weight and height changes in 12-, 15-, 18-, and 24-month-old children.
6. What developmental milestones should 12-, 15-, 18-, and 24-month-old children exhibit?
7. What are the red flags in development of 12-, 15-, 18-, and 24-month-old children?
8. What screening should be done for 12-, 15-, 18-, and 24-month-old children?
9. When should a toddler receive his or her first dental check-up?
10. When is fluoride recommended for 12-, 15-, 18-, and 24-month-old children?
11. Discuss the immunizations toddlers should receive.
12. What changes in physical development are seen in 12-, 15-, 18-, and 24-month-old children?
13. What safety hints should be given to the parents of 12-, 15-, 18-, and 24-month-old children?
14. Discuss thumb sucking, toilet training, protodeclarative behavior, and rapprochement in 12-, 15-, 18-, and 24-month-old children.
15. Discuss nutrition issues seen in 12-, 15-, 18-, and 24-month-old children.

16. Discuss discipline and parenting concerns with 12-, 15-, 18-, and 24-month-old children.

17. What symptoms would lead you to do lead testing?

 ## BIBLIOGRAPHY

Algranati, P. S. (1998). Effect of developmental status on the approach to physical examination. *Pediatric Clinics of North America, 45,* 1–22.

American Academy of Pediatrics, Committee on Environmental Health. (1998). Screening for elevated blood lead levels. *Pediatrics, 101,* 1072–1078.

Colson, E. R., & Dworkin, P. H. (1997). Toddler development. *Pediatrics in Review, 18,* 255–259.

Dixon, S. D., & Stein, J. T. (2001). *Encounters with children.* St. Louis: Mosby.

Green, M. (2000). *Bright futures.* Arlington, VA: National Center of Education in Maternal and Child Health.

Johnson, C. P., & Blasco, P. A. (1997). Infant growth and development. *Pediatrics in Review, 18,* 224–242.

Mills, M. D. (1999). The eye in childhood. *American Family Physician, 60,* 907–916.

Nelson, W. E. (Ed.) (2000). *Textbook of pediatrics.* Philadelphia: W. B. Saunders.

Sanchez, O. M., & Childers, N. K. (2001). Anticipatory guidance in infant oral health: Rationale and recommendations. *American Family Physician, 61,* 115–120.

Zitelli, B. J., & Davis, H. D. (1997). *Atlas of pediatric physical diagnosis.* St. Louis: Mosby.

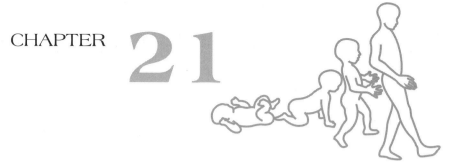

CHAPTER 21

Preschoolers

Ages 3 to 5 Years

MARGARET R. COLYAR

OBJECTIVES
- *Become familiar with the components of the examination of pre-school children.*
- *Develop physical examination skills used with preschool children.*
- *Ascertain appropriate anticipatory guidance for parents of preschool children.*

The preschool period is one of many developmental and cognitive changes. Preschoolers face many new situations and challenges. Well-child visits occur yearly during this period, with a continued emphasis on history, review of systems, physical examination, and anticipatory guidance. Common parental concerns for preschool children are poor appetite, night-mares, night terrors, enuresis, thumb sucking, aggressiveness, and sexual exploration.

PERIODICITY TABLE

The important components of the well-child visit for the preschool child are shown in Table 21–1. They include history, screening, physical examination, laboratory/diagnostic testing, immunizations and anticipatory guidance.

338

TABLE 21–1. PERIODICITY TABLE FOR PRESCHOOL WELL-CHILD VISITS

Areas of Examination	Age 3 Years	Age 4 Years	Age 5 Years
History	X	X	X
Measurements	X	X	X
Height	X	X	X
Weight	X	X	X
Head circumference			
Blood pressure	X	X	X
Sensory screening			
Vision	X	X	X
Hearing	X	X	X
Developmental/behavioral assessment	X	X	X
Cognitive	X	X	X
Ego	X	X	X
Physical examination	X	X	X
Hereditary or metabolic screening*			
Immunizations†			
Tuberculosis test‡			
Hematocrit or hemoglobin§			
Urinalysis§			
Lead level§			
Sickle cell screening¶			
Anticipatory guidance	X	X	X

*Perform by age 1 month.
†Refer to Centers for Disease Control and Prevention's guidelines.
‡Perform at least once during this time period.
§Perform at least once between ages 15 months and 5 years.
¶Only if appropriate.

HISTORY

Ask about the history of infections, diseases (common childhood diseases and others), accidents, hospitalizations, emergency room visits, and surgeries. Note any allergies to food, drugs, or the environment. Ask if the child is taking any medications (prescribed, over-the-counter, or herbal). Ask to see the immunization record, note the dates the immunizations were received, and note if any complications occurred.

Do a complete review of systems. Specific areas of interest are the head, eyes, ears, nose, and throat (HEENT); gastrointestinal (GI); neurologic; respiratory; cardiovascular; genitourinary; and musculoskeletal systems, and skin. Ask the parent specifically if the child has had ear infections, sore throat caused by group A beta-hemolytic streptococci, or changes in vision or hearing. For the GI system, ask about constipation, diarrhea, enuresis, and encopresis. For the neurologic system, ask about the occurrence of seizures (petit mal, grand mal, jacksonian), speech, and coordination problems. Asthma is the main problem with the respiratory system for this age group.

TABLE 21–2. NORMAL VITAL SIGNS FOR PRESCHOOL CHILD				
Age, Years	Temperature, °F	Heart Rate, bpm	Respiratory Rate, breaths/minute	Blood Pressure, systolic/diastolic
3–4	99.0	73–137	21–27	72/110–40/73
5	98.6	65–133	18–24	75/116–40/75

Note any episodes of syncope, shortness of breath, or stopping to rest. Ask about the occurrence of urinary tract infections. Determine whether the child has any bone or joint problems. Find out if the child has had any rashes or has developed eczema.

CURRENT HEALTH

Ask the parents if they have any concerns about the child. Determine what the child eats during a typical day. Note any nutritional supplements (e.g., vitamins, herbals, iron) provided to the child. Find out the last time the child visited a dentist, either for prevention or to fix a cavity. Determine whether the child has difficulty falling to sleep or is difficult to awaken in the morning. Ask how much sleep the child gets. Ask what time the child goes to bed and when he or she gets up. Note the need for extra nap times, and check the child's behavior patterns. This is a good time to determine whether the parent is using appropriate discipline. Ask about the use of day-care or preschool services.

SCREENING

HEIGHT, WEIGHT, AND HEAD CIRCUMFERENCE

Measure the child's height and weight. Head circumference is not measured in children of this age group because the fontanels are closed, and the skull has slowed in growth to approximately 1 inch/year. Check the percentiles on the growth chart to determine the child's growth pattern. Compare with previous growth measurements.

VITAL SIGNS

Measure the heart rate, respiratory rate, temperature, and blood pressure at each well-child visit. Normal ranges for vital signs for children ages 3 to 5 years are shown in Table 21–2.

HEMATOCRIT OR HEMOGLOBIN

Hematocrit or hemoglobin should be measured at least one time between ages 15 months and 5 years. The normal hematocrit values for 3- to 5-year-old children are 35% to 45%; hemoglobin is 11.5 to 14.5 g/dL.

LEAD SCREENING

Lead screening should be performed at each well-child visit. Lead levels should be checked only if they are indicated from the screening checklist or if the child has unexplained symptoms.

TUBERCULOSIS

A purified protein derivative (PPD) test should be checked at this age if tuberculosis is suspected.

URINALYSIS

A urinalysis should be performed one time between ages 15 months and 5 years.

DENTAL ISSUES

The first dental examination is recommended by the American Pediatric Association to be completed by age 3 years. Encourage parents to locate a dentist who is accomplished at pediatric dental examination.

VISION

Visual acuity should be checked using the Snellen pictorial chart. Make sure the child is oriented to the shapes, or a false result will be given. Perform the cover/uncover test to screen for strabismus.

HEARING

Perform a whisper test in the office. If you think a central or peripheral hearing deficit is occurring, check for conductive and sensorineural hearing loss by doing the Weber and Rinne tests (see Chapter 5). The most common causes of hearing problems in preschoolers are otitis media and cerumen impaction. Tympanometry and audiometry testing should also be done.

GROWTH AND DEVELOPMENT

Plot the child's gross motor, fine motor, language, and social and behavior development on the Denver Development II chart. Compare with previous results if available.

EGO DEVELOPMENT

Evaluate the child's ego development at each visit. Erikson's bipolar crisis of 3- to 5-year-old children is initiative versus guilt. Positive resolution is the development of a sense of purpose and direction. This can be developed by receiving praise, accomplishing small tasks, being allowed to make small decisions, and becoming more independent. Negative resolution is a sense of unworthiness.

COGNITIVE DEVELOPMENT: PREOPERATIONAL

Piaget noted that thinking in children of this age group is concrete and literal. At this age, children use symbols (words) to represent people, objects, and actions in the environment. They are developing the ability to represent the external world by means of arbitrary symbols that stand for objects. They tend to make inappropriate generalizations and attribute feelings to inanimate objects. For example, clouds "cry" when it rains. They are prone to magical thinking. Because they associate one event with a simultaneous event, they believe that thoughts are all-powerful. For example, if their pet cat scratches them and they wish the cat dead and then the cat is run over by a car, they believe their thoughts caused the death of the pet. Their inability to logically reason the cause and effect of illness or an injury makes it especially difficult for them to understand such events.

DEVELOPMENTAL MILESTONES

Growth and development are outlined on the Denver Developmental II testing tool, which includes fine motor, gross motor, language, and social and behavior development. Fine motor skills vary from 3-year-old to 5-year-old children. Three-year-old children can copy a circle and draw a person with two or three parts. Four-year-old children can copy a cross. By 5 years of age, children can copy a square and draw a person with six parts. Beginning at age 3 years, children should be able to pick the larger line of two lines that are side by side.

Gross motor skills also vary from age 3 to 5 years. Three-year-old children can hop and broad jump. They should be able to ride a tricycle, stand on one foot for 3 to 5 seconds, wash and dry their hands, and dress and undress with supervision. Four- and 5-year-old children can skip, walk on their heels and tiptoes, and use alternating feet when descending stairs.

Three- to 5-year-old children have a vocabulary of 1000 words or more. They are able to use well-formed sentences. Comprehension of speech should be at 90%. Stuttering and baby talk occur frequently in this age group.

Behaviorally, preschool children have a fear of disruption of bodily integrity. They understand social rules but cannot always initiate self-control; however, they are capable of feeling guilty about bad behavior. Preschoolers live in a rich imaginary world, and play is an important outlet for aggression. During this age, children are developing gender identity and self-esteem.

APPROACH

For 3-year-old children, position them on the parent's lap. Four- and 5-year-old children usually feel comfortable on the examination table by themselves. Be very slow, patient, and deliberate in approaching the child. Respect the child's privacy and modesty. Use short, simple explanations. Talk to the child and explain the steps of the examination.

Allow the child to make choices. Do *not* allow choices when there are none. For example, do not ask the child, "Can I look in your ears?" Ask instead, "Which ear do you want me to look in first?" The child will be an active participant in the examination. Gain cooperation by seeking the child's help. Allow the child to feel a sense of control by helping with the examination. Holding the stethoscope on the chest will provide the child with a sense of control and not disrupt the examination. Allow the child to play with equipment to decrease fears. Use games such as "blow out the light." Give feedback on what you find. Compliment the child on his or her cooperation.

PHYSICAL EXAMINATION

EYES

Assess visual acuity using the Snellen E or pictorial chart. Refer the child to an ophthalmologist if there is a two-line difference in visual acuity. Screen for strabismus by looking at the corneal light reflections, extraocular muscle tests, and cover/uncover test (see Chapter 6).

After the age of 5 years, the development of amblyopia is unlikely. Check for color vision in boys starting at age 4 years using the Ishihara color blindness test.

EARS

Perform an otoscope examination of the canals and tympanic membranes. By age 4 years, children can hear 1000 to 2000 at 20 dB. Conduct the whisper test. If hearing loss is suspected, perform the Weber and Rinne tests for conduction and sensorineural hearing loss. Tympanometry and audiometry testing also should be done.

NOSE

Look inside the nares for color and condition of the mucous membranes and turbinates, color of mucus, and presence of polyps. Do not forget to look for foreign bodies if unilateral nasal drainage is present.

ORAL

Check the number and condition of the teeth. Note the condition of the gums, mucous membranes, and tongue. Note the tonsils and posterior pharynx. Tonsils are often enlarged, and the epiglottis may be visible in children at this age.

NECK

Observe to determine if the child can complete full range of motion of the neck. Note the absence of torticollis, and palpate the thyroid.

CARDIOVASCULAR

Auscultate the heart for murmurs, clicks, rubs, and regularity. Check blood pressure, pulses, and capillary refill bilaterally.

ABDOMEN

Perform a basic abdominal examination. First auscultate for bowel sounds in all four quadrants. Then palpate for liver and spleen enlargement, rigidity of the abdomen, and tenderness and masses. Give children control by having them place their hand on top of yours. This position also helps if the child is ticklish.

MUSCULOSKELETAL

Observe the child as he or she walks and runs, checking for genu varum (bow-legged), genu valgum (knock-kneed), and abnormal gait. Check for strength and tone. This can be fun for the child. For upper extremity strength and tone, have the child hold your fingers. Then have the child push and pull. For lower extremity strength and tone, have the child push your hands away with his or her legs and pull them back to the examination table. Also instruct the child to dorsiflex and plantarflex the feet and toes.

GENITALIA

Always check for labial adhesions and undescended testes. The foreskin should be fully retractable at this time. Also check for signs of enuresis and encopresis. Enuresis may present as excoriated perineum. Encopresis may present as an irritated anus or evidence of stool staining on the external perineum.

NEUROLOGIC

Check the cranial nerves while doing the head and neck examination. Elicit the deep tendon reflexes (Fig. 21–1). Children often enjoy this part of the examination and may start to giggle. At this age, you may be able to assess proprioception (Romberg test). Explain and make a game of checking position sense, rapid alternating movements, and coordination. Assess memory by giving the child three words to remember and asking the child to repeat the words later in the examination.

FIG. 21–1. Deep tendon reflex testing on a 5-year-old boy.

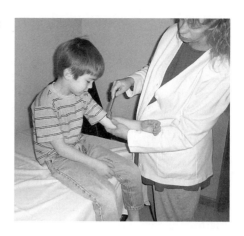

PSYCHOSOCIAL

Observe the child's interaction with the caregiver. Table 21–3 outlines findings the healthcare provider should be concerned about if detected.

ANTICIPATORY GUIDANCE

Anticipatory guidance for this age group includes growth and development, safety, dental issues, nutrition, and parenting and discipline.

GROWTH AND DEVELOPMENT

Sleep

At this age, children still sleep a good deal. Ten to 12 hours per night with naps is the norm. If not already started, advise the parents to develop bedtime rituals so the child knows that it is time for bed and rest. Preschoolers have many fears, and you should be aware of what they are. Advise parents to show the child that there is nothing to fear. Parents may leave a nightlight on if necessary.

TABLE 21–3. PSYCHOSOCIAL EXAMINATION: FINDINGS OF CONCERN IN PRESCHOOLERS

- Is timid, withdrawn, fearful
- Has trouble relating to or communicating with people
- Eating, sleeping, or toilet training difficulties
- Moody, irritable, oversensitive
- Too passive, aggressive, or impulsive
- Cannot complete tasks
- Has speech, language, or motor difficulties

Bedwetting (Enuresis)

Bedwetting is a big concern. Teach the parent that there are nonpathogenic (97%) and pathogenic (3%) causes for this condition. The four top nonpathogenic causes are that the child drinks too much before bedtime (evening polydipsia), is not able to wake up, has an inability to delay urination, and has a small bladder capacity with inability to delay urination. For a child who drinks too much, limit the intake of fluids to less than 2 oz 2 hours before bedtime. Small bladder capacity or the inability to delay urination is the problem if the child frequently urinates during the day and is wet every night or several times per night. The child's normal bladder capacity is the child's age plus 2 oz. Therefore, if the child is 4 years old, he or she has a bladder capacity of 6 oz (180 mL). Encourage the caregiver to teach bladder-stretching exercises during the day.

For a child who has trouble waking up, have the caregiver practice waking the child up. Have the child lie in bed with the eyes closed and pretend he or she needs to urinate. Then the child should get up and go to the bathroom. The other alternative is to wake the child 3 hours after going to sleep the first night, then 2.5 hours the second night, then 2 hours the third night, and so on. On the fifth night, tell the child to wake up himself or herself.

Always provide positive reinforcement when the child does not wet the bed. If the child is still bedwetting by age 8 years, consider a bedwetting alarm and medication (desmopressin).

SAFETY

At this age, children are more independent but still unable to make logical decisions. Drowning is the most prevalent accident in children at this age. Encourage the caregiver always to watch the child closely around water, including the bathtub. The use of water wings or a life jacket when the child is near or in a swimming pool or lake is imperative.

For preschool children, there is a greater incidence of burns from fires. Teach the child and parents fire safety. Teach children to always use helmets and kneepads when skateboarding, rollerblading, rollerskating, or biking.

Instruct parents to be aware of the location of the child when starting up the car. This age group is capable of opening the car door and trying to get out of a moving or stationary motor vehicle without the parent's knowledge. Childproof door locks are necessary. Teach the child never to talk to or get close to a car with a stranger. Continue the use of seat belts.

DENTAL ISSUES

Continue to use fluoride if it is not already added to the water supply. Brush twice daily using only a small amount of toothpaste. If this is not already done, the American Pediatric Association recommends the first dental visit by age 3 years.

TABLE 21–4. TIPS FOR SCHOOL READINESS

Parents should:
- Let the child know what his or her day's schedule at school will be like.
- Ask the child how he or she feels about starting school.
- Visit the school and meet the teacher.
- Meet a classmate.
- Point out positive aspects of starting school, including that it is a chance to have fun and make new friends.
- Let the child know that all children are nervous about the first day of school.
- Let the child know that if he or she encounters any problems, you will help to resolve them.
- Arrange for the child to walk to school or ride the bus with another child in the neighborhood.

NUTRITION

Look at nutrition from a weekly perspective, *not* a daily or per-meal perspective. Children of this age may get on food jags and only want to eat certain foods on a particular day. If the child has a balanced diet each week, he or she will have adequate nourishment. Do not force the child to eat. The child should get three meals per day plus nutritious snacks. Offer small portions. The rule of thumb is 1 tablespoon per year of age of each of three foods. Do not use food as a reward. Be aware of nutrition information the child is watching on television or getting through media exposure.

PARENTING AND DISCIPLINE

Preschoolers are generally people pleasers. Provide clear limits. Explain the consequences if they break the rules. Point out the feelings of others. Praise positive actions. Catch the child being good and give lots of positive verbal reinforcement.

Make the child responsible for his or her things; have the child hang up clothes, clean his or her room, and put away books and toys. Establish balance between the need for independence and the need for limits.

Ignore "mouthy" behavior and reward good behavior. Time-outs of 1 minute per year of age are appropriate.

GENERAL BEHAVIOR

Limit television viewing to 1 hour of nonviolent programming per day. Educational programs are best. Play educational board and card games with the child. Prepare the child for starting school. Starting school can be a difficult time for children. All children are hesitant to go somewhere new and see people they have never met before. Table 21–4 provides tips for school readiness.

SEX EDUCATION

Sexual curiosity is normal at this age. Answer questions factually and simply. Use correct terms for the genitalia. Redirect overt sexual play without shaming the child or creating anxiety.

 # BIBLIOGRAPHY

Algranati, P. S. (1992). *The pediatric patient*. Baltimore: Williams & Wilkins.

Muscari, M. E. (2001). *Advanced pediatric clinical assessment*. Philadelphia: Lippincott.

Siberry, G. K., & Iannone, R. (2000). *The Johns Hopkins Hospital. The Harriet Lane handbook*. St. Louis: Mosby.

Whaley, L. F., & Wong, D. L. (2000). *Essentials of pediatric nursing*. St. Louis: Mosby.

TEST YOUR KNOWLEDGE OF CHAPTER 21

1. What are the components of the well-child visit for preschool children?
2. What are the components of the history and review of systems for preschool children?
3. What current health practices should be assessed for preschool children?
4. What screening should be done with preschool children?
5. In what stage of ego development and cognitive development are preschool children?
6. What developmental milestones would you expect preschool children to exhibit?
7. Describe the approach to preschool children.
8. What physical assessment differences would you expect to find with preschool children?
9. How can the physical examination be made fun for preschool children?
10. What areas of anticipatory guidance should be discussed with parents of preschool children?
11. Discuss the nonpathogenic causes and treatments for enuresis.
12. What safety instructions should be given to the parents of preschool children?
13. Discuss the dental and nutrition guidance you should give to the parents of preschool children.
14. Discuss parenting concerns with preschool children.
15. What findings should alert you to psychosocial problems in preschool children?
16. What are some practical tips for school readiness?

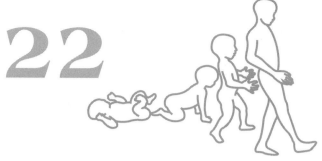

Assessment of School-Age Children

Geeta Maharaj

The school-age years (ages 6 to 12 years) mark the time when the child's world expands to include the school environment and the influence of peers and teachers. Children are now able to think more logically and can understand instructions and procedures. School-age children are generally more willing to cooperate in the physical examination than younger children unless there is a history of unpleasant visits and the child is fearful. Ask the child simple social questions to enhance rapport. Communication with the child gives insight into the child's personality and cognitive abilities. You will get more cooperation if the child's level of maturity is acknowledged and if the child is included as well as the parents. During the assessment, telling the child what you are going to do and why acknowledges his or her developing cognitive level and lets the child know that he or she is important. Six- to 8-year-old children may still have difficulty expressing themselves verbally, but they can usually draw a picture accurately depicting their families or what is wrong with them. Older school-age children (i.e., 10 to 12 years of age) should be offered the chance to talk to you without the

349

parents in the room. At this age, some children might find it easier to discuss their pubertal changes without the presence of their parents.

The child's modesty also must be considered when you assess him or her. Younger school-age children may be comfortable in underwear for the examination, but usually older children welcome wearing a gown and having to expose only the parts of the body being examined.

SCREENING

VITAL SIGNS

The vital signs of school-age children are gradually becoming closer to the normal adult values. The temperature can now be taken in the mouth because the child understands how to hold the thermometer. Average temperature ranges from 98°F to 98.6°F. Respiratory rate decreases between the ages of 6 and 12 years as the lung capacity increases and the amount of air exchanged with each breath increases. The normal respiratory rate for this age group should be between 16 and 25 breaths per minute. As the child grows, the heart is also growing, resulting in an increasing blood pressure. The average systolic pressure is 96 to 112 mm Hg, and the average diastolic pressure is 56 to 66 mm Hg. It is important to select an appropriately sized cuff for the child's size. A cuff that is too large may produce low readings, and one that is too small may produce high readings. Increasing heart size also results in a decreasing heart rate. Additionally, there are several factors that can influence heart rate, including medications, activity, fever, pain, and fear. Acutely, hemorrhage, respiratory distress, and increased intracranial pressure may affect the heart rate. The average heart rate for this age group is 70 to 80 beats per minute, with a resting rate of 60 to 76 beats per minute.

HEMOGLOBIN, HEMATOCRIT, AND CHOLESTEROL LEVELS

Hemoglobin or hematocrit levels should be measured every 2 years during the school-age years. Normal hematocrit levels should be between 33 and 47 million cells/mm^3, and hemoglobin should be between 11.5 and 15.5 gm/dL. African-American children generally have lower hemoglobin levels than those of white children. Children with a history of pica and those whose history reveals a poor diet should also be screened for iron deficiency. Cholesterol also should be measured at least once during the school-age years; levels should fall below 170 mg/dL.

LEAD POISONING

Children with a history of pica and those who live in urban areas with houses built before 1978 should be screened for lead exposure. Children with levels greater than 10 µg/dL are at increased risk for neurobehavioral problems and cognitive development. Research studies have shown that children with high lead levels during the elementary school years are more likely to have reading problems and drop out of school.

Early screening can detect high lead levels, and subsequent treatment can prevent unnecessary learning problems.

DENTAL CARE

Between ages 6 and 7 years, the exfoliation of the primary teeth begins and permanent teeth start erupting. The rate of loss and replacement of primary teeth is four teeth per year until approximately age 12 years. After all four of the permanent first molars have erupted, the child can be evaluated for braces. Fluoride in drinking water can help reduce tooth decay. In areas where fluoride concentration is less than 0.7 ppm in the drinking water, the provider should recommend supplements. Children in areas with fluoride concentration of 0.3 to 0.7 ppm in the drinking water should get fluoride supplements of 0.5 mg/d. In areas where fluoride concentration is less than 0.3 ppm, supplements should be 1.00 mg/d.

VISION

You should ask the child if he or she has difficulty seeing the blackboard at school, watching television, or reading. A normal farsighted preschool child usually has 20/20 vision by age 8 years. Yearly visual acuity is screened using the Snellen chart standardized at 20 feet. A tumbling E chart should be used if the child does not recognize the letters of the alphabet. Color vision also should be tested at least once during the school-age years.

GROWTH AND DEVELOPMENT

During the school-age years, growth may slow until puberty, when a growth spurt occurs. Secondary sex characteristics also appear toward the latter part of the school-age years. Average growth is 2 inches/year and 4 to 6 lb/year.

GROSS MOTOR SKILLS

At the beginning of the school-age period, children should have reasonably good gross motor skills. At age 6 years, most children can skip, hop, roller-skate, and catch a bounced ball. In the next few years, gross motor skills continue to improve. By age 10 years, eye-hand coordination is good enough for children to play games such as softball.

FINE MOTOR SKILLS

At age 6 years, most children can write (print) neatly. By age 8 years, most can use script. Six-year-old children can eat neatly but may need help to cut their meat. They should be able to dress themselves; draw a circle touching a square; tie their shoes; and draw a person with 12 parts, including a head with facial features and trunk.

LANGUAGE

School-age children are developing the ability to express their feelings as well as their thoughts. A 6-year-old child can usually express his or her feelings and follow at least three commands. As children get older, they can follow five or more serial commands. By age 8 to 10 years, most children have developed language patterns. Children who have difficulty with expressive or receptive skills often present with impaired social interactions. They are unable to use language to settle differences and consequently they may fight, have temper tantrums, ignore, back talk, or clown around.

COGNITIVE DEVELOPMENT

According to Piaget, during the school-age years, children move from pre-operational thinking to concrete operations, meaning thinking becomes more organized and rational. In this stage, children become less egocentric and more flexible in thinking and are able to see the viewpoints of others. During the school-age years, children acquire the skills of conservation, transformation, reversibility, seriation, and decentration. Acquisition of these skills enables children to add and subtract, learn to write, spell, read, and understand and solve problems mentally. Children have increased attention spans, ask questions, seek cause and effect, and categorize based on size and other characteristics, and can trace steps from point A to point B and vice versa.

EGO DEVELOPMENT

Erickson identifies the psychosocial crisis of school-age children as industry versus inferiority. Children in this age group become increasingly competent at attempting a variety of tasks and projects and completing them. Children's independence and self-esteem are boosted by their success in attempted projects, especially when they receive recognition from their parents, teachers, and peers. Their sense of industry makes it easy for them to become bored and irritable if they are not participating in some meaningful activity. Erickson proposed that if a child is unable to learn new skills and perform tasks successfully, then feelings of inferiority could develop and the child may lose interest in learning. A child who feels inferior might become passive, afraid to try new tasks, and lack self-esteem and self-confidence. If this sense of inferiority is not resolved, the child—and eventually the adult—will exhibit a variety of behavior problems.

IMMUNIZATIONS

By age 6 years, if the child's immunizations were not completed in the preschool years, then the fifth DTaP (diphtheria, tetanus, and acellular pertussis vaccine), the fourth IPV (inactivated poliovirus) vaccine, and the second MMR (measles, mumps, and rubella) vaccine should be given. At the 11- to 12-year well-child visits, the child should be given a tetanus diphtheria (Td). If the second MMR was not completed, then it should be given. The varicella vaccine also should be given if it has not been received before and if there is no history of chickenpox. The hepatitis B vaccine should be given if the child does not have the series. Consider the flu vaccine if the child has a chronic illness.

PHYSICAL EXAMINATION

School-age children should be measured at each well-child visit. Weight and height should be plotted on the growth chart and should stay along the growth curve normal for that child. As discussed previously, the child's modesty must be taken into consideration, and a gown should be provided or the child should be allowed to stay in his or her underwear. Wash your hands before beginning the examination. The physical examination of school-age children may be done in a head-to-toe format because these children are more cooperative than younger children. Nevertheless, to foster a sense of control, children should be offered choices and informed of what will happen as the examination proceeds.

HEAD AND NECK

Inspect the head and neck for shape and symmetry. Inspect the scalp carefully by parting the hair from the front to the occipital region. Observe for lesions, scaliness, nits, lice, and alopecia. Ask the child if any itching or tenderness is present. The hair may become oily as the child approaches puberty.

Alopecia, or loss of hair, may be noted. Traction alopecia is often found in school-age girls from wearing tight braids and hair holders. Tinea capitis, a fungal infection of the scalp, also results in alopecia. Alopecia areata is hair loss in which the scalp is totally smooth; it may be caused by systemic illness or may be idiopathic.

Palpate the skull from the front to the back. It should feel smooth and symmetrical. Palpate the temporal artery, and inspect the neck from the front. Check for symmetry, lymph nodes, enlarged thyroid gland, alignment of the trachea, masses, skin folds, and jugular vein distention. Palpate the neck for lymph nodes. Note their size, consistency, tenderness, temperature, and mobility. Palpable, small, nontender, mobile nodes are commonly found in the necks of school-age children. Palpate the trachea for midline position. Place the thumb on one side of the trachea and the index finger on the other side, and palpate along the trachea with the child's neck slightly hyperextended. The trachea should be midline. Next palpate the thyroid gland (Fig. 22–1), but be aware that in normal children, the thyroid may not be palpable. Stand in front of the child and observe the area of the thyroid gland. Rest both of your thumbs or forefingers over the gland and ask the child to swal-

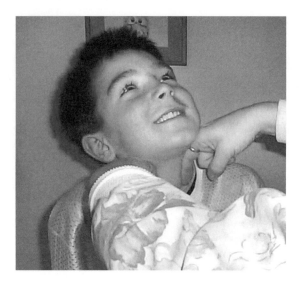

FIG. 22–1. Palpating the thyroid in a school-age child.

low. Move your thumbs or forefingers over the thyroid as the child swallows. Feel for size, nodules, or irregularities. Record the size and any abnormalities.

INTEGUMENT SYSTEM

The entire skin surface should be assessed. The skin of school-age children normally appears smooth and even. Apocrine sweat glands are not functioning yet; therefore, the skin is less oily and perspiration does not have a strong odor. The presence of body odor may be an indicator of early puberty.

Observe the skin for color, turgor, bruises, rashes, and odor. Ensure adequate light for inspection. Remember that school-age children are very active, so it is common to find bruises on their shins, knees, and elbows. Pallor may indicate anemia or may only be inherited coloring. Inspect the face, mouth, conjunctiva, and nail beds to assess for pallor. Inspect the skin for dryness. Normally, skin should be slightly dry, and the mucous membranes should be moist.

Inspect and palpate skin for lesions. Note location, size, color and distribution of lesions. Sometimes, it is helpful to draw a picture in the chart to show location on the body and to show size and shape of the lesions. Common childhood disorders that result in rashes include scabies, tinea corporis, and scarlet fever.

Scabies is caused by a small mite that burrows into the skin and deposits eggs and excrement. The lesions of scabies are usually papules, pustules, or tiny vesicles. In school-age children, the lesions are found from the neck down but are mostly concentrated on the hands, wrists, and webs of the fingers; in the axillae and gluteal cleft; and on the belt line. The parents and child report intense itching that seems worse at night. Diagnosis of scabies is confirmed by examining a scraping of one of the lesions under a microscope and identifying a mite, eggs, or feces.

Tinea corporis is a superficial fungal infection caused by *Trichophyton tonsurans*. The lesions are generally ringlike and red. Often, there is a border with central clearing. Usually, the border is scaly and slightly elevated, and may contain tiny vesicles and pustules. The child may experience itching but usually is asymptomatic.

Scarlet fever presents as a fine, rough papular rash on an erythematous base. This is caused by a strain of group A beta-hemolytic streptococci that produces an erythrogenic toxin. The rash starts on the face and neck, and then spreads to the shoulders and upper chest. The rash feels like fine sandpaper to the touch. Infrequently, circumoral pallor is present, and pastia lines or erythematous accentuation of the flexural creases can be seen. The rash also may appear as a white coating of the tongue that then turns red; this is called red strawberry tongue. One to 2 weeks after the infection, desquamation of the hands and feet may be seen, and the rest of the body may exhibit a fine scale.

VISUAL SYSTEM

Inspect the eyes for shape, symmetry, placement, and size. Observe for tearing, redness, cloudiness, protrusion, and jittery eyes (i.e., nystagmus). Observe the eyelids for proper placement. Normally, the eyelid rests between the upper border of the iris and the upper border of the pupil. If the eyelid is red, edematous, and tender to the touch, assess for the presence of a stye. A nontender node may indicate a chalazion. A sunken periorbital area may be suggestive of dehydration, and shadows under the eyes, also known as allergic shiners, may indicate allergies. Observe the eyelashes for distribution and condition. The eyelashes should curl outward; if they do not, they can cause irritation of the eye.

Inspect the pupils for size, shape, equality, and response to light. To test the pupil's response to light, shine a penlight directly on the pupil and note the reaction. Note consensual reaction by observing the pupil of the opposite eye react simultaneously with the pupil into which the light is shone. To test for accommodation, ask the child to look at an object in the distance and then to look at your finger held about 10 cm from the child's nose. When the child's eyes focus on your finger, the pupils should constrict.

To check for strabismus and compare vision between the two eyes, the corneal light reflex test and the cover/uncover test should be routinely performed. To perform the corneal light reflex, shine a light directly into the eye from about 16 inches away. The light should be reflected symmetrically on both pupils normally. To do the cover test, ask the child to look at an object held straight ahead about 16 inches away. Cover one eye and observe the uncovered eye for movement as it focuses on the object; then observe the covered eye for movement as it is uncovered. This test should be performed on both eyes. Any movement observed may indicate strabismus. Often if a child sees only from the covered eye, he or she tries to regain vision by moving away the cover.

Test for visual acuity using the HOTV or Snellen chart. For the HOTV test, the child must stand 3 meters away, and for the Snellen chart test, the distance is 20 feet. Both eyes should be tested at the same time, and then each eye should be tested separately. Normal visual acuity from age 6 years is 20/20. If there is a two-line difference between the eyes, then the child should be referred to an ophthalmologist for further testing.

To assess extraocular movement, ask the child to keep his or her head still while following your light through the six cardinal fields of gaze.

To assess the fundus, ask the child to focus on an object behind you and not to focus on your light. Tell the child that even though your head would obstruct his or her view of the object, he or she should still keep looking at it. Observe the red retinal reflex from about 12 inches from the child and then focus on the fundus. You should be able to see the disc margin, which is normally sharp and well defined.

RESPIRATORY SYSTEM

Assess the respiratory system with the child sitting on the examining table. Begin by counting the respirations. In school-age children, the normal rate is 16 to 25 breaths per minute. Inspect the child's color, assessing for cyanosis. Look for nasal flaring, accessory muscle use, retractions, and chest wall shape and deformity. By age 6 years, a child's chest should have a ratio of anteroposterior to transverse diameter of 1:1.36. Note any pectus excavatum (i.e., funnel chest) and pectus carinatum (i.e., pigeon breast). Observe for equal movement of the chest wall by observing respirations from the child's side. A child older than age 7 years should exhibit thoracic rather than abdominal breathing. Note the size of the child's breasts. Enlarged breasts may be indicative of gynecomastia in prepubertal boys. Enlarged breasts in children younger than age 8 years may indicate precocious puberty.

Palpate the breast for any abnormal masses. Normal young breast tissue has firm elasticity. Inspect the nipples and areolas for color, size, shape, and discharge. Breast buds are palpated under the nipple; they are tender and are normal findings in both boys and girls.

If respiratory problems are suspected, palpate to assess respiratory excursion, tactile fremitus, and position of the trachea. Percuss the anterior and posterior chest using the indirect method. Resonance should normally be heard over all lung surfaces. The chest in thin children may be hyperresonant.

Auscultate over each lobe, comparing the two sides of the chest. Using the diaphragm of your stethoscope, assess whether breath sounds are normal, diminished, or increased. You can encourage the child to breathe deeply by asking him or her to blow away a cotton ball, by pretending to blow out candles, or by asking the child to blow out the light on your otoscope. If you suspect that the sound is referred from the upper respiratory tract, place the stethoscope diaphragm near the child's mouth. Referred sound would be loudest at the mouth. If the child is thin, the breath sounds normally seem louder.

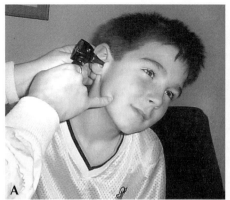
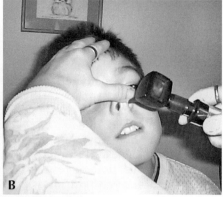
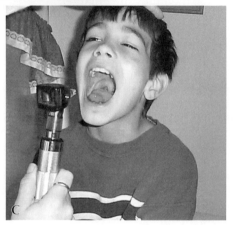

FIG. 22–2. Examination of the ear, nose, and mouth in a school-age child. (*A*) Ear examination. (*B*) Nose examination. (*C*) Mouth examination.

EARS, NOSE, AND THROAT

Inspect and palpate the external ear. The child should not feel any pain on palpation unless he or she has otitis externa. Assess the ear canal and the tympanic membrane using a size four speculum on your otoscope (Fig. 22–2). The pinna should be pulled up and back. The tympanic membrane should be assessed for translucency, color, and landmarks. Mobility of the drum is assessed with the use of an insufflator. Tell the child he or she will feel a puff of air. Assess hearing by using the whisper test, Weber test, and Rinne test.

Inspect the nose, looking for scarring, discharge, odor, and excoriation. Inspect the turbinates and septum using a light. The mucosa should be firm and pink. Pale and boggy mucosa is seen in children with allergic rhinitis. A nasal pleat or allergic crease is a horizontal crease on the nasal bridge seen in children with allergic rhinitis. This develops from frequent wiping of the nose in an upward motion, called the allergic salute. The septum should be midline; note any deviation.

357

Inspect the mouth for color and moisture. Normally, the oral membranes are pink and moist. Assess for halitosis, which may indicate sinusitis, pharyngitis, dental cavities, or a foreign body in the nares. Inspect the teeth for loss of primary teeth and growth of secondary teeth. At age 6 years, children begin to loose primary teeth, and secondary teeth erupt throughout the school-age period. Assess for malocclusion by asking the child to bite down hard. Ask the child to say "aah" to assess the size of the tonsils, tongue, palate, uvula, and posterior pharynx. The tonsils usually enlarge to their peak size by age 6 to 8 years. A "strawberry tongue" may be seen when a streptococcal infection is present. The uvula should be midline, and no deviation should be seen with movement. If the adenoids can be seen during assessment of the tonsils, then they are enlarged.

ABDOMEN

Begin assessing the abdomen by carefully inspecting for bulges, distention, and asymmetries. Second, auscultate for bowel sounds in all four quadrants. The stethoscope also can be used to assess for peritoneal irritation. After listening to bowel sounds, press the stethoscope more firmly in all four quadrants and at the umbilicus and observe the child's face for any sign of pain. Check for rebound tenderness by pressing deeply with the stethoscope and then quickly withdrawing the pressure. If pain is felt, then rebound tenderness may be present.

Last, palpate the abdomen to check for masses and to assess the spleen, liver, and kidneys. First palpate lightly in all four quadrants with a warm, flat hand. If the child is ticklish, have the child place his or her hand on the abdomen and cover his or her fingers with your hand (Fig. 22–3). As the child self-palpates, move your fingers slowly onto the abdomen, still resting on the child's hand, and palpate all four quadrants. Perform deep palpation to assess size of the liver and spleen and to check for any abdominal masses. In school-age children, the liver spans from 8 to 10 cm in the midclavicular line, and the lower edge may be palpated 1 to 2 cm below the right costal margin. The tip of the spleen may be palpable 1 to 2 cm below the left costal margin. A sausage-shaped mass palpated in the left lower quadrant represents feces in the sigmoid colon and may indicate constipation.

CARDIOVASCULAR SYSTEM

Begin the cardiovascular assessment by taking the blood pressure and observing the skin color. Note any cyanosis, pallor, or mottling. Observe for any respiratory distress signs such as grunting, retractions, or nasal flaring. Observe the anterior chest for symmetry of chest movement and visible pulsations such as lifts or heaves. Observe the fingernails for clubbing, which may indicate hypoxia.

Palpate the point of maximal impulse (PMI). In children older than age 7 years, the PMI should be felt in the fifth intercostal space to the right of the

FIG. 22–3. (A) and (B) Examination of the abdomen in a ticklish child.

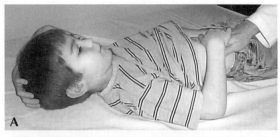

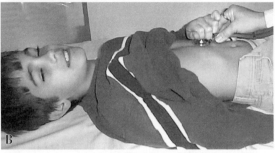

midclavicular line. Sinus arrhythmia is a normal finding in children. Feel for vibratory thrills or rubs.

Auscultate the heart with the child upright and then lying down, using both the bell and the diaphragm. Note the heart rate, rhythm, and sounds. S_3 may be heard at the apex at times in school-age children. It is best heard with the child lying on the left side. If it is not associated with a pathologic murmur, then it is considered a normal finding. Innocent murmurs do not increase over time or affect growth. Usually, they are first heard in school-age children. Organic murmurs that occur before age 3 years are usually related to congenital heart disease. After age 3 years, organic murmurs are often related to rheumatic heart disease.

Finally, palpate the radial, femoral, popliteal, and dorsalis pedis artery pulses. Normally, pulses should be palpable and symmetrical.

MUSCULOSKELETAL SYSTEM

A major part of the evaluation of the musculoskeletal system in school-age children is accomplished by observing the child as he or she walks into the office and throughout the examination. Observe the child's gait for limping or any sign of foot, knee, or hip problems. Observe the child's coordination as he or she climbs up and down from the examination table. School-age children have increasing muscle bulk, strength, and coordination. Observe the curve of the spine for lateral curvature or scoliosis. Observe for any asymmetry of the scapulae and the hips. Idiopathic scoliosis most commonly begins in older school-age children as they enter puberty. Early identification of scoliosis is extremely important to prevent expensive surgery and long-term consequences of the problem.

Full range of motion (ROM) should be carried out on all joints. Assess for swelling and tenderness. Assess for genu valgum (knock-knee) and genu varum (bow-legged). Normally, genu valgum may be present in children younger than age 7 years. A space of more than 3 inches between the knees of a child older than age 7 years indicates genu valgum.

Assess for strength of the upper and lower extremities. To test strength in the upper extremities, ask the child to squeeze your crossed fingers tightly. To test strength in lower extremities, ask the child to push against your hand with the soles of his or her feet. Strength should be symmetrical in the upper and lower extremities.

Common musculoskeletal problems that may occur in school-age children are transient synovitis, Legg-Calvé-Perthes disease, and "growing pains."

Transient synovitis is an acute transient disorder of the hip that causes unilateral hip pain. The cause of the disorder is unknown, and the condition is self-limited. Most common in early school-age and preschool children, it also occurs in older children. When the symptoms are experienced, septic arthritis, osteomyelitis, and Legg-Calvé-Perthes disease should be ruled out. Treatment for transient synovitis consists of analgesic and bedrest for 2 to 7 days.

Legg-Calvé-Perthes disease is idiopathic necrosis of the femoral head. It may be associated with hip pain, stiffness, and a limp. Pain also may be referred to the thigh and knee. It is most commonly seen in boys between the ages of 5 and 9 years. Only one side is usually involved, and fever and systemic illness are not present. In the progressive stage of the disease, the pain decreases, but the ROM is markedly decreased and there is leg length difference. Treatment may include bracing, traction, surgery, or bone reconstruction.

Growing pains may be seen in early school-age children who are normally active. Children may complain of pain in the knee area, in the shins or thighs, or in the entire leg. The child usually experiences the pain at night after being very active during the day. Treatment may include ice or heat, massage, and analgesic agents.

GENITOURINARY SYSTEM

To make the genital examination comfortable for school-age children, special attention must be paid to providing the child with privacy. The child should be appropriately draped, and you should reassure the child in a soft, soothing voice.

Girls

Have the child lie in the frog-legged position (see Chapter 14) with assistance using a gentle manner. Palpate femoral pulses bilaterally and feel for femoral hernia. Inspect the labia majora, labia minora, and clitoris for size, color, skin integrity, and lesions. The labia should be pink and moist. The labia enlarge as puberty begins. Swelling and redness of the labia may indicate infection, masturbation, or sexual abuse. Inspect the urethra and vaginal vault for swelling, redness, blisters, pimples, chancres, or warts, which may indicate venereal disease and sexual abuse. In prepubertal girls, it is normal to have a small amount of clear, odorless watery or mucous discharge. Development of pubic hair should begin between ages 8.5 and 14 years. Soft downy hair seen on the labia majora indicates early sexual maturation. Every child enters puberty at a different age; therefore, sexual characteristics should be assessed and Tanner stage of sexual maturity noted (see Chapter 3). Assess the anus for redness, rash, and fissures. Scratch marks may indicate itching caused by pinworm infestations, and fissures may indicate passage of hard stools.

Boys

Inspect the penis, urethra, scrotum, testes, and anus. The prepubertal penis is approximately 6 cm long. In obese boys, the penis appears smaller because it is hidden by a fat pad. Penile enlargement normally occurs between ages 10.5 and 14.5 years. Precocious puberty may be the reason for a penis that is large relative to the child's stage of development. Onset of puberty before age 9 years is considered as precocious puberty. Attempt to retract the foreskin if the child is not circumcised. If the foreskin is not easily retracted, it may indicate phimosis. The urinary meatus should be slitlike and slightly ventral at the tip of the penis. The size of the testes before puberty should be about 1.5 to 2 cm, and the left testis is usually lower than the right. Use "testicle beads" for accurate measurement if they are available in your practice. You should be able to palpate each testicle in the scrotum. If unable to palpate, ask the child to sit with legs crossed "Indian style" on the examination table.

Testicular enlargement is the first sign of puberty in boys (Tanner stage II) and occurs between ages 9.5 and 13.5 years. Scrotal skin thinning occurs together with testicular enlargement. Growth of pubic hair usually begins 6 months after testicular enlargement begins.

Palpate femoral pulse bilaterally and assess the inguinal area for hernias. Assess the anus for redness, rash, and fissures. Palpate the prostate to assess its size. The normal size before age 10 years is 1 cm; after puberty, the size may be 2 to 3 cm.

NEUROLOGIC SYSTEM

Assessment of the neurologic system should include assessment of mental status, motor function, sensory function, cranial nerve function, level of consciousness, and deep tendon reflexes (DTRs). School-age children are normally able to follow directions and cooperate, thus making it fun and easy to successfully complete a neurologic examination.

Mental status can be assessed throughout the history and the examination. Observe if the child appropriately responds to directions. Note the child's speech and if he or she is easily understood. Note the child's behavior during the examination and if he or she cooperates or is easily distracted and readily interrupts while you or the parent is talking. Also assess the child's cognitive level by asking about his or her performance at school. Ask specifically what grades the child gets in school and whether the child has had to repeat any grade. School-age children should have improved speech and understanding. Reasoning and reading skills are noticeably more refined as the child gets into the older school-age period.

A major part of motor function assessment is done during the musculoskeletal assessment. Check muscle strength and symmetry. Perform ROM on all joints to check for flaccidity or spasticity. Six-year-old children should be able to skip, walk on their toes, walk heel to toe in a straight line, and balance on each foot for 6 seconds. Fine motor abilities should include copying a square, tying their own shoelaces, and drawing a six-part human. Eight-year-old children should be able to perform rapid alternating movements such as touching the thumb to each successive finger on the same hand as fast as they can. Normally, 8-year-old children should be able to do this in 5 seconds. They should also have good handwriting skills and developed eye-hand coordination.

Assess cerebellar function with the Romberg test. To perform the test, ask the child to stand with the eyes closed and arms at the side. School-age children should be able to do this without leaning, but you should stand close to catch the child if he or she leans.

Some of the assessment of sensory function is done when the cranial nerves are assessed. The cranial nerves are assessed when the eye, head, and neck are assessed. By age 6 years, with eyes closed, children should be able to identify common objects you place in their hands (i.e., stereognosis) and use two-point discrimination. By age 8 years, they should be able to identify shapes you draw in their open hands (i.e., graphesthesia).

Level of consciousness is assessed using the pediatric version of the Glasgow Coma Scale (see Chapter 3). A normal child's score is 15; a score of 8 or less may indicate coma.

The biceps, brachioradial, triceps, patellar, and Achilles DTRs should be assessed in school-age children. If reflexes are hyperactive, test for ankle clonus because upper motor neuron disease is associated with sustained clonus.

ANTICIPATORY GUIDANCE

GROWTH AND DEVELOPMENT

Parents should be taught that growth of school-age children normally follows the child's growth curve but deviates at the growth spurt. Girls need to be prepared for menarche, and boys need to be prepared for pubertal changes. Sex education books and videos may be suggested to help parents discuss these changes with their children. Emphasize the need to keep communication open between parent and child. Teach the child about the body changes that are going to take place. For girls, breast enlargement occurs between ages 8 and 11 years, axillary hair and pubic hair growth begins between ages 10 and 14 years, and menarche occurs between ages 10 and 16 years. For boys, testicular enlargement occurs between ages 10 and 12 years, axillary hair growth begins between ages 12 and 14 years, facial hair growth begins between ages 11 and 14 years, and pubic hair growth occurs between ages 12 and 15 years. Advise parents that sexually oriented play and masturbation are common in this age group, but children should be taught that masturbation should be done in private. Discussions about alcohol, tobacco, and drug use should be included and emphasized more as children reach puberty.

SAFETY

School-age children are more independent, but their motor and cognitive skills are often inadequate to protect them from injury and death from accidents. In fact, more children in this age group die from injuries than from all other diseases combined, according to the American Academy of Pediatrics. Most of these accidents are preventable, so parents should be made aware of steps they can take to protect their children. Anticipatory guidance must include sports safety, water safety, stranger safety, car safety, and firearm hazards.

Sports Safety

Children should be encouraged to participate in sports to prevent the growing problem of obesity and to promote a healthy lifestyle. Safety equipment must be used to prevent injury. Children always should wear a helmet when rollerblading or riding a bike, skateboard, or scooter. Children should avoid riding in the dark. Protective kneepads and elbow pads also should be used for rollerblading and riding scooters and skateboards.

Water Safety

Children should never swim or play in water without the supervision of parents or a responsible adult. They should be taught to always enter the water feet first and to never swim in canals or fast-moving water.

Stranger Safety

Parents must warn their children about the risk of being lured away by strangers. They should practice scenarios of what their children should do and say if approached by a stranger. School-age children also should know to dial 911 in case of an emergency.

Car Safety

Parents should be advised that the safest place for school-age children to ride is in the back seat. Both lap and shoulder belts should be used, and everyone should buckle up before the car is started.

Firearm Hazards

Parents should be told that the best prevention for accidents with a firearm is not to keep one in the home. If a gun must be kept in the home, then the gun and ammunition should be locked in separate locked cabinets. Parents also must counsel their children on what to do if they encounter a gun at a friend's house or at school. Parents should be reminded to ask the parents of the child's friends whether there are guns kept in the home.

DENTAL CARE

At this age, children should be establishing good dental hygiene with yearly visits to a dentist. Children should be able to brush their own teeth but still need help from the parent with flossing until age 8 years, when they will have the motor skills required. Fluoride supplementation also should be given to children without adequate fluoride levels in the water supply to prevent tooth decay.

NUTRITION

The school-age years are a time when healthy or unhealthy dietary habits can become ingrained. Parents and school-age children should be reminded of the importance of a healthy, balanced diet to facilitate normal growth and prevent obesity. Children should be taught to distinguish between nutritious food and junk food and taught to avoid non-nutritious, high-calorie, high-fat, and high-sugar snacks and foods. They should have no more than 2 to 3 cups of skim milk per day and regular balanced meals with foods from the four basic food groups. Children should have three nutritious meals and two healthy snacks a day. At this age, children should be encouraged to become involved in planning, shopping for, and preparing meals. Table 22–1 indicates the recommended daily nutrition for school-age children.

DISCIPLINE AND PARENTING

School-age children are becoming more independent of their parents and have a wider sphere of influence that includes peers and teachers. Parents need to understand the importance of providing opportunities for their children to become more independent while simultaneously adding new responsibilities. Parents should praise and support the child's activities, get to know the child's friends and their families, and communicate with their teachers. Active time must be spent with the child, teaching how conflicts should be resolved and actively listening when the child speaks.

TABLE 22-1. RECOMMENDED DAILY NUTRITION FOR SCHOOL-AGE CHILDREN	
Nutrient	Daily Recommendation
Fats	Use sparingly
Breads and cereals	Four or more servings
Fruits and vegetables	Five or more servings
Milk	2 to 4 cups
Meat and eggs, beans, and lentils	Two or more servings

Established rules in the home provide guidance for children and help parents maintain discipline. Reasonable limits must be set, and discipline techniques such as loss of privileges and grounding must be discussed. Limit the amount of television viewing, time spent on video and computer games, and high-fat and high-sugar foods. Encourage reading, adequate sleep, and extracurricular activities such drama, music, and sports. Provide an allowance and guidance in spending it. Parents also should make arrangements for adult supervision when they are absent and always supervise activities that may be potentially dangerous.

TEST YOUR KNOWLEDGE OF CHAPTER 22

1. What is the best approach to physical examination for school-age children?
2. What are the components of screening school-age children?
3. What is the expected cognitive development of school-age children?
4. What is the expected ego development of school-age children?
5. How is the thyroid palpated in school-age children?
6. What differences in physical assessment of each body system would you expect to find in school-age children?
7. What differences are seen in neurologic development in children at different ages?
8. Why is anticipatory guidance necessary?
9. What anticipatory guidance should be given to the parents of school-age children?

BIBLIOGRAPHY

Algranati, P. S. (1992). *The pediatric patient. An approach to history and physical examination.* Baltimore: Williams & Wilkins.

American Academy of Family Physicians. (1999). *Summary of policy recommendations for periodic health examinations.* Washington, DC: American Academy of Family Physicians.

American Academy of Pediatrics (1997). *Guidelines for health supervision III*. Elk Grove Village, IL: American Academy of Pediatrics.

Andrews, J. (1997). Making the most of the sports physical. *Contemporary Pediatrics, 14*(3), 183–205.

Boyton, R. W., Dunn, E. S., & Stephens, G. R. (1998). *Manual of ambulatory pediatrics* (4th ed.). Philadelphia: J. B. Lippincott.

Burns, C., Brady, M. A., Dunn, A. M., & Starr, N. B. (2000). *Pediatric primary care: A handbook for nurse practitioners* (2nd ed.). Philadelphia: W. B. Saunders.

Engel, J. (1997). *Pediatric assessment. Mosby's pocket guide series*. St. Louis: Mosby.

Goldbloom, R. B. (1999). *Pediatric clinical skills*. New York: Churchill Livingstone.

Graham, M. V., & Uphold, C. R. (1994). *Clinical guidelines in child health*. Gainsesville, FL: Barmarrae Books.

Green Hernandez, C., Singleton, J. K., & Avonzon, D. Z. (2001). *Primary care pediatrics*. Philadelphia: Lippincott, Williams & Wilkins.

McMillan, J. A., DeAngelis, C. D., Feigin, R. D., & Warshaw, J. B. (1999). *Oski's pediatrics. Principles and practice*. Philadelphia: Lippincott Williams & Wilkins.

Murray, R. B., Zentner, J. P., & Pinnell, N. N. (2001). Assessment and health promotion for the school child. In R. Beckman Murray & J. P. Zentner (Eds.). *Health promotion strategies through the life span* (7th ed.). New Jersey: Prentice Hall.

Muscari, M. E. (2001). *Advanced pediatric clinical assessment. Skills and procedures*. Philadelphia: J. B. Lippincott.

Schor, E. L. (1998). Guiding the family of the school-age child. *Contemporary Pediatrics, 15*, 75–94.

Seidel, H. M., Ball, J. W., Dains, J. E., & Benedict, G. W. (1999). *Mosby's guide to physical examination* (4th ed.). St. Louis: Mosby.

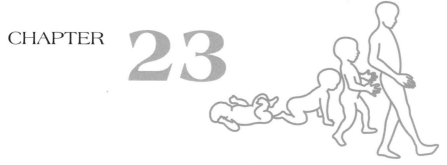

CHAPTER **23**

Assessment of Adolescents

Wendy Whitney

Objectives
- Identify the stages of adolescence.
- Develop an approach to the assessment of adolescents.
- Understand special issues of adolescent assessment.
- Establish major categories of adolescent anticipatory guidance.

The word *adolescence* is derived from the Latin word *adolescere*, which means "to grow up." This new growth refers not only to physical and sexual growth but also to social and psychologic growth. This period of life is a confusing passing from childhood to adulthood. Adolescence begins at age 11 to 12 years with the appearance of secondary sex characteristics, and ends with the cessation of somatic growth around age 19 years. Most adolescent clients are at a physical peak, but they may struggle with emotional, social, and cognitive development. The passage to adulthood encompasses at least four phases: (1) completion of growth, including sexual development; (2) completion of school; (3) becoming an individual, enabling the adolescent to separate from the family; and (4) setting goals for a way to make money through a career or vocation.

 ## STAGES OF ADOLESCENCE

EARLY ADOLESCENCE

Early adolescents (ages 11 to 13 years) have a rapid growth spurt. Sexual organ and axillary and pubic hair growth may cause self-concept changes and cause these adolescents to be unsure of themselves. Peer acceptance affects adolescents throughout this period. Teens who are delayed or accelerated in sexual characteristics may have shattered self-concepts if their peers do not accept them or if their peers comment negatively on the body changes. These teens are in Piaget's stage of concrete thinking and may not develop realistic goals about their future unless they are helped by an adult. Piaget believes adolescents are searching for self-identity and depend on cognitive skills, which enable them to see life through abstract thinking. At times, early adolescents may struggle with the loss of innocence. They question adults and themselves about their place in a world that is no longer a child's world. To most teens, the world opens up new opportunities to explore without an adult watching over them so closely.

MIDDLE ADOLESCENCE

Middle adolescents (ages 14 to 16 years) may still struggle with their new bodies. Emotionally immature teens with adult bodies and the emotional skills of a child experience wide mood swings. This is the period when children start to think abstractly, according to Piaget. Abstract thinking is defined as the ability to make decisions by using logic and eliminating unsupported ideas to achieve a workable solution to a problem.

LATE ADOLESCENCE

Late adolescents (ages 17 years and older) show a decline in narcissistic thinking and openness to others. These adolescents start to look outside the peer group to focus on creating more intimate relationships. Nearly 50% of all teens in America have had a sexual relationship by age 18 years of age.

🏐 STAGES OF PSYCHOSOCIAL (EGO) DEVELOPMENT

Erickson believes that individuals develop according to the individual's capabilities and the environmental demand. According to Erickson, the adolescent years are full of psychosocial crises. The central focus for adolescents is discovering who they are. Role confusion promotes conflict within adolescents. Teens try to redefine their self-concept by shifting into different roles. These roles are often defined by their peers because peers are the main focus at this time in adolescents' lives. If these roles are nonproductive in society, teens often discover further conflict with life. If the role is productive according to society, the teens progress toward adulthood. Our society expects teens to be productive, excel in school, and not cause trouble in society.

In some societies, the roles of teens are already defined. There is no specific conflict, but the defined passage may cause similar turmoil. An example of this is teens of the Masai tribe in Kenya, Africa. Before becoming men, the function of young teens is to tend cattle and practice their "jump" (a dance).

The warrior who can jump the highest is valued. Jumping high also enables warriors to see farther distances for game or dangerous animals. When teens are circumcised, they wear a black skin and ostrich feathers and are in a period called "Imugit of the arrows." Their only job is to shoot birds for a few months. Afterward, these teens become warriors. This passage is expected and followed so that adolescents only have to wait for the event to happen.

 ## STAGES OF MORALITY

Concepts of right or wrong should be solidly established by the time a child reaches adolescence. Kohlberg believes that adolescents have developed morality judgments by progressing through three stages: preconventional, conventional, and postconventional. The preconventional, or premoral, stage includes punishment and the need for the child to conform to the rules through punishment. The conventional, or moral, stage bases moral judgment on the "good boy, nice girl" roles. The child has an obligation to conform to authority and respect law and order. The concept of punishment for wrong and reward for good and right is reconfirmed in this stage. Adolescents are in the postconventional stage, which is based on the idea that correct behavior is a decision of conscience with self-chosen ethical principles. Moral principles, which govern relationships such as empathy and resolving conflict, begin as norms when applied between young friends, according to Kohlberg.

 ## PEERS

Peers have tremendous input into adolescents' identity because of their need to belong to groups. How one dresses and behaves, and even moral decisions, are often directed by peers. It has been found that physically mature boys and girls tend to be more popular and leaders in the group. Socioeconomic affluent teens have an advantage with most mature male leaders and other teens in the group because access to money often opens doors. Peers may use coercion to force teens into violence. Many gang members are forced into association, and it is often difficult, even potentially deadly, to break away (Table 23–1).

 ## CULTURE

Culture is also a factor that binds some teens together. Some gangs are specific to cultures, and some gangs are made up of teens in similar neighborhoods or sections of cities. Other gangs are formed from adolescents who are similar in culture or ethnicity. Mixed groups may have different requirements for popularity than same-culture or same-socioeconomic status groups. Parents and caregivers need to listen to teens and influence them before a gang does. After a teen is caught up in the lifestyle of violence, drugs, and money, he or she is, for the most part, "lost forever." In *Oliver*

TABLE 23–1. REASONS TO JOIN GANGS

Reason	Discussion
Coercion	Gangs are stronger with more people. Many teens convince other teens to join, which creates a stronger gang. There is always a threat that teens who do not want to join or want to quit may be harmed or killed.
Money	Teens who live in poverty find that money gives them power and respect. Some contribute this money to their families. Others purchase cars, clothing, or jewelry. Even young teens can earn thousands of dollars by becoming lookouts or making drug or weapon deliveries.
Identity and power	Becoming a part of a group of people that is feared and respected establishes power, identity, and belonging. This force behind the teen can create a shield to protect him or her from authority and other gangs.
Familiarity	Adolescents may want to emulate an older brother or someone who is looked up to.
Unstable home life	The gang has rules and safety that may be lacking in the adolescent's life. It provides community ties and clear values to follow with established punishments if they are not followed.
Limited opportunity	If life is a dead-end with no support from family, no chance in school, and unavailable employment, involvement with a gang, which always has money, parties, and friends, may seem inviting.

Twist, Dickens describes a pack of young boys roaming the streets of London and picking pockets in 1830. In the story, Fagin offers these young boys a place to stay, some money, and a sense of "family." Youths who join gangs today are often alienated and feel powerless because they lack a traditional support system such as family. Gangs give teens a sense of belonging and become a source of identity for its members. Activities of the gang also can be an outlet for anger.

APPROACH

The main reason adolescents seek medical care is because of an injury or the need for a school or sports physical examination (see Chapter 26). Adolescents seeking an identity frequently reject adults' beliefs and values and take risks. When treated as a partner in their health care, some teens are receptive to healthcare teachings. The guidelines from the American Medical Association (AMA) for adolescents suggest yearly examinations, which include health guidelines (Table 23–2), and evaluation of physical and psychosocial development.

Adolescents are very sensitive, and need to be treated with respect and not like little children. You need to develop relationships with adolescents that will establish trust so the adolescent and the parent will provide infor-

TABLE 23–2. GUIDELINES FOR ADOLESCENT PREVENTIVE SERVICES

Recommendation	Description
1	All adolescents ages 11 to 21 years have annual routine health visits.
2	Preventive services should be age and developmentally appropriate. The visits should be sensitive to individual and sociocultural differences.
3	Care providers should establish office policies regarding confidential care for adolescents and the way parents will be involved in the care. Policies should be made clear to adolescents and their parents.
4	Care providers should give parents and other adult caregivers information about health guidance for adolescents at least once during early adolescence, once during middle adolescence, and once during late adolescence.
5	Care providers should provide information for health guidance to the adolescent annually. This is to promote better understanding of the adolescent's physical growth and psychosocial and psychosexual development as well as the importance of actively involvement in decisions concerning their health care.
6	Adolescents should receive guidance annually to promote the reduction of injuries.
7	Annual health guidance about dietary habits and a healthy diet should be reviewed with adolescents. Benefits and ways to achieve a healthy weight should be addressed.
8	All adolescents should receive health guidance annually about the benefits of exercise. Adolescents should be encouraged to participate in safe exercise on a regular basis.
9	Annual information about responsible sexual behavior, including abstinence, should be given to all adolescent patients. Latex condoms to prevent sexually transmitted diseases (STDs) should be made available with instructions on how to use condoms effectively (unless the state you are practicing in disallows this).
10	Annual guidance to promote avoidance of tobacco, alcohol, and other abusable substances and anabolic steroids should be provided to adolescent clients.
11	Annual screening for hypertension according to the protocol developed by the National Heart, Lung, and Blood Institute's Second Task Force on Blood Pressure Control in Children should be done.
12	Adolescents at risk for hyperlipidemia should be screened for high cholesterol level and adult coronary heart disease. Providers should follow the protocol developed by the Expert Panel on Blood Cholesterol Levels in Children and Adolescents.
13	All adolescents should be screened annually for eating disorders and obesity by determining weight and stature and asking about body image and dieting patterns.

(continued)

TABLE 23–2. GUIDELINES FOR ADOLESCENT PREVENTIVE SERVICES (Continued)

Recommendation	Description
14	All adolescents should be asked annually about their use of tobacco products, including cigarettes and smokeless tobacco.
15	All adolescents should be asked annually about their use of alcohol and other abusable substances and about their use of over-the-counter and prescription drugs, including anabolic steroids, for nonmedical purposes.
16	The care provider should provide information annually about involvement in sexual behaviors that may result in unintended pregnancy and STDs, including HIV infection.
17	Sexually active adolescents should be screened for STDs.
18	Adolescents at risk for HIV infection should be offered confidential HIV screening with the ELISA and a confirmatory test.
19	Female adolescents who are sexually active and women age 18 years and older should be screened annually for cervical cancer by use of a Papanicolaou test.
20	Annual inquiries should be made about behavior or emotions and then explored if they indicate recurrent or severe depression or risk of suicide.
21	All adolescents should be asked annually about history of emotional, physical, and sexual abuse.
22	Inquiries about learning and school problems should be asked annually.
23	Adolescents should receive a tuberculin skin test if they have been exposed to active tuberculosis, have lived in a homeless shelter, have been incarcerated, have lived in or come from an area with a high prevalence of tuberculosis, or currently work in a healthcare setting.
24	All adolescents should receive prophylactic immunization according to the guidelines established by the federally convened Advisory Committee on Immunization Practices.

ELISA = enzyme-linked immunosorbent assay.
Adapted from Montalto, N. J. (1998). Implementing the guidelines for adolescent preventive services. *American Family Physician, 57,* 2181–2190.

mation and allow you to teach healthy guidelines. It is best to greet the adolescent before greeting the parent. You should lead the interview by showing interest in the teen. Gear the conversation to the appropriate level for the teen. Chat about interests and how things are going in general.

The visit flows better if there is an understanding with the parent and the teen about confidentiality at the start of the visit. The adolescent must understand that the interview will be confidential unless there is a problem that needs to be addressed for health. If there is a medical need, the adolescent should be informed that the parent must be told. The parent and the adolescent should come to an agreement that you will do two interviews, one with the parent and the adolescent and one with the adolescent alone. The information received in such interviews allows you to gather information about how each perceives the other and allows you to stay somewhat neutral You need to be open to both parties. Your focus should be to take in information from both sides, give helpful information, stay neutral, and resolve conflicts.

You should make an effort to understand how the adolescent perceives the problem and the relationships with important people in the teen's life. The adolescent may not want to have the parent involved with health concerns. You need to be astute to this and somehow fulfill the wishes of the parent and the teen. Psychological problems that may cause future problems also must be shared with the parent. Young adolescents may be timid and not want to communicate any needs to the caregiver. Adolescents also may not allow the parent to speak for them, and the parent's knowledge of the problem can be very limited.

State law determines whether the adolescent can be treated without the consent of the parent. Teens often ask questions about sex and birth control. Each state dictates legalities about birth control and adolescent patients. You can answer questions but should defer from prescribing unless the laws of the state define otherwise. Each state has laws that affect your ability to give confidential evaluations to adolescents. Information that is crucial to the well-being of the teen legally needs to be shared with the parent because the parent is legally responsible for the teen until he or she is 18 years old. Suspicion of any criminal offense, such as child abuse, should be reported to the authorities.

You may open conversation better by not appearing overwhelming to the client. Try to present yourself as just a person who has special skills and is eager to find out about the adolescent's interests. You should focus on the needs of the client and remember that the developmental age may not be the same as the chronologic or emotional age. Begin the interview with broad questions and move to specific ones. Ask nonthreatening questions first, such as, "What do you like to do? Tell me about your friends. What are they like?" Do not start the conversation with invasive questions such as, "Do you do drugs or smoke cigarettes? Are you sexually active?" It is important to ask for clarification of abstract phrasing or words if they are unclear. Watch for nonverbal communication. Body language outside the teen's awareness helps you open up the conversation when it is described. You do not need to tell the adolescent your perception of the problem. Simply ask questions to elicit the adolescent's perceptions. For example, "I noticed when I asked you about your brother, you clenched your fists and frowned. What's going on with your brother?"

Learning to pause and use silence is important to allow the teen time to process information and give a response. Sometimes just pausing and asking, "What are you thinking of?" may encourage a response.

HISTORY

In addition to the medical, surgical, and family history, a good sexual, social, and substance use history should be obtained. Use the HEADSS (home, education, eating behaviors, activities, drugs, sex, and suicide) as a guideline for history taking with adolescents. Sexual history is very important and gives you an opportunity to do anticipatory guidance (Table 23–3). Social history includes friends, family, school activities, grades, extracurricular activities, employment, and the formulation of plans or goals (Table 23–4). If an adolescent indicates the use of substances, ask which substances are being used, the age of first use and most recent use, the occurrence of blackouts, the most recent intoxication, and the time of day the adolescent starts using the substance (Table 23–5). If the adolescent is female, do not omit the menstrual history. Include the age of onset, last menses, frequency, regularity, flow, pain, and if school absenteeism occurs because of menstrual pain.

TABLE 23–3. COMPONENTS OF THE SEXUAL HISTORY

- Onset of intercourse
- Age of first partner
- Number of partners in lifetime
- Number of partners in past 6 months
- Pregnancy
- Sexually transmitted disease
- Contraceptive history
- Current partner
- Gender of partner

TABLE 23–4. COMPONENTS OF THE SOCIAL HISTORY

- Friends
- Family
- School
- Grades in school
- Extracurricular activities
- Employment
- Plans and goals

TABLE 23–5. COMPONENTS OF SUBSTANCE ABUSE HISTORY*

- Age of onset
- Most recent use
- Blackouts
- Most recent episode of intoxication
- Time of day use begins

*Including nicotine, alcohol, marijuana, steroids, inhalants, cocaine, lysergic acid diethylamide (LSD), phenylcyclohexyl piperidine (PCP), stimulants, prescription drugs, gamma-hydroxybutyrate (GHB), methamphetamine, and ecstasy.

TABLE 23–6. REVIEW OF SYSTEMS FOR ADOLESCENTS

- Diet
- Exercise
- Sleep
- Mood
- Weight change and ideal weight
- Stress
- Absenteeism
- Menstruation

REVIEW OF SYSTEMS

To uncover issues specific to the adolescent, do a review of systems that focuses on activities, mood, and health habits (Table 23–6).

MEDICAL QUESTIONNAIRES

Medical questionnaires that adolescents can fill out alone are useful and save time in the clinic setting. The questionnaire should contain items that identify at-risk teens (Table 23–7). Many times, parental assistance is necessary.

IMMUNIZATIONS

At present, adolescents should receive a tetanus (Td) booster and the second measles, mumps, and rubella (MMR); hepatitis B (if the adolescent was not previously immunized); hepatitis A (if in an area of high prevalence of the disease), varicella (if the adolescent did not have the disease); and meningococcal (if the adolescent is preparing for college) vaccines. If an adolescent has chronic health problems, consider Pneumovax and flu vaccines. Check the Website of the Centers for Disease Control and Prevention (*www.cdc.gov*) for updates on immunization recommendations.

TABLE 23–7. AT-RISK ADOLESCENT BEHAVIORS IDENTIFIED ON MEDICAL QUESTIONNAIRE

- Cutting school
- Changing friends or involvement with a gang
- A change in behavior, violent behavior, or boredom with life
- Having a problem with the law; getting arrested
- Conflicts with parents, rebellious behavior, or changes in personality
- Drug and alcohol abuse
- Running away from home
- Sexual acting-out behavior

Hay, W. W., Hayward, A. R., Levin M. J., & Sondheimer, J. M. (1999). *Current pediatric diagnosis & treatment.* New York: McGraw-Hill.

PHYSICAL EXAMINATION

PHYSICAL GROWTH: HEIGHT AND WEIGHT

Adolescents have growth spurts that usually peak at age 12 years in girls and age 14 years in boys. Adolescents nearly double in weight during puberty. The organs double in size except for lymphoidal tissue, which decreases in mass. Before puberty, boys and girls have about the same amount of muscle mass. In boys, muscle mass enlarges with the increase in testosterone level, which elevates by a factor of about 20 late in puberty. Coordination of the muscles increases with strengthening of the muscles. Evaluating an adolescent's growth chart is very important in determining normal progression. A careful evaluation of the parents is also important so as not to miss what is normal for this teen's genetics. If a teen is below the 50th percentile and the parents are small, this is most likely normal growth for this teen's genetic makeup. A genogram of three generations should be explored if a child is large or small for his or her age group. Refer to *www.ormedassoc.org* for guidelines for adolescent services.

VITAL SIGNS

Temperature

The normal temperature for adolescents is 98.6°F. The temperature for young women who are ovulating can increase 0.5 to 1.0°F. Some young women do not ovulate in the first 1 to 2 years after starting menses. Fluctuations in temperatures include diurnal changes of 1.0 to 1.5°F. These changes are different for each person. Some peak in the morning, and others peak in the afternoon or evening. Temperatures also fluctuate with illness, dehydration, strenuous exercise, and stress.

Pulse

The radial artery pulse should be used for adolescents. The normal pulse for teens depends on age (Table 23–8). Fluctuations in heart rate may be caused by activity, illness, or even eating disorders. Adolescents who are devoted athletes may have a resting heart rate of 50 to 60 beats per minute. Immature teens may continue to have variations of heart rate with the respiratory cycle; that is, the heart rate increases with inspiration and decreases with expiration. Teens who have eating disorders may have bradycardia (a pulse of ≤ 60 beats per minute).

Respiration

The respiratory rate for teens is 12 to 20 breaths per minute. Alterations in respiration are the same as in adults, including disease process and autonomic nervous system effects on respiration.

TABLE 23–8. NORMAL PULSE RATES FOR TEENS	
Age, Years	Beats per Minute
12–13	70–110
14–15	Girls: 65–105
	Boys: 60–100
16–17	Girls: 60–100
	Boys: 55–95
18–21	Girls: 55–95
	Boys: 50–90

Blood Pressure

Blood pressure should be monitored yearly after the age of 3 years. Remember to use the correct width of blood pressure cuff, which covers 50% to 75% of the upper arm. The cuff bladder should not overlap the arm, just encircle it. The upper thigh and popliteal artery may be used instead of the brachial artery in the arm. The normal blood pressure for adolescents is a systolic range of 100 to 120 mm Hg and diastolic range of 50 to 70 mm Hg.

HAIR

Adolescents may show independence and peer pressure with their hairstyles. It seems that anything goes, from shaving the entire head to dreadlocks (Fig. 23–1). Coloring encompasses every color in the rainbow from black to black with white roots, white with black roots, to multicolored hair. Coloring chemicals can harm the hair and scalp. Coloring products also can be food substances such as Jell-O, Kool-Aid, and fruit jellies. Teens may quickly lengthen their hair by applying hair extensions, which are long pieces of either human or synthetic hair glued on the existing hair shaft. This process usually causes hair loss because it is difficult to comb through the hair extensions without pulling out some of the natural hairs. African-American adolescents may have dry hair that easily breaks and tangles and may want to cornrow their hair to eliminate tangles or to make natural dreadlocks. Cornrows are tight braids that are close to the scalp. With these braids, the hair may be pulled out, causing alopecia. Examine the scalp closely to check for lesions or breakage. Persistent dandruff may be caused by tinea or seborrhea. Dandruff may be caused by teens' washing their hair too frequently and drying out the scalp.

EYEBROWS

Eyebrows may be pierced or shaved. Shaved eyebrows may never grow back. Also, scars from piercing may interfere with the normal growth of eyebrow hair.

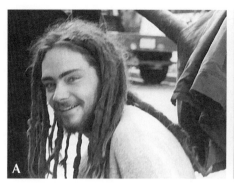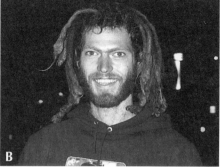

FIG. 23–1. Examples of dreadlocks.

NAILS

The nails can provide clues about diseases. Renal, dermatologic, hematopoietic, respiratory, or hepatic conditions may be evident in the nails. Inspect the nails for shape, color, size, brittleness, grooves, transverse lines, increased white lines, and hemorrhages (see Chapter 15).

SKIN AND FACE

With increasing hormones, adolescents' sebaceous and apocrine glands enlarge and become more active. Axillary sweat and body odor increase. Eccrine glands are fully developed and respond to heat and emotions. Androgen and other hormones cause the sebaceous glands to increase sebum production, causing acne. Facial hair increases because of testosterone and androgen changes. You should evaluate acne for scarring and adjust therapy as necessary. A referral to a dermatologist may be required for difficult acne.

Adolescents may mark, brand, or pierce their bodies (Fig. 23–2) to be accepted by peers or to show independence from their parents. Tattooing (Fig. 23–3) often links gangs or peers and is often a form of identification. Document any tattoo, branding, or piercing, and evaluate it for any infection. Ask the teen about the meaning of and feelings about tattoos. Also ask the teen about piercing of the genitals. Examination and documentation of the piercing for infection or possible injury are needed. Some penile piercing may cause vaginal damage with coitus. Consult with the patient and the parent if the piercing seems dangerous to others.

EYES

Assess teens for problems with their vision. Ask if the client can see the blackboard at school or participate in sports. Adolescents may need to wear glasses but not want to because of not feeling attractive to peers or the opposite gender. Adolescents may opt to wear contact lenses. Care of the teen's corneas should be evaluated if contact lenses are being used. Teens sometimes wear contact lenses just to change the color of their eyes. Ask the teen

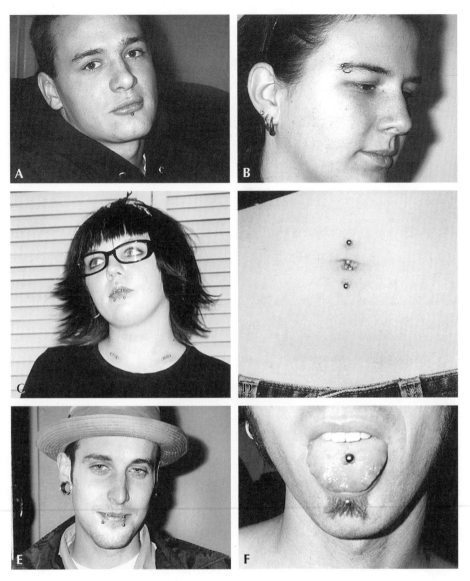

FIG. 23–2. Examples of body piercing.

about cleaning their contact lenses. Give guidance to the teen and the parent about safety glasses when participating in sports. Visual acuity should be evaluated with a standard Snellen eye chart. Evaluate the eyelid for fasciculations or tremors, which can be a sign of hyperthyroidism. Make sure the eyelid closes completely and can open wide without lag. If one eyelid covers more of the iris than the other or extends over the pupil, ptosis may be present. A weakness of the levator muscle may indicate a congenital or

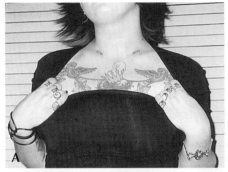

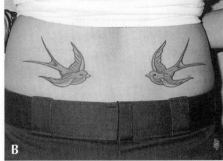

FIG. 23–3. Examples of tattooing.

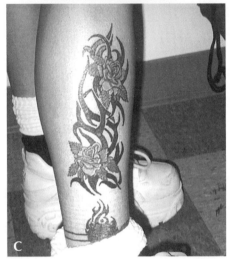

acquired weakness or a paresis of the third cranial nerve. Record the differences of the eyelids in millimeters. Drawing a picture of the differences helps to record the abnormality.

EARS

Examine adolescents' ears with an emphasis on acuity by using the whisper test. If there is a question of decreased hearing acuity, perform the Weber and Rinne tests (see Chapter 5). Listening to loud music may cause some hearing loss. Some music is accentuated by speakers purchased for extreme decibels, enclosed in cars or "boom boxes," which the teens turn up to attract other teens.

NOSE

During puberty, the nose grows as well as the sphenoid sinuses. Usually, the nose reaches its full size by age 16 years in young women and age 18 years in young men. Frontal sinuses can be transilluminated in clients after age 10 years.

MOUTH

The incidence of malocclusion, which is any deviation from absolutely straight teeth, can be as high as 90% in adolescents. Crooked teeth occur only in 10% to 15% of patients. Abnormal dental occlusion may predispose teens to caries or periodontal disease, or increase their susceptibility to trauma of the mouth, root resorption, temporomandibular joint disorders, muscular dysfunction, speech defects, or masticatory disturbances. Orthodontic treatment is usually sought because of appearance or because other peers have braces. Suspect malocclusion if a teen is a "mouth breather," "was a thumb or finger sucker," or used a pacifier as an infant or child. Ask the parent about early childhood pacifiers, and examine the teen's teeth for crowding, crooked bite, and trauma to the mucosa.

Teens who have orthodontic corrective braces need to be assessed for caries and trauma to the lips and inner mouth. An orthodontist usually does this, but it is a good practice to ask teens about their braces and how they are tolerating the treatment.

Some teens pierce their tongues or lips, or even between their teeth. A tongue piercing is a device that has a bar left inside the tongue with a ball of different sizes, usually on the top of the tongue and a screw on the end under the tongue. Adolescents who have tongue piercing are susceptible to infection because of the normal bacteria in the mouth and may experience pain caused by using a muscle that moves often to eat, drink, and talk. The threat of the metal device's tapping the hard palate and teeth is a constant problem. Often teens acquire the piercing without the permission of the parent. Advise parents to accept the teen's piercing unless the teen has an infection, trauma, or handicap because of it. You may need to give comfort to the parents about passing fads and ways to repair piercings if or when the teen decides to remove the piercing device.

Evaluate the mouth and neck for evidence of bulimia. The inside of the teeth may be eroded because of constant vomiting. The parotid glands also may be enlarged with constant vomiting. Additionally, a scar on the dorsal surface of the chosen finger may be present.

TONGUE

Dryness of the tongue may be caused by chronic mouth breathing. The texture of the tongue is important because it may indicate disease. A red or strawberry tongue is seen in individuals with scarlet fever. Herpes, which includes blisters and ulcers, may involve the tongue. A geographic tongue, in which the surface has an appearance of several borders, may indicate that the teen has an underlying allergic disease. Fine tremors of the tongue indicate that the adolescent needs to be evaluated for a central nervous system disease.

NECK

The neck needs to be examined for range of motion and tenderness. The thyroid gland is rarely palpable in normal children, so the thyroid may not be palpable in early and middle adolescents. Late or more mature adolescents' thyroid glands should be examined as an adult's would be. The thyroid gland increases approximately 10 times in weight from birth to puberty, and most of the growth occurs during puberty. The thyroid cartilage increases in boys more than in girls.

The trachea should be midline but can be within 4 mm to the right. It is best to inspect the trachea at the end of inspiration with the teen taking a deep breath. Examine the trachea for tracheal tug by inspecting the trachea while the teen is seated. Examine the teen with his or her mouth closed and chin fully elevated. Hold the cricoid cartilage between your thumb and index finger, and press upward. Have the teen take a breath and evaluate for a tug.

The lymph nodes need to be evaluated for lymphadenopathy. By the end of adolescence, the tonsils decrease in size to adult dimensions. Anterior cervical nodes are associated with upper respiratory infections and dental infections. Adenopathy found in posterior nodes is seen in individuals with infections of the middle ear and scalp. Viral disease such as measles, rubella, or mononucleosis is seen as generalized adenopathy. When checking the supraclavicular nodes superiorly, have the teen perform a Valsalva maneuver, which increases intrathoracic pressure and exposes the nodes more.

CHEST AND LUNGS

Examine the chest and lungs to evaluate size, symmetry, movement with respiration, tenderness or masses, and breast characteristics. Evaluate by observation, percussion, and auscultation. Adolescents can be examined with a regular adult stethoscope. Teens may have episodes of inadequate oxygenation because the respiratory system seems to grow slower than the rest of the body. Boys' lungs mature slower than girls' lungs but also have a greater vital capacity because boys have a greater chest size. Teens reach adult vital capacity by age 17 to 18 years. Ask the adolescent if he or she has problems when playing sports. If symptoms of asthma are mentioned, the teen should be evaluated by having him or her run in a hallway or around the building to evaluate for symptoms of exertional asthma.

BREASTS

Development of breast tissue is stimulated by estrogen. The shape of the breast is caused mostly by fat deposits. If a child is very thin, the fat may be deposited slower than in a child who is obese. Female breasts often develop asymmetrically and progress in several stages. A total of 25% of women have asymmetrical breasts, even into adulthood. Usual causes of this pattern include unilateral breast hypoplasia, absence of the pectoralis major muscle, and a unilateral hypertrophy or massive enlargement of breast tissue during adolescence. The areolar diameter starts to enlarge usually between ages 8 and 13 years and is completed by ages 12 to 19 years. Enlarging breasts usually exhibit an "achy" pain when developing. Adolescent boys may develop transient unilateral or bilateral firmness. Sometimes, painful subareolar masses occur that disappear within 1 year of onset. Teens must be reassured that this is temporary and will resolve. Boys who develop breast tissue after onset of puberty may be using marijuana or anabolic steroids, which can increase breast mass. The Tanner scale is used to describe sexual maturity with breasts and pubic hair (see Chapter 3).

HEART

During adolescence, the heart grows faster than the blood vessels. Some teens may develop chest pains during activity because of this lack of vessel growth. Sinus arrhythmia is normal during the adolescent years. Athletic teens may have a heart rate in the range of 40 to 60 beats per minute. Murmurs need to be evaluated to determine whether they are innocent or pathologic. Innocent murmurs occur in 50% of the adolescent population. These innocent murmurs are unassociated with any radiographic, electro-cardiographic, or symptomatic evidence of heart disease. They have several characteristics in common. They are best heard with the bell of the stethoscope because they are low-pitched sounds. They are musical or vibratory, and their intensity is no greater than I/VI to II/VI. They are heard most commonly at the second left interspace or the lower left sternal border and at the apex. The murmurs are heard early in systole and are short in duration. Another common location to listen to innocent murmurs is to have the child sitting and listen above or beneath the clavicles. This murmur is called a venous hum.

An adolescent with hypertension should be evaluated for renal disease. Anxiety needs to be ruled out because the teen simply may be anxious in the office or anxious in general.

A review of family hypertension should be completed because essential hypertension may be more prevalent than was previously believed. If available, have the school nurse or another healthcare provider check the teen's blood pressure in a noninvasive setting. Children with pectus excavatum need to be evaluated yearly to ensure that the heart is not crowded by the misshaped sternum and limited thoracic space.

ABDOMEN

Young adolescents may still exhibit scaphoid abdomen unless they are obese. In adolescents, the abdomen changes to an adult shape. The capacity of the stomach reaches 1.0 to 1.5 L, and the amount of gastric acid increases. Appetites increase or decrease, depending on peer influence. If a teen believes that he or she is overweight, an eating disorder may appear during the adolescent years. A patient who complains of stomach pain should be evaluated for anxiety, gastric ulcers, constipation, and sexual abuse.

During adolescence, the liver reaches adult size. Liver enlargement and tenderness need to be evaluated to determine whether the adolescent has a serious, life-threatening disease. The size of the liver is evaluated by estimating the span and height in the right midclavicular line and using the edge of the ribcage as a borderline. Acceptable margins are one to two finger-breadths below the right costal margin.

The scratch test is valuable for obese adolescents. This is a test to determine the lower portion of the liver by auscultation. The stethoscope's diaphragm is placed just above the right costal margin in the midclavicular line. Starting below the umbilicus, scratch the skin upward. The sound of the scratching becomes dull when you reach the edge of the liver.

The edges of the liver may be altered with hyperinflation of the lungs, pneumothorax, retroperitoneal mass, or perihepatic abscess. Structural abnormalities, such as narrow costal angles, flared costal margins, pectus excavatum, and accessory lobes, also can displace the liver. Hepatomegaly can be found in asymptomatic teens. Information about nutrition, exposure to hepatotoxins, and geographic exposure to possible infections should be explored.

In girls, some abdominal pain may be caused by dysmenorrhea. Adolescents who are starting menstruation may have anxiety monthly if menstrual cramping is severe. A total of 80% of cases of primary dysmenorrhea occur in teens and women in their early 20s. The pain occurs the first day or two of menstruation and is associated with diarrhea, nausea, and vomiting. The pain is located in the suprapubic area and radiates to the back. Even though this is considered a gynecologic problem, many teens and parents describe this pain as abdominal rather than pelvic. The teen should be assessed for primary and secondary dysmenorrhea. Primary dysmenorrhea is painful uterine contractions that are caused by prostaglandin release. Primary dysmenorrhea does not have pelvic pathology. Secondary dysmenorrhea is painful uterine contractions caused by several identifiable causes. The pain may be caused by problems that are external to the uterus as in endometriosis, tumors, adhesions, and nongynecologic causes. Secondary dysmenorrhea may be caused by leiomyomas or adenomyosis, which occur within the wall of the uterus. Polyps and infections can cause pain within the cavity of the uterus and are also considered causes of secondary dysmenorrhea. Sometimes ovulation can cause severe enough abdominal pain (Mittelschmerz) to send an adolescent to the hospital with suspected appendicitis.

Because of the erratic eating behavior of teens, constipation often occurs. Fast foods and fatty, high-sugar, and salty foods are devoid of most fiber. Busy adolescents often do not take the time to have a bowel movement and may become constipated. Bowel movements should be discussed at each visit for frequency, amount, and consistency of the stools.

MUSCULOSKELETAL SYSTEM

The growth of the trunk and extremities in the child will predict growth of bone, muscle, and adipose tissue. Stature growth predominates first in the lower extremities before puberty and then in the trunk during puberty. The trunk needs to be assessed for scoliosis, which is usually best observed in children between the ages of 6 and 12 years (see Chapter 12). Scoliosis is most often found in pubertal girls.

The distal extremities achieve adult size before the proximal extremities. This is one reason preadolescent children have feet that appear too large for their bodies. Ossification of growth cartilage and union of the epiphyses and diaphyses of long bones are completed by age 25 years of age. Shin splints, which produce extreme leg pain and inflammation, are caused by overuse of the muscles originating from the shaft of the tibia. This happens more often in adolescents who are not properly conditioned and do not warm up before exercising. Shin splints are a problem for teens who run on hard or uneven surfaces, wear improper shoes, or have an anatomical abnormality. The teen will complain of an aching pain over the medial tibia that increases with exercise and decreases with rest.

The muscles increase in number, size, and length throughout childhood. The ratio of muscle mass to body weight is 1:4 to 1:5 at birth, 1:3 at early adolescence, and 2:5 in early maturity. Muscle mass increases earlier in girls to age 10 years. Boys catch up and surpass girls after age 14 years. Boys have greater shoulder width, and longer arms and legs compared with their trunks. Growing pains have unknown etiology but are possibly caused by edema of muscles within tight fascial sheaths during periods of activity or overuse.

The gait of the teen should be evaluated for deviations. The normal gait is divided into phases: heel strike, flat foot, midstance, and push off. The width of a normal base measures about 2 to 4 inches from heel to heel. The normal forward step measures about 15 inches, depending on the length of the leg. The hip, or center of gravity, oscillates vertically approximately 2 inches. If this center of gravity is more than 3 to 4 inches, the teen will limp. Limps should be evaluated early in a child's progression. If an adolescent has a limp that was not recognized in childhood, a sports injury should first be suspected. Children between the ages of 9 and 16 years who present with knee pain and a limp should be examined for slipped femoral capital epiphysis. This problem is most common in sedentary, obese male adolescents. The main complaint is aches and pains in the groin or referred pain in the knee, along with a limp. The teen may have a dislocation of the head of the femur, which can be rather sudden. To test for this disorder, examine abduction, internal rotation, and flexion of the hip to evaluate whether they are limited. If the diagnosis is missed, there is a poor prognosis because of the high risk of avascular necrosis.

Osgood-Schlatter disease is a degeneration of the tibial tubercle at the insertion site of the quadriceps ligament. This disease is associated with overuse and rapid growth spurts, which can result in micro stress fractures. Osgood-Schlatter disease can be evaluated by palpation over the tibial tubercle, which reveals painful swelling and point tenderness over the anterior aspect of the tubercle. Have the teen resist knee extension, which is painful if Osgood-Schlatter disease is present. Pain occurs with strenuous activity, which includes using the quadriceps muscles. After the injury has healed, recurrence of the pain can arise in 60% of adolescents until they have reached bone maturity at age 25 years. The teen may have permanent prominence of the tibial tubercle into adulthood.

Patellofemoral pain syndrome (PFPS) is the most common report in sports medicine, especially in teens who run. PFPS occurs more often in girls because of the increased width of the gynecoid pelvis, which exaggerates a "Q" angle with the knees. The teen will complain of dull, aching knee pain, which may be associated with popping and clicking of the knee when moving. The pain is often localized and is usually bilateral. The teen may report extreme pain, especially when sitting in class, running, climbing stairs, or going downhill. No erythema or swelling is present. You can elicit pain by palpating over the patella in the femoral groove or moving the patella laterally. Evaluate for femoral anteversion, external tibial torsion, ankle valgus, and excessive foot pronation. If PFPS is not diagnosed, the adolescent may develop chondromalacia patellae and patellofemoral degenerative arthritis as an adult.

If the teen presents with painful heels, the shoe always should be evaluated to ascertain if the shoe is the problem. The Achilles tendon also should be evaluated to rule out a partial avulsion if there is pain in the heel.

NEUROLOGIC SYSTEM

During the adolescent years, the brain continues to grow, and teens' cognitive development progresses (see Chapter 11). The number of neurons does not increase, but the cells that support and nourish them do increase. You should evaluate the adolescent's reading and cognitive abilities. An adolescent's mental status (see Chapter 28) should be evaluated with expectation of mood swings, confused thought, and resistance to authority.

SEXUAL CHANGES

Gonadotropin and sex steroid levels increase during preadolescence and early adolescence. Growth of the sexual organs and axillary and pubic hair may cause self-concept changes and doubts. Teens who are delayed or accelerated in sexual characteristics may have a shattered self-concept if their peers' comments about body changes or lack of body changes taunt the teen. During early adolescence (ages 11 to 13 years), the secondary sexual characteristics develop.

Girls

The earliest sign of puberty in girls is the widening of the pelvic girdle and breast budding, followed by pubic hair growth. Menarche occurs on the average of 12.7 years. Delayed adolescent development is defined for girls as the absence of breast buds by age 13 years or a lack of menses 4 years after the development of breast buds.

Boys

At the average age of 11.5 years, boys develop testicular growth. The testicles grow in length more than 2.4 cm and in volume 4 mL. This is followed by penile length growth and then pubic hair growth. These sexual growth spurts are followed by height growth spurts. For boys, delayed adolescent development is defined as the lack of testicular growth or phallic enlargement by age 14 years.

 # NUTRITIONAL HEALTH ISSUES

ANOREXIA NERVOSA AND BULIMIA

Eating disorders can start as a temporary way to eliminate calories. It has been found that if the pattern of bingeing, purging, or dieting is established, it can be difficult to alter. Some adolescents become addicted to using the eating disorder as a coping mechanism to eat what they want but not alter their bodies. One study of girls in Iowa found that 46% of the girls interviewed wished they were thinner. This study showed that 21% of the girls often felt guilty when they ate foods that could make them fat. A study of 1599 girls in a South Carolina middle school showed that the girls tried to lose weight by dieting (43%), fasting (11%), vomiting (6%), using laxatives (2%), or taking diuretics (2%).

Both anorexic and bulimic adolescents have the same negative self-image, which is influenced by weight and body shape. Teens with eating disorders also may be perfectionists and want a body that American society believes is beautiful. Another reason teens develop eating disorders is that they have a sense of personal ineffectiveness and have had difficulties with communication and conflict resolution. Teens with anorexia or bulimia are often girls, but boys do participate in this practice, especially if they compete in sports that have a weight requirement that is difficult to achieve. Questions to ask during the history are provided in Table 23–9.

OBESITY

The best measurement is underwater weight, but using the triceps skin fold is the most practical way to measure obesity in teens. To evaluate an adolescent at risk for obesity, ask how long the adolescent has been overweight and about the history of family obesity. Also ask how much time is spent exercising, watching television, playing video games, or using the computer. Determine whether there have been any previous attempts to lose weight, if the attempts were successful, if the teen is ready to lose weight, and if the teen's friends comment about the weight problem. Also consider type 2 diabetes as a source of the obesity.

VEGETARIAN OR VEGAN ADOLESCENTS

Approximately 2% of the adolescent population in America claims a "meat-free" diet. Most vegetarians in America are ovolactovegetarians who eat egg

TABLE 23–9. QUESTIONS TO ASK REGARDING ANOREXIA AND BULIMIA

1. Do you feel good about your body?
2. Do you think you eat too much?
3. What do you do when you are over your goal weight? When you have eaten too much? When you have eaten high-calorie foods?
4. Do you like to eat alone?
5. Do you need to take laxatives? How often?
6. Do you have a sore throat most of the time?
7. How often do you exercise?

Examination of these clients includes observation of:

- Height and weight
- Mouth and throat examination: palatal trauma (i.e., pharyngeal stimulation)
- Parotid gland examination (the gland usually inflamed if the client is constantly vomiting)
- Dental erosion because the enamel is chemically "eaten" by hydrochloric acid from the stomach
- Metacarpal-phalangeal bruises or calluses, which are constant abrasions, even scars, on the base of the index finger or finger used in purging
- Vital signs, bradycardia (a resting heart rate of ≤ 60 beats per minute is often found in anorexics), bradypnea, hypotension, hypothermia, and poor capillary refill
- Evaluate hydration state
- Scaphoid abdomen or organomegaly
- Skin edema of extremities (loss of protein)
- Mental state, including apathy, psychomotor retardation, depression, anxiety, obsessive-compulsive traits

and dairy products; however, vegans eat no animal products. The advantage to this is that vegetarian/vegan adolescents usually have lower weight, blood pressure, and cholesterol than in nonvegetarian/nonvegan teens. Vegetarians seem to get adequate protein and calorie contents as well as fiber. Some nutrients that are lacking in the vegetarian diet are iodine, vitamin B_{12}, vitamin D, and some essential fatty acids. It is wise for vegetarian adolescents to take a multivitamin and mineral supplement daily. Vegans are more at risk for deficiencies because of the dairy limitation. These teen should be guided to produce that is high in calcium such as dark, leafy vegetables, especially broccoli; calcium-enriched orange juice; and soymilk. Herbs such as horsetail or molasses also may be used as calcium supplements. General nutritional requirements for adolescents are listed in Table 23–10.

PREGNANT ADOLESCENTS

Pregnant adolescents have twice the mortality rate of nonadolescent expectant mothers because the mother is still growing herself. The growth of the mother and the fetus is hindered because they compete for the nutrients. The weight gain for adolescent mothers should be 25 lb if the woman is over-

TABLE 23–10. NUTRITIONAL REQUIREMENTS OF ADOLESCENTS

Nutrient	Age	Daily Requirement
Water	11–19 y	50 mL/kg
Protein	≤19	30 mL/kg
	All ages	45–56 g
Calories*	Girls 11–14 y	2200 cal
	Boys 11–14 y	2700 cal
	Girls 15–18 y	2400 cal
	Boys 15–18 y	3000 cal
Calcium[†]	All ages	1200 mg
Iron[†]	Boys 11–18 y	12 mg
	Girls 11–24 y	15 mg
Zinc[†]	Boys 11–18 y	15 mg
	Girls 11–18 y	12 mg
Iodine	All ages	150 mg
Phosphorus	All ages	1200 mg
Selenium	Boys 11–14 y	40 mg
	Girls 11–14 y	45 mg
	Boys 15–18 y	50 mg
	Girls 15–18 y	50 mg
Vitamin A	Boys 11–18 Y	1000 mg
	Girls 11–18 y	800 mg
Vitamin D	All ages	10 mg
Vitamin E	Boys 11–18 y	10 mg
	Girls 11–18 y	18 mg
Vitamin K	Boys and girls 11–14 y	45 mg
	Boys 15–18 y	65 mg
	Girls 15–18 y	55 mg
Vitamin C	Boys and girls 11–14 y	50 mg
	Boys and girls 15–18 y	60 mg
Thiamin	Boys 11–14 y	1.3 mg
	Girls 11–18 y	1.1 mg
	Boys 15–18 y	1.5 mg
Riboflavin	Boys 11–14 y	1.5 mg
	Girls 11–18 y	1.3 mg
	Boys 15–18 y	1.8 mg
Niacin	Boys 11–14	17 mg
	Girls 11–14 y	15 mg
	Boys 15–18 y	20 mg
	Girls 15–18 y	15 mg
Vitamin B_6	Boys 11–14 y	1.7 mg
	Girls 11–14 y	1.4 mg
	Boys 15–18 y	2.0 mg
	Girls 15–18 y	1.5 mg
Folate	Boys and girls 11–14 y	150 mg
	Boys 15–18 y	200 mg
	Girls 15–18 y	180 mg
Vitamin B_{12}	All ages	2 mg

*Adjust calories for degree of activity or pregnancy.
[†]Note: Girls are susceptible to decreased calcium, zinc, and iron because of menses and dieting.

weight and 40 lb if she is underweight. Another requirement is 60 g of protein per day. Requirements for vitamins (except vitamins A and D) are increased during pregnancy. Folic acid, 1 mg a day, should have been started before the pregnancy to reduce neural tube defects.

ADOLESCENT ATHLETES

The caloric intake of adolescent athletes must contain 60% to 75% of calories from carbohydrates, 15% to 20% of calories from protein (1.5 g/kg/d), and less than 20% to 30% fat intake.

Hydration is very important for adolescent athletes. Athletes should drink 1 quart of caffeine-free fluid for every 1000 calories consumed and 2 cups of water or sport drink 2 hours before exercise. After exercise, 16 oz of fluid should be consumed for every pound lost.

CHOLESTEROL SCREENING

Cholesterol, a sterol (not a fat), is important in metabolism and the production of bile acid, vitamin D, adrenocortical steroids, and sex hormones. Diets that are high in cholesterol produce heart disease. The Committee on Nutrition of the American Academy of Pediatrics recommends that adolescents with a family history of high cholesterol need to be screened for high blood pressure and high cholesterol. The American College of Physicians does not believe that adolescents need to be screened until age 25 to 30 years for men and age 35 to 40 for women. Diseases that may increase cholesterol are diabetes mellitus, hypothyroidism, chronic renal failure, nephrotic syndrome, biliary atresia, and cholestatic liver disease. Medications also may increase cholesterol, and teens taking them may need to be screened, especially if they are at risk for high cholesterol. These medications include anabolic steroids, oral contraceptives, anticonvulsants, cyclosporine, and 13-*cis*-retinoic acid.

The clinical decision to test the child for high cholesterol may be because of medication taken, a disease process, or family history of cardiac disease. Other reasons include identification of hypertension, obesity, planar cutaneous xanthomas (often at the site of injury), and thickening of the Achilles tendon. The child should be tested two to three times, and hypercholesterolemia should be confirmed before treatment is started. Fasting total cholesterol or low-density lipoprotein values are most accurate for initial testing. If the adolescent is to be considered for dietary management because the fasting total cholesterol is elevated, he or she should first be screened for high-density lipoprotein cholesterol (HDL-C) and triglycerides. Treatment is based on total cholesterol (TC) and low-density lipoprotein cholesterol (LDL-C). The adolescent should be treated with changes in the diet if he or she is in the 75th to 90th percentile (Table 23–11). A child in the 95th percentile and up should receive more intensive treatment with consideration of anticholesterol medications. Anticholesterol medications are limited

TABLE 23–11. LIPID REFERENCE VALUES (mg/dL) FOR CHILDREN AGES 3–19 YEARS				
Lipid Component	Value by Percentile			
	50%	75%	90%	95%
Cholesterol	155	175	190	200
LDL-C	95	110	125	135
HDL-C	52	60	68	73
Triglycerides	60	80	100	115

HDL-C = high-density lipoprotein cholesterol; LDL-C = low-density lipoprotein cholesterol.

in children because of dangers to the liver and growth enzymes. They are usually only considered if the child has a history of heterozygous familial hypercholesterolemia.

 # OTHER HEALTH ISSUES

SUBSTANCE ABUSE

Adolescents usually first use illicit drugs or alcohol because of experimentation or peer pressure. One factor that may encourage teens to use illicit drugs is the prior use of alcohol or tobacco, although it has been found that a number of teens initiate marijuana use without prior use of either alcohol or tobacco. Drug and alcohol use should be questioned at every visit. Some teens come forward without prodding because they may believe they are hurting their bodies. Others do not because they fear punishment or disappointment from their parents. You need to be concerned if a teen is having behavioral problems or deterioration in family life, athletic endeavors, or school performance. Physical problems related to drug use include sore throat, fatigue, cough, chest, abdominal pain, and headache. Chronic drug abuse may cause such problems as hepatitis, streptococcal arthritis, anorexia, weight loss, bacterial endocarditis, osteomyelitis, fever, convulsions, and renal disorders.

SUICIDE

Suicide is the third leading cause of death in adolescents aged 15 to 24 years. Girls make suicide attempts three to four times more often than boys. Approximately 25% of high school students think about suicide each year, 15% have a plan, 8% make some kind of attempt, and 2% get medical attention because of the suicide attempt. Most adolescents who think about or attempt suicide are overcome with stress or anger. Some are overachievers who have failed or are rejected. The majority of teens who commit or threaten suicide give clues to their distress. More than 60% of teens who state their suicidal wishes attempt to kill themselves within a 24-hour period. In one study, 70% of teens who did complete their suicide experienced a loss of

TABLE 23–12. SUICIDE INTERVIEW

- How have you been feeling lately?
- Have you been discouraged lately? For how long? How often?
- Do these down feelings interfere with your life?
- Do you have sleep or appetite disturbances?
- How is your schoolwork?
- How is your family life?
- How are your friends?
- Do you participate in sports?
- Do you feel helpless, hopeless, or worthless or want to give up?
- Are the feelings strong, and does life seem not worth living anymore?
- Do you have thoughts of suicide?
- Do you have a plan?
- Do you have the means to carry out the plan?
- How strong are these feelings?
- Does it take a lot of effort to resist the feelings?
- Can you tolerate the pain you are feeling?
- What deters you from carrying out your plan?
- If the feeling to commit suicide is subsiding, can you resist the temptation if it returns?
- Who is there for you if you need help?
- Has this idea of taking your life come up in the past? When? How often?
- What happened during those times?
- Can we make a contract that you will not hurt yourself now and you will ask for help if you need it?

Adapted from Hay (2001). p. 177. Hay, W. W., Hayward, A. R., Levin M. J., & Sondheimer, J. M. (1999). *Current pediatric diagnosis & treatment*. New York: McGraw-Hill.

some kind such as rejection by a person, girlfriend, or boyfriend; an arrest; or failure of some kind. Questions to ask teens regarding suicide are provided in Table 23–12.

DEPRESSION

Similar to suicide, depression is usually caused by a loss. Losses include the loss of support through separation, divorce, or moving to a new school. Additionally, loss of friendships as a result of quarrels, fights, or even death can cause depression. The loss may be caused by a failure such as the inability to maintain a grade or status. You should look for signs of academic deterioration or changes in behavior. Teens may be withdrawn from friends and family or even change friends abruptly. Questions about drugs, arrests, sexual acting-out behavior, rebellious behavior, and running away from home need to be explored. Somatic complaints need to be evaluated, sometimes with laboratory tests. A complete blood count, sedimentation rate, thyroid function tests, and Venereal Disease Research Laboratory Test (VDRL) need to be considered. Symptoms of depression are given in Table 23–13.

TABLE 23–13. SYMPTOMS OF MAJOR DEPRESSION

- Depressed mood
- Markedly diminished interest in normal pleasurable activities
- Significant weight loss or gain
- Insomnia or hypersomnia
- Psychomotor agitation or retardation
- Fatigue or loss of energy
- Indecisiveness
- Feelings of worthlessness or excessive or inappropriate guilt
- Diminished ability to think or concentrate; problems at school
- Recurrent thoughts of death; recurrent suicidal ideation

Adapted from American Psychiatric Association, Committee on Nomenclature, *Diagnostic and Statistical Manual of Mental Disorders* (3rd ed., rev.). Washington, DC: American Psychiatric Association; 1987. Reproduced by permission of the publisher.

ANTICIPATORY GUIDANCE

Anticipatory guidance for adolescents should include growth and development (along with pubertal events), parenting, mortality and violence, sexuality issues (e.g., contraception, sexually transmitted diseases), and risk behaviors (e.g., bulimia and anorexia, drugs, depression).

GROWTH AND DEVELOPMENT

Present information to parents about the normal development of adolescents. This is usually the simplest form of intervention and often eliminates anxiety parents may have about their adolescent daughters and sons. Changing needs of teens need to be discussed with parents. Just as a teen may lock the bathroom or bedroom door at home to permit privacy, the parent needs to be aware that the adolescent may no longer want a parent present during the physical examination. The teen's maturing body may be a source of shame until the teen has come to grips with enlarging breasts or penis or the growth of pubic hair.

Explore parents' understanding about the normal progression of adolescents. Parents are often frustrated because they do not see the child as a "preadult" who demands to be treated differently from a child. Normal adolescent developmental progression is as follows:

1. To be separate from the parents
2. To be comfortable with a developed body and sexual identity
3. To formulate lasting relationships
4. To achieve a vocation and to become socially accepted and economically independent
5. To evaluate and develop a moral value system
6. To develop a relationship with one's parents that is based on equality

Parents' need to separate from the teen is also crucial. Parents usually want to prevent their children from making the same mistakes they have made. Often the parents' approach may be presented strongly, so it is rejected by the youth. You should explore the parents' feelings of mortality or loss or the destroyed dreams of their youth, which may be the source of conflict that blocks communication. Parents' conflicting feelings of loss, envy, hostility, and inability to know the future may coexist with love, pride, and satisfaction of what the youth is achieving. Some parents use their children to live out the part of their lives they could not achieve. For example, a parent who was not an athlete may encourage his or her child to be the captain of the team. In that way, the parent can live that part of life over again with achieved victory as a parent rather than as an athlete. You should listen for hidden messages from parents. With this information, the provider can guide the parent toward a better understanding of the adolescent's development and goals.

The adolescence period is a time of rapid growth. Teens gain 50% of their adult weight, 20% of their adult height, and 50% of their skeletal mass during puberty. Girls deposit twice as much fat as boys. Male teens double their lean body mass during this period. Specific nutritional deficiencies in calcium, iron, riboflavin, thiamin, and vitamins A and C commonly occur during adolescence. Obesity is part of the American culture, with more than one third of Americans being obese. Obesity is defined as 20% above normal guidelines. For typical American adolescents, dietary fat makes up one third of all calories consumed. One fourth of all vegetables consumed are French fries. The intake of sugars in processed products exceeds the intake of complex carbohydrates and fiber. Children who are obese and enter adolescence have a 1 in 4 chance of being obese as adults. If an adolescent is obese by age 18 years, the chance of being an obese adult is 1 in 28. Just before adolescence in girls, a "sorting out" process takes effect. Obesity is more prevalent in girls from higher socioeconomic classes. The opposite is true of boys; that is, boys from higher socioeconomic classes tend to be more obese than boys from lower socioeconomic classes. Boys of lower socioeconomic class and their fathers tend to be leaner.

PARENTING

You can guide parents toward understanding teens by providing information and encouraging reflection on how the parents felt when they were teens. To achieve productive guidance, be aware of communication skills, attitudes, and areas of personal conflict that may block information. The parent and the teen must come to a cohesive decision about activities with peers. The parent must try not to make arbitrary rules about dress, curfews, leisure time, and matters that may prevent the teen from taking part in the group activities unless the child could be harmed or forever altered by the activities, such as with tattoos, piercing, or eyebrow shaving.

Good friends help show teens when to plunge ahead and when to stop. It is almost impossible to choose the teen's peers. One way to determine what

is going on in school is to volunteer time in the classroom to evaluate interactions with teachers and peers at school.

MORTALITY AND VIOLENCE

A report from the Surgeon General provides guidelines (Table 23–14) to parents to help buffer the risk of violence and other problem areas adolescents
face. Parents should explore the adolescent's friendships and group pres-
sures at school. Parents should look for changes in eating or sleeping habits
or increasing violence in the teen.

A comprehensive study conducted in 1977 by the Harvard School of
Public Health found that one in five high-school teenage girls is a victim of
violence. Girls reported being "hit, slapped, shoved, or forced into sexual
activity" by boys they were dating. Often, girls do not tell their parents about
date violence because of the fear that they might be banned from seeing the
abusive person or their peers. Parents should inform their daughters that
they are still vulnerable when a person is bigger and stronger and that violence is unacceptable. Information that friendship also involves respect
should be taught throughout girls' lives.

Experimentation with speed, sports, sex, and weapons does not seem so
threatening to adolescents because of narcissistic ideas that nothing can hurt
them. The leading causes of death in teens include unintentional injury
(46.3% from motor vehicle accidents), homicides (18.3%), and suicides
(12.6%). The Youth Risk Behavior Surveillance Survey, a study of students in
grades 9 to 12, found that 72% of all deaths for school-aged youth were from
motor vehicle accidents or other unintentional injuries, homicide, and suicide.

Acting-out behavior is as normal for adolescents as nursing is for infants.
At least 20% of teens carry a weapon to school. Weapons in school can be as
common as nail files. Many schools check students for weapons. All
weapon-like items can be confiscated at the front door depending on the
nature of the weapon, and the adolescent may be expelled.

The American lifestyle has a profound effect on teens today. Television,
movies, and video games do not hesitate to show severed arms gushing out
blood or unspeakable mutilation of human beings in full color. Studies of the
effects of televised violence are consistent: Children learn aggression by
watching aggression. A study done in Canada showed that children were
more aggressive 2 years after television was introduced to their town. One
problem was that the children became more fearful because they believed
that aggression and violence were acceptable in the world just as it is on television. Violence is not a secret kept from the young, impressionable minds
of adolescents; even small children laugh at gore when they view it in
movies.

Some adolescents are inquisitive about death and what it really looks and
feels like to kill. Desensitization to what is real in life by video games may
actually train children to commit violence. The "point-and-shoot" video
games are similar to military training tools that condition soldiers to fire

TABLE 23–14. SURGEON GENERAL'S SUGGESTIONS OF PROPOSED PROTECTIVE FACTORS TO SAVE CHILDREN AND ADOLESCENTS FROM VIOLENCE

MONITOR THE INDIVIDUAL

- Develop an intolerant attitude toward deviant behavior. Any violent behavior is avoided. Develop an attitude of being a protector to the less fortunate.
- Encompass interests in education. It has been found that people with high IQs exhibit qualities such as curiosity and creativity. They develop artistic qualities and look for cultural experiences. A high IQ helps adolescents benefit from educational, creative, and cultural experiences, which may open doors to alternative values and lifestyles.
- Girls seem less impulsive and not as daring. Maybe the lower testosterone level helps create less aggression. (One factor suggesting that this is not true is that girl gang members seem to want to please their male counterparts by acting tough and more like aggressive gang members.)
- Being committed to school helps adolescents to be less tolerant of deviant behavior. Adolescents who are oriented into the school program have most likely adopted the traditional values and norms of the community.
- Peer disapproval of deviant behavior is important to adolescents. The risk of not being accepted by peers who have the belief that violence will not be tolerated usually stops individuals from being violent.

FAMILY

- Infants who experienced secure attachment to a parent or adult who met the infant's needs helps the adolescent develop trust and progress through stages of growth and development. This loving, supportive relationship helps the adolescent develop conventional behavior and disapproval of delinquent behavior.
- Supportive behavior before adolescence helps the teen make choices, but it has been found that this may be only an indirect pull from a choice for nondeviant behavior. Parents' positive evaluation of the adolescent's peers seems to help reduce the risk of delinquency.
- Parents must monitor and supervise activities as a protection against antisocial behavior and deviant behavior.

SCHOOL

- Develop a commitment to school. Teens who are committed to school develop goals and values to achieve success. Violence would jeopardize their achievements in school and compromise their goals.
- Teachers' approval is important to adolescents' development. Teachers who encourage teens help them seek continued education or job skills training.
- Extracurricular activities in music, art, drama, and school publications give adolescents opportunities to participate in constructive group activities, which may help them achieve recognition for their efforts.

PEER GROUP

- Friends who behave conventionally and do not believe in deviant behavior are a proposed protective factor that reduces the risk of delinquency. Teens who disapprove of violence may inhibit violence.

reflexively to overcome natural inclinations *not to kill*. An extreme example of violence occurred when two preteens dragged a toddler 2 miles through to a railway line, where they beat him with metal bars and bricks, put paint in his eyes, and placed him on the train tracks, where a train cut him in half. It was found that these teens wanted to kill the toddler to see if killing is as it is seen in the movies.

SEXUALITY ISSUES

Explore the adolescent's sexual history. If the teen is sexually active, discuss contraception options and sexually transmitted diseases. Access the laws for your state to determine what information can be given and to find out about treatment options and confidentiality issues.

RISK BEHAVIORS

Risk behaviors in adolescents include bulimia and anorexia, drugs, and bowing to peer pressure. Appropriate guidance for parents and children are needed to deal with these problems. See information previously discussed in this chapter for tips to give to families.

TEST YOUR KNOWLEDGE OF CHAPTER 23

1. What are the four phases that adolescents go through in passage into adulthood?
2. How do the three stages of adolescence differ?
3. What are stages of ego development and morality that adolescents should achieve?
4. How do peers affect adolescents' behavior, self-concept, and health?
5. What are the components of the approach to the health care of an adolescent?
6. What are the components of the health history of adolescents?
7. How does the review of systems differ with an adolescent?
8. What immunizations should adolescents receive?
9. Describe the changes in height, weight, and vital signs in adolescents.
10. How do body piercing, tattooing, and changing hair color and styles affect the health of adolescents?
11. What endocrine changes can be expected in adolescents?
12. What cardiovascular problems can occur in adolescents?
13. What are the components of a musculoskeletal examination of adolescents, and what problems frequently occur?
14. Explain the nutritional health issues of adolescents.

15. Describe the issues of suicide, depression, and substance abuse in adolescents.
16. What components should be addressed in the anticipatory guidance of adolescents and their parents?

BIBLIOGRAPHY

American Medical Association. (1995). *Guidelines for adolescent preventive services (GAP). Clinical evaluation and management handbook.* Chicago: American Medical Association, 54–55.

Burnett, G., & Walz, G. E. *Clearinghouse on Urban Education, http://Eric-web.tc. columbia.edu/digests/dig 99.htm*

Callahan, L. R. (2000). The evolution of the female athlete: Progress and problems. *Pediatric Annals, 29,* 149–153.

Dershewitz, R. A., (1993). *Ambulatory pediatric care* (2nd ed.). Philadelphia: J. B. Lippincott.

Dickens, C. (1998). *Oliver Twist.* New York: Tom Doherty Associates.

Fiera, M., & Pisco, J. D. (2000). *Field guide to the American teenager, a parent's companion.* Cambridge, MA: Perseus Publishing.

Goldbloom, R. B. (1997). *Pediatric clinical skills* (2nd ed.). New York: Churchill Livingstone.

Greif, J., & Hewitt, W. (1998). The living canvas, health issues in tattooing, body piercing and branding. *Advance for Nurse Practitioners,* June, 26–31.

Guiterrez, Y., & King, J. C. (1993). Nutrition during teenage pregnancy. *Pediatric Annals, 22,* 99–1908.

Hay, W., Hayward, A. R., Levin, M. J., & Sondheimer, J. M. (1999). *Current pediatric diagnosis & treatment.* New York: McGraw-Hill.

Halmi, K. A., Halmi, Mitchell, J. E., & Rigotti, N. A. (1995). Recognizing and treating eating disorders in adolescents. *Contemporary Adolescent Gynecology,* Winter, 13–22.

Hobbs, W. L., & Johnson, C. A. (1996). Anorexia nervosa: An overview. *American Family Physician,* Sept. 15, 1273–1279.

Hoekelman, R. A., Stanford, F. B., Nicholas, N. M., & Henry, S. M. (1987). *Primary pediatric care* (2nd ed.). St Louis: Mosby.

Jacobs, E. A., Copperman, S. M., & Joffe, A. (2000). Indications of management and referral of patients involved in substance abuse. *Pediatrics, 106,* 143–147.

Kirschmann, G. J., & Kirschmann, J. D. (1996). *Nutrition almanac* (4th ed.). New York: McGraw-Hill.

Kohlberg, I. (1976). Moral stages and moralization: The cognitive developmental approach. In T. Likma (Ed.). *Moral development and behavior: Theory, research, and social issues.* New York: Holt, Rinehart and Winston.

Konopka, G. (1973). Requirements for healthy development of adolescent youth. *Adolescence, 7,* 1–26.

Kreipe, R. E., & Dukarm, C. P. (1999). Eating disorders in adolescents and older children. *Pediatrics in Review, 20,* 410–420.

Ledigham, J. (2001). The effects of media violence on children. The National Clearinghouse on Family Violence, *http://www.media-awareness.ca/eng/med/ home/resource/famvlnc.htm*

Metzl, J. D. (2000). Sports medicine in pediatric practice: Keeping pace with the changing times. *Pediatric Annals, 29,* 146–148.

Montalto, N. J. (1998). Implementing the guidelines for adolescent preventive services. *American Family Physician, 57,* 2181–2190.

Muscari, M. E. (2001). *Advanced pediatric clinical assessment skills and procedures.* Philadelphia: J. B. Lippincott.

Newman, T. & Garber, A. (2000). Cholesterol screening in children and adolescent. *Journal of the American Academy of Pediatrics, 103,* 637–638.

Oski, F.A. (1994). Pubertal events and Tanner stage diagrams. In *Principles and practice of pediatrics.* Philadelphia: Lippincott.

Sankan, O. S. S. (1995). *The Maasai.* Kenya Literature Bureau: Nairobi.

Spock, B. (2001). The school years. In *The emotional and social development of children.* New York: Pocket Books.

Stashwick, C. (1996). When you suspect an eating disorder. *Contemporary Pediatrics, 13,* 124–153.

Wahl, R. (1999). Nutrition in the adolescent. *Pediatric Annals, 28,* 107–111.

Walz, G. (1999). *Gangs in schools*—ERIC Clearinghouse on Urban Education. *http://eric-web.tc.columbia.edu/digests/dig99.html.*

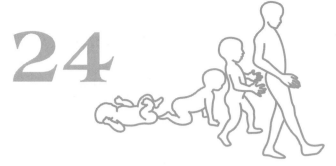

International Adoptees: Special Issues

TERRY GESULGA

OBJECTIVES
- List pertinent concerns to screen for in the examination of internationally adopted children.
- Obtain a broad health history of internationally adopted children.
- Follow a systematic approach in physical assessment of internationally adopted children.
- Confidently assess and refer adoptive families to resources as needed.

Adoption of international infants and children has increased to approximately 15,000 children per year. Recent media coverage of the joys and health problems of these children has made healthcare providers and families more aware of international adoption issues. The needs of internationally adopted children and their families are unique and are challenging for healthcare providers. A confident healthcare provider with knowledge of the adoption process and the importance of focused assessments and care can improve the quality of life for the child and his or her family. It is the responsibility of healthcare providers to feel confident in their counseling, physical assessment, and care of these adopted children and their families. This chapter highlights health concerns of internationally adopted children and helps focus the assessment of these children (Fig. 24–1).

HISTORY

The child's health history is often nonexistent. Existing information may be false or inaccurate because of numerous factors (Table 24–1). You must use

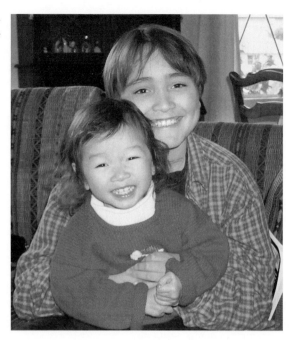

FIG. 24–1. International adoptee from Vietnam with adoptive mother.

existing resources to develop a thumbnail history that will help in planning care.

The credible medical health history often begins with you. The adopting parents should be urged to obtain any information they can by using a general guide during their interviews with the adoption agency, the orphanage, or the foster parents. Obtaining information using the health history guidelines in Table 24–2 will augment new healthcare providers' assessment and diagnostic skills. Actual and hypothetical information can be gathered by observing the child's natural setting and country of origin, and by interviewing the caretakers and agencies involved. Prospective parents should, however, be urged to use sensitivity and caution while obtaining data. They should explain their purpose and be open, accepting, and composed while collecting information. Prospective parents must not be disappointed if information is unobtainable and should be aware that some terms will be difficult for an interpreter to translate.

TABLE 24–1. INACCURATE HEALTH HISTORY

- Incomplete documents
- Lost documents
- Out-of-date information
- Falsified records, dates, treatments, names, information: Parents may not want to be identified
- Inaccurate records: Dates, medications, immunizations
- Language translation errors or unusual terminology
- Tests, examinations: Inefficient, without depth, faulty equipment or results

Date of birth: _____ Birth length: _____ Birth weight: _____ Gestational
   age at birth: _____
Present length and height: _____ Weight : _____ Age: _____
Occupation or socioeconomic status of Mother: _____ Father: _____
Parents' religion: _____
Siblings of child: _____
Diseases in the child's country of origin: _____
Diseases or health conditions often seen in children from this orphanage or region:
_____
_____

Prenatal history (actual, country or population norm): _____
Intrapartum history (vaginal, surgical C-section, complications): _____
_____

Postnatal care: _____
Reason for giving child for adoption: _____
Length of stay in institution or foster home: _____
Condition of institution:
   Physical facilities: _____
   No. of children at institution: _____
   Ages of children at institution: _____
   Caretaker-to-child ratio: _____
Feeding:
   Formula or food, type: _____
   Brand name of formula or food: _____
   Food supplements: _____
   Child food preferences: _____
   Times fed: _____ Usual amount: _____ Bottle prop: Y N
   Feeding concerns: Easy ___ Difficult ___ Slow ___ Fast ___ Regurgitation ___
   Strong or weak suck reflex ___ Colic ___ Time of day _____
GI Stools: How often ___ Amount ___ Loose ___ Formed ___ Hard ___ Soft ___
   Color_____ Mucus ___ Blood ___ Other_____
GU Urine: How often ___ Amount ___ Color _____ Odor ___ Clear ___
   Sediment ___ Blood ___ Mucus ___ Urgency ___ Pain ___
   ACTIVITY
Usual activities of daily living routine: _____
Describe child's usual routine: _____
Describe play time: What _____ When _____ How long _____
Child's activity preferences: _____
Evidence of sensory deprivation: Listless ___ Flat affect ___ No eye contact ___
Sleeping situation: Hours/day _____ Position _____
Sleep routine (describe): _____
Sleeping environment or condition (describe): _____

(continued)

IMMUNIZATION HISTORY

Immunizations are frequently not given or are poorly documented.
Sometimes when the forms are filled out too perfectly, they may be fraudu-
lent. Carefully analyze immunization records, including dates of immuniza-

LANGUAGE DEVELOPMENT: SHOULD BE ASSESSED BY SOMEONE FLUENT IN CHILD'S PRIMARY LANGUAGE

Is language age-appropriate? For example:

- Receptive language: 0–3 months: Attends to voice; turns head or eyes
  - 24 months: Seems to understand what is being said.
- Expressive language: 0–3 months: Undifferentiated but strong cry, coos, gurgles
  - 24 months: Names some body parts; imitates one or two words
- Intelligibility milestones: 1–2 years < 25% unintelligible to unfamiliar listener
  - 3 years: 70% to 80% in context

IMMUNIZATION HISTORY

Include the dates of these specific injections:

DTP/DtaP: _____

Hib: _____

IPV/OPV: _____

HBV: _____

HAV: _____

MMR: _____

Tetanus: _____

Varicella: _____

BCG for TB: _____

Allergies: Food _____ Drugs _____ Seasonal _____ Eczema _____

Lab test history (circle all that have been done; record results if available):

- CBC with differential (screen for hemoglobinopathy, anemia, infection): _____

- PKU (screen for metabolic disorder): _____
- Thyroid (screen for metabolic disorder): _____
- Lead (screen for lead exposure): _____
- Blood type (screen for risk for Rh incompatibility): _____
- ELISA/PCR (screen for HIV): _____
- Hepatitis A, B, and C surface antigen (screen for hepatitis): _____
- VDRL test, fluorescent treponemal antibody: _____
- Absorption test (FTA-ABS; screen for syphilis): _____
- Ova and parasites (O & P; screen for stool parasites): _____
- Mantoux PPD (screen for tuberculosis): _____

GROWTH AND DEVELOPMENT

Assess Dubowitz (gestational age): _____

Denver II Development Screening (ages 1 month–6 years): _____

(continued)

tion, spacing of immunizations, and age of the child. If immunization administration intervals are not appropriate, the immunization may not stimulate adequate antibodies. It is also possible that the immunization solution used lacked potency because of poor storage, solution expiration, or inaccurate dosing. It is safer to repeat the immunizations or draw the more expensive immunization blood titers if the records are questionable or if the children are from orphanages in Eastern Europe, China, or Russia. The Hib (*Haemophilus influenzae* type b), measles-mumps-rubella (MMR), and varicella vaccinations are the ones that are commonly missing. Additionally, a

REVIEW OF SYSTEMS

- EENT: Otitis media, visual problems, hearing problems
- Respiratory: URI, bronchiolitis, RSV infection, pneumonia, wheezing, cough
- Cardiovascular: Heart murmur, cyanotic spells, chest pain, palpitations, arrhythmia, anemia
- GI: Bowel movement, how often, consistency, diarrhea, constipation, GERD, parasites, colic
- GU: Urinary stream strong—boys, UTI, abuse, lesions and signs of abuse
- Neurological: Cognitive, reflexes, gait, trauma, head injury, head circumference, seizure
- Musculoskeletal: Gross and fine motor skills (these are almost always delayed, but catch-up is common), muscle tone, trauma, rickets
- Endocrine: Delay in growth and development, sleeping pattern, early puberty in girls, age assessment; referral after 12-month growth catch-up transition period
- Psychosocial: Bonding and affection; reactive attachment disorder
- Behavioral problems: Autistic-like, growth and development delays, physical, cognitive
- Language and developmental tasks, repetitive movements, obsessive, intolerant to change

BCG = Bacille Calmette-Guérin; CBC = complete blood count; DtaP = diphtheria, tetanus, acellular pertussis; ELISA = enzyme-linked immunosorbent assay; GERD = gastroesophageal reflux disease; GI = gastrointestinal; GU = genitourinary; HAV = hepatitis A vaccine; HBV = hepatitis B vaccine; Hib = *Haemophilus influenzae* type b; IPV = injectable polio vaccine; MMR = measles, mumps, and rubella; OPV = oral polio vaccine; PCR = polymerase chain reaction; PKU = phenylketonuria; PPD = purified protein derivative; Rh = rhesus; RSV = respiratory syncytial virus; TB = tuberculosis; URI = upper respiratory infection; UTI = urinary tract infection; VDRL = Venereal Disease Research Laboratories.

high percentage of internationally adopted children studied were not protected adequately against tetanus, diphtheria, and poliomyelitis. Be cautious when administering live low-dose virus immunization in chronically ill children or if a child's human immunodeficiency virus (HIV) status is unknown.

SCREENING TEST HISTORY

Many screening tests and examinations are performed routinely, and others should be performed as indicated based on the child's presentation or on the incidence of disease in the child's country of origin. Table 24–3 provides a list of recommended screening tests and examinations. Prescreening tests should not be encouraged before adoption if there is a risk of blood being drawn with contaminated needles. If possible, adopting parents should observe blood draws and supply sterile equipment. Many tests may have to be repeated for accuracy. Sometimes only the hematocrit, hemoglobin, HIV, and hepatitis surface antigen tests are performed in the child's country of origin (Table 24–4). The gold standard for medical evaluation of internationally adopted children is the American Academy of Pediatrics' *2000 Red Book: Report of the Committee on Infectious Diseases*, which has updated information

TABLE 24-3. RECOMMENDED SCREENING TESTS AND EXAMINATIONS FOR ALL INTERNATIONAL ADOPTEES

Test ALL children for the following:
- Urinalysis with microbiology
- CBC with differential and red blood cell indices*
- PKU if age <3 months
- Thyroid panel or TSH if developmental delay
- Lead screen (especially China)
- Mantoux intradermal skin test (PPD). Vaccination with BCG is not a contraindication because immunization from the BCG is not consistent. A follow-up PPD 12 months after arrival should be considered. Many false-negative results occur because of recent exposure or anergy secondary to chronic malnutrition or other infections.
- HbsAg,* especially Asia, Africa, Europe, Russia, Romania, China
- Stool for ova and parasites* if child shows growth delay (common parasites include *Giardia lamblia*, *Ascaris lumbricoides*, and *Trichuris trichiura*)
- Stool cultures if diarrhea is present (common organisms include *Salmonella* spp., *Shigella* spp., *Yersinia* spp., *Campylobacter* spp., *Escherichia coli*, and *Giardia* spp. [use *Giardia* antigen assay]); retest three times after treatment
- Metabolic panels, *Helicobacter pylori* if child shows growth and development delay
- Syphilis serology*: Rapid reagin test, RPD, VDRL; yaws and pinta can give false-positive VDRL result

ELISA for HIV, PCR if age <15 months or + ELISA*

Skin scraping: Scabies, lice, tinea corporis, tinea capitis, impetigo

Iron-deficiency anemia (Hgb/HCT, serum ferritin)

Vision, hearing, and dental examination

CMV if someone in the family is pregnant

Malaria screen if child shows febrile (common non-intestinal parasite): Giemsa-stained thick and thin smears of blood

---

Adapted from American Academy of Pediatrics (2000). Medical evaluation of internationally adopted children. In Pickering, L. (Ed.). *2000 Red Book: Report of the Committee on Infectious Diseases*. (25th ed.). Elk Grove Village, IL: American Academy of Pediatrics; 147–152.

BCG = Bacille Calmette-Guérin; CBC = complete blood count; CMV = cytomegalovirus; ELISA = enzyme-linked immunosorbent assay; HbsAg = hepatitis B surface antigen; Hgb/HCT = hemoglobin/hematocrit; PCR = polymerase chain reaction; PKU = phenylketonuria; PPD = purified protein derivative; RPD = reactive protein derivative; TSH = thyroid-stimulating hormone; VDRL = Venereal Disease Research Laboratories.

and practice guidelines for pediatric care providers. Another source of updated information on specific countries is the Website of the Centers for Disease Control and Prevention (*www.cdc.gov*).

PREADOPTION VISIT

During the preadoption visit, prospective parents may have photographs or a video of their adoptee that they received in the mail and will ask for an assessment of the media for any unusual child behaviors (Fig. 24–2). The preadoption visit gives you the chance to give the prospective parents emotional support and educate them about the health screening and physical examination process.

TABLE 24–4. SPECIFIC TESTS TO BE DONE, BY COUNTRY

Country	Hepatitis C	Hepatitis D	Thalassemia	Sickle Cell HgbSS/HgbS	Hgb E	G6PD
China	X				X	
Asia						X
Southeast Asia	X		X			
Philippines						X
India				X	X	
Russia	X					
Eastern Europe	X	X				
Africa		X	X	X		X
South America		X				X
Central America		X				X
Middle East		X	X	X		X
Mediterranean		X	X	X		X

G6PD = glucose-6-phosphate dehydrogenase; Hgb E = hemoglobin E ; HgbSS/HgbS = hemoglobin SS/hemoglobin S.

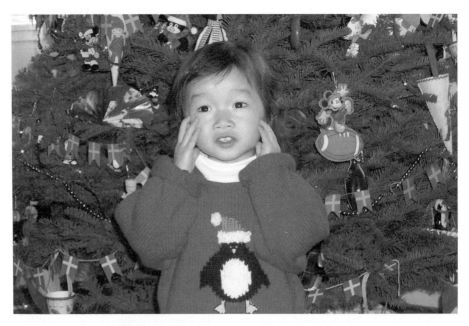

FIG. 24–2. International adoptee at Christmas.

PHYSICAL EXAMINATION

Unless the adoptive parents report symptoms that need urgent attention or the child has a known chronic disease, the child can be examined within 14 days of arrival to his or her new home. Waiting several days before the initial examination allows the child and family to adjust to the new setting and possible time zone differences. It also gives the parents time to learn more about the child's behavior, temperament, and needs. Parents should be encouraged to get to know their child and be prepared to share their observations in moderate detail during the history and physical examination. Be aware that out-of-country visa medical physical examinations are often inadequate. Your examination will establish a baseline from which the child's health, growth, and development will be monitored. Perform the usual comprehensive history and physical examination (Table 24–5). Focus on and screen for problems that are unique to internationally adopted children in general and specific to the child's country of origin.

The following common conditions should be screened for in international adoptees: fetal alcohol syndrome, Turner's syndrome, reactive attachment disorder, rickets, cerebral palsy, anemia, cardiac myopathy, and cystic fibrosis (Table 24–6). A complete head-to-toe physical assessment should be performed with each visit. Diagnoses of major disorders are often missed on the first examination because the symptoms are masked by anemia and other acute problems. A physical assessment that focuses on common problems found in internationally adopted children is extremely important. Refer to the chapters in this book for physical assessment detail by body system.

PSYCHOSOCIAL ASSESSMENT

A psychosocial assessment of the child is essential during the physical examination to screen for common problems related to attachment in children who experienced prolonged neglect from institutionalization. Some children avoid many negative effects of institutionalism because they are social, outgoing, or able to attract favorable attention, and some countries place prospective adoptees in foster homes, where they receive more attention.

REFERRAL AND RESOURCES

A complete history and physical examination of the internationally adopted child determines what resources and referrals are needed. Specialists can assist in the diagnosis and treatment of children with complex infectious diseases and conditions as needed. The Internet has vast resources and support groups such as *www.adoptivefam.org*, which is a national parent advocacy group for domestic and international adoption information; *www.rcic@po.cwru.edu*, which is the Rainbow Center of International Child Health, Cleveland, Ohio (216-844-3224); and *www.rainbowkids.com*, which is by and for adoptive parents.

TABLE 24–5. FOCUSED PHYSICAL ASSESSMENTS

Birth Age: _____ Length: _____ cm _____ % Weight: _____ cm _____%
  OFC: _____ cm _____%
Present Age: _____ Length: _____cm _____ % Weight: _____ cm _____%
  OFC: _____ cm _____%

PERCENT GROWTH CURVE

Standard U.S. growth charts are used for all children to assess growth pattern. Ask about the common stature, body type, and physical condition of people in the child's country of origin.

PSYCHOSOCIAL

Child temperament: Easy-going, slow to warm up, difficult, outgoing, shy, attention span, distractibility, intensity, maladaptive behaviors (stranger anxiety at age 6 to 30 months is normal), reactive attachment disorder (see Table 24–6)

HEENT

- Head circumference, microcephaly, hydrocephaly, fontanel, sutures, and head shape
- Eyes: Vision screening, including red eye reflex, strabismus, light reflex, cover/uncover test, extraocular movement, color blindness
- Ears: Hearing test (if otitis media or externa is not present)
- Nose: Patent, drainage, lesions
- Throat: Tonsils, uvula, palate, tongue mobility, lesions, thrush
- Dental: Count teeth (teeth and bone development may be delayed)

INTEGUMENT

Document all skin lesions: Mongolian spots, hemangioma, lesions, scars, bruises, signs of abuse (e.g., bruises in unusual places and in varied levels of healing, unusual skin lesions, bone pain and fractures), lice (head), scabies (check between fingers and toes, scattered lesions), tinea corporis or capitis, impetigo, eczema, dermatitis, diaper rash, herpes simplex I or II, chicken pox, purpura

RESPIRATORY

URI, bronchiolitis, RSV, asthma, pneumonia, tuberculosis, cystic fibrosis

CARDIOVASCULAR

Congenital heart defects (pathological murmurs), coarctation of the aorta (brachial and femoral pulse asymmetry), anemia (pale, lucent skin, weakness, fatigue), hemoglobinopathy (HgbE, HgbSS/HgbS), alpha- and beta-thalassemia (Hgb, MCV), iron-deficiency anemia (HCT/Hgb, serum ferritin) and thrombocytopenia (platelet count)

GASTROINTESTINAL

Intestinal parasites (eosinophilia, bloating, diarrhea, weight loss, lactose intolerance, failure to thrive), HPS, GER, stool characteristics (steatorrhea, amount, mucus, blood), abdominal distention, hernias, signs of abuse

GENITOURINARY

Hypospadias, epispadias, retractile or undescended testicles, phimosis, circumcision, UTI, genitalia, yeast infection, signs of abuse

MUSCULOSKELETAL

Muscle strength, crawl, gait, developmental dysplasia of the hip (Ortolani/Barlow sign), asymmetrical leg length and gluteal folds, rickets (decreased PO_4, elevated alkaline phosphatase, hypotonia, growth failure, bowing of legs), torticollis (injury to the sternomastoid muscle—wryneck), clubfoot, internal tibial torsion, scoliosis, signs of abuse (e.g., multiple bruises in different stages of healing, fractures, lesions)

(continued)

TABLE 24–5. FOCUSED PHYSICAL ASSESSMENTS (Continued)

NEUROLOGICAL

Spina bifida, facial droop, head shape and circumference, symmetry of reflexes and cranial nerves, tics, paralysis, Erb's palsy—shoulder, upper arm paralysis (C5, C6 nerve damage), Klumpke's paralysis—forearm, wrist, hand (damage C7, C8, T1), cerebral palsy—head lag > 4–5 months, asymmetry in motor function, scissoring of legs, early hand preference.

ENDOCRINE

TSH, decreased or elevated thyroid hormone levels, decreased or elevated adrenal activity, signs of precocious puberty (girls), polyuria, polydipsia, polyphagia

Immunity: HIV, malaria, fever of unknown origin, leukemia, infection, PPD

GROWTH AND DEVELOPMENT

Denver II Developmental Screening: Gross and fine motor, cognitive, social and emotional, and language ability

COMMON SYNDROME FEATURES

Fetal alcohol syndrome, Down syndrome (epicanthal fold and slanted eyes, flat nasal bridge), Turner's syndrome, reactive attachment disorder

---

HEENT = head, eyes, ears, nose, and throat; Hgb = hemoglobin; HgbE = hemoglobin E ; HgbSS/HgbS = hemoglobinSS/hemoglobinS ; HPS = hypertrophic pyloric stenosis; HCT = hematocrit ; MCV = mean corpuscular volume; OFC = occipital-frontal circumference; PPD = purified protein derivative; RSV = respiratory syncytial virus; URI = upper respiratory infection; UTI = urinary tract infection.

TEST YOUR KNOWLEDGE OF CHAPTER 24

1. How is a routine pediatric patient history similar to and different from a history obtained for an internationally adopted child?

2. In what manner should a healthcare provider cluster and list various diseases or conditions for which internationally adopted children should be screened?

3. What immunizations are often missed or inadequate for international adoptees?

4. What diseases or conditions can be missed if there is only one initial assessment or clinic visit?

5. What characteristics accompany fetal alcohol syndrome?

6. What are the signs of cerebral palsy? What other factors or disorders could account for these signs?

7. How and when should the PPD be administered to international adoptees? What considerations must be made for those who have had a BCG?

8. Based on the specific healthcare needs of international adoptees, what kind of resources or referrals will be needed?

TABLE 24–6. SCREENING FOR SYNDROMES AND CONDITIONS IN INTERNATIONAL ADOPTEES

Disorder	Cause	Clinical Presentation
Reactive attachment disorder	Neglect, abuse, traumatic separation from primary caregiver, trauma, prolonged deprivation in an institution	Feels need to be in control; internalized rage and distrust of parents; takes care of self-need; decreased affection reciprocity; decreased regulation of emotion; decreased sense of conscience, self-esteem, empathy, and logical thinking; pushes parents away; intense battles, bossy, argumentative, defiant, angry; resists affection on parents' terms; decreased eye contact; manipulative in a superficial, charming, and engaging manner; indiscriminately affectionate with strangers; poor peer relations; hypervigilant or hyperactive; food issues, including hords, gorges, refuses to eat, hides food; fascination with fire, blood, weapons
Fetal alcohol syndrome	Teratogen exposure, maternal alcohol consumption, and maternal chronic alcoholism	Flat nasal bridge; upturned nose; elongated, less prominent philtrum; low-set ears; thin upper lip; sharp chin; high incidence congenital heart defects, neural tube defects, and microcephaly
Turner's syndrome	Genetic: 45,X chromosome anomaly	Older girls and women: Short stature, shieldlike chest, wide-spaced nipples, puffy hands and feet, low posterior hairline, webbed neck
Rickets	Vitamin D deficiency, renal or hepatic disease, certain medication overuse (e.g., antacids), and rare diseases	Elevated alkaline phosphatase and low phosphorus levels; low serum 1,25, dihydroxycholecalciferol, bowing legs, fractures, growth failure, enlargement of the knees and wrists
Cerebral palsy	10% perinatal hypoxia caused by in utero cord strangulation, birth trauma, high-risk pregnancy, low birth weight, and premature birth; etiology unknown	Increased muscle tone and movement asymmetry, spasms or spasticity, head lag > 4 months, motor asymmetry—crawl, early hand preference, scissoring of legs, late sitting, late ambulation, and mild to moderate cognitive delay (caution: transient developmental delay may enhance or mask findings; e.g., an infant may spend most of the time supine or confined in a crib where motor development is impeded)

✪ BIBLIOGRAPHY

Algranati, P. S. (1992). *The pediatric patient: An approach to history and physical examination.* Baltimore: Williams & Wilkins.

American Academy of Pediatrics. (2000). Medical evaluation of internationally adopted children. In Pickering, L. (Ed.). *2000 Red Book: Report of the Committee on Infectious Diseases* (25th ed.). Elk Grove Village, IL: American Academy of Pediatrics; 147–152.

Aronson, J. (2000). Medical evaluation and infectious consideration on arrival. *Pediatric Annals, 29*(4), 218–223.

Barnett, E. D., & Miller, L. C. (1996). International adoption: The pediatrician's role. *Contemporary Pediatrics, 13*(8), 29–46.

Chamberlain, L. J. (2001). Children adopted abroad could face life-long psychological problems. *Infectious Disease in Children, 14*(1), 20.

Faber, S. (2000). Behavioral sequelae of orphanage life. *Pediatric Annals, 29*(4), 242–248.

Filipkowski, A. M. (2001). Become familiar with international adoption issues. *Infectious Disease in Children, 14*(1), 16–17.

Giorgi, A. Z. (2001). AAP says international adoptees need careful vaccination screening. *Infectious Disease in Children, 14*(1),12.

Glascoe, F. P. (2000). Early detection of developmental and behavioral problems. *Pediatrics in Review, 21*(8), 272–280.

Havlik, K. (2000). Care of the internationally adopted child. Presented at the Pediatric Pharmacology Conference Presentation, Yarrow Hotel, Park City, UT, September 8, 2000.

Iovino, L. A., Jr. (2001). There are many considerations when adopting children from abroad. *Infectious Disease in Children, 14*(1),18.

Jenista, J. A. (2001). Infectious disease and the internationally adopted child. Available at: *www.rainbowkids.com.*

Jenista, J. A. (2000). Preadoption review of medical records. *Pediatric Annals, 29*(4), 212–215.

Johnson, D. E. (2000). Long-term medical issues in international adoptees. *Pediatric Annals, 29*(4), 234–241.

Johnson, D. E., & Hostetter, M. (1996). Adopted children. *Pediatric Basics, 77* (Summer), 10–17.

Kirsche, M. (2001). ACIP updates vaccination guidelines for children adopted from overseas. *Infectious Disease in Children, 14* (1), 19.

Kronemyer, B. (2001). Providing care for internationally adopted children proves rewarding. *Infectious Disease in Children, 14*(1), 15.

Lears, M. K., Guth, K. J., & Lewandowski, L. (1998). International adoption: A primer for pediatric nurses. *Pediatric Nursing, 24*(6), 578–586.

Miller, L. C. (2000). Initial assessment of growth, development, and the effects of institutionalization in internationally adopted children. *Pediatric Annals, 29*(4), 224–232.

Miller, L. C., Kiernan, M. T., Mathers, M. I., & Klein-Gitelman, M. (1995). Developmental and nutritional status of internationally adopted children. *Archival Pediatric Adolescent Medicine, 149*(January), 40–44.

Mitchell, M. A. S., & Jenista, J. A. (1997). Healthcare of the internationally adopted child. Part 1: Before and at arrival into the adoptive home. *Journal of Pediatric Healthcare, 11*(2), 51–59.

Mitchell, M. A. S., & Jenista, J. A. (1997). Healthcare of the internationally adopted child, Part 2: Chronic care and long-term medical issues. *Journal of Pediatric Healthcare, 11*(2), 117–127.

Quarles, C. S., & Brodie, J. H. (1998). Primary care of international adoptees. *American Family Physician, 58*(9), 2025–2039.

Stephenson, M. (2001). Pediatricians can assess medical records of adopted children. *Infectious Disease in Children, 14* (1), 11–12.

CHAPTER 25

Cultural Assessment: Special Issues

MARGARET R. COLYAR

OBJECTIVES
- *Competently assess cultural variations and orientation to health care.*
- *Competently assess children of various cultures.*

As any nation becomes more linguistically and culturally diverse, healthcare providers have a responsibility to understand how best to meet the healthcare needs of children and their families. Individuals from racial and ethnic subgroups comprise a majority of the population in the United States. A total of 51% of the current United States population comes from culturally diverse backgrounds. As a healthcare provider, you will need to assess foreign visitors, students studying abroad, immigrants, refugees, members of diverse ethnic groups, and Native Americans.

To intervene with culturally accurate, sensitive, and meaningful care, you must include cultural considerations during health assessment. When performing an assessment of a child of culturally diverse background, a knowledge of certain terminology is necessary (Table 25–1).

The four basic characteristics of culture are that culture is learned, shared, adapted, and dynamic (Table 25–2). This chapter focuses on the following areas of cultural assessment: dominant value orientation, relationships, health-related customs and practices, health-related beliefs, communication styles, space, and value orientation. Use these concepts to become more culturally sensitive and to provide healthcare to children and their parents that is more meaningful to them. The goal is that children and parents will be

TABLE 25–1. TERMINOLOGY

Term	Definition
Acculturation	Adaptation to and adoption of the values, traits, and behaviors of another group; rarely are the values of the original culture completely rejected
Custom	Habit or pattern of responses to given occasions; usually passed on from one generation to another
Ethnic group	A group of the same race or nationality, with a common culture and distinctive traits
Minority	A group with a religion, color, race, or ethnic origin different from the majority of the population
Nationality	Belonging to a particular nation by origin, birth, or naturalization and having common traditions
Race	A distinct group differentiated by genetically transmitted physical characteristics, including identifiers such as skin color, head shape, and stature
Subculture	A group or subgroup within a larger culture that has values and behavioral patterns or other distinctive traits that differentiate it from other groups or subgroups; different gangs could be considered subcultures

more apt to understand and follow healthcare plans, attain positive health outcomes, and develop favorable relationships with you and other healthcare providers.

In addition, you must be aware of your own cultural orientation. You must acknowledge the assumptions and biases you have about children's cultural predispositions. You must overcome these assumptions and biases when caring for children from different cultural environments.

CULTURAL VARIATIONS

Healthcare providers need to be aware of the cultural context and norms of specific groups to assess health problems, interventions, and prevention

TABLE 25–2. CHARACTERISTICS OF CULTURE

Characteristic	Description
Learned	Cultivated from birth through language acquisition and socialization
Shared	Collective or common knowledge and beliefs mutual to all members of the same cultural group
Adapted	Modified to specific conditions of environmental and technical factors and availability of natural resources
Dynamic	Ever-changing

strategies in children and youth. Table 25–3 provides considerations concerning space, communication, relationships, health-related beliefs, and health-related customs and practices of selected populations. For further information on specific cultures, see the *Mosby's Pocket Guide Series: Cultural Assessment* by E. M. Geissler.

CHILDREN AND CULTURE

Parents and healthcare providers must recognize that children actively attempt to understand their world through their own language and culture. Thus, children learn best when they acquire skills in a meaningful context. Identifying what a particular child already knows about healthcare issues and building on his or her prior learning helps promote an environment that engages the child in learning.

You have a responsibility to respect the child and family. At the same time, you must realize that parents rely on caregivers to honor and support their children in the cultural values and norms of the family. Children are cognitively, linguistically, and emotionally connected to the language and culture of their homes. Thus, separating a child from his or her culture is virtually impossible.

Children who are growing up in a country different from their parental homeland have added responsibilities and conflicts, including the responsibility learning a new language, fitting in at school, and role reversal. These children usually learn the new language and behavior patterns of the new country before the older members of the family group learn them. These children possibly adopt values, attitudes, and behaviors of the new community, which are often at odds with the traditions of the older generation. This may pose extra problems for these children that could result in frequent somatic complaints, such as headaches, stomachaches, and the development of ulcers and other stress-related illnesses, such as anxiety and depression. If a child has recently migrated from a country at war or persecution in which the child experienced struggle for survival, torture, life in a refugee camp, or separation from family and friends, or loss of security and home, psychological problems may develop.

Newly immigrated children may develop other problems such as identity crisis, school problems, and drug and alcohol abuse problems. They also may experience domestic violence. Defining self, values, beliefs, and sexuality becomes more difficult when a child is a product of two cultures. There can be conflict between the desire to be part of the family's culture and the newly acquired desire for independence. School problems may manifest because the child is teased about his or her accent and cultural background. A child's difficulties at school may also reflect anxiety or depression that is hidden within the family. Rebellion against parental authority and peer pressure to join the new culture may result in an added risk of drug and alcohol abuse. Increasing risk of domestic violence may be experienced in homes in which both parents are struggling to find work and suffering from stress

TABLE 25–3. CHARACTERISTICS OF CULTURE

Concept	African-American	Asian-American	Native American	Hispanic-Latino	European	Russian
Space	Close personal space	Noncontact space	Space very important and has no boundaries	Touch, handshake, embrace	Noncontact, aloof Value social distance	Touch is important
Communication	Direct eye contact Verbal and nonverbal must match High level of caution for majority of group	Use of silence No finger pointing; this is a sign of disrespect Do not look directly into eyes	Use of silence and body contextual cueing Unwavering eye gaze is insulting. Pause after a question and give thought. Must develop trust	Sustained direct contact is rude or dangerous Small talk with initiating actual topic. Like open-ended questions Father should be present with male child	Frequent quick eye contact Verbal rather than nonverbal Handshake is OK, although is infrequent	Direct eye contact Sustained eye contact
Health-related beliefs	Illness is natural due to conflict or disharmony, or sent by God as a punishment	Magicoreligious orientation Eastern and herbal medicine Sick care only Self-medication and polypharmacy Injections more often than PO	Natural and magicoreligious folk medicine Health results from disharmony with nature and universe Believe that illness is price paid for something in the past or future	Matter of chance or God's will Disease influenced by hot and cold imbalance Focus—curative Prevent illness by being good, eating proper food, doing good works, and spending the proper amount of time in prayer with religious amulets	Active involvement Health promotion is important Get to immediate issue No small talk View asking questions as challenging authority	Passive role Emphasis on health prevention

(continued)

Concept	African-American	Asian-American	Native American	Hispanic-Latino	European	Russian
Health-related customs and practices	Proper diet, rest, and clean environment produce good health Folk medicine First-aid and home remedies	Ying-yang Hot-cold balance	Healer or medicine man or woman Regain harmony and health through sweat lodges, immersion in water, and special rituals	*Mal ojo* ("evil eye") *Mal puesto* ("hex") Curandero or curandera (healer) Homeopathic, naturopathy, spiritism For severe problems, use scientific system in conjunction with promises, prayers, and use of medals and candles	Self-care and over-the-counter medications Intolerance of healthcare delays Tend to accept healthcare professional's medical judgment	
Relationships	Many single-parent families Woman is head of household Large extended family networks Strong church association	Large extended family networks Devoted to tradition Traditional family—oldest man makes the decisions	Family oriented Children taught to respect tradition	Extreme modesty Patriarchal nuclear families Collective needs of family take precedence over individual Strong church association Respect wisdom of elders	Patriarchal nuclear families Extended families Man and woman share in decision making	

417

because of changing circumstances. Be aware of the responses of children to these potential circumstances. Children may feel powerless to seek help outside the family.

 APPROACH

The approach to the examination of a child from another culture must be varied based on the cultural orientation and age of the child. Table 25–3 presents the preferred communication approach for various cultural groups. Actively involve the parent and the child in the healthcare examination. The parent is probably more ingrained in the cultural traditions, and the child is most likely a mixture of the traditional culture and culture learned from interactions with other children. Both the cultural beliefs of the parent and the age of the child must be taken into account. For example, Jose, a 7-year-old Hispanic child, and his father come in for a well-child examination. Because the Hispanic culture traditionally views sustained eye contact as rude and dangerous, you should not fixedly stare at the child or the father. The Hispanic culture also likes small talk. Be polite and ask about the family, school, grades, and other relevant social issues. Remember that Hispanics are very modest; therefore, structure the physical examination so that modesty is preserved. Last, remember that the child is 7 years old, so explain what you are doing to the child, allow the child to check out your instruments, and answer questions in a matter-of-fact manner.

 SCREENING

Perform all screening examinations as required by the age group, region, and area of rearing. Always check vital signs, the teeth, hearing, vision, and overall growth and development. For children of African-American descent, consider screening for sickle cell anemia. For children of Jewish descent, consider screening for thalassemia. See Chapter 24 for other diseases of concern in different newly immigrated cultural groups.

EGO DEVELOPMENT AND COGNITIVE DEVELOPMENT

Erikson and Piaget do not differentiate between culture backgrounds. Their research was based on white northern European children and families. However, children in certain age groups are expected to develop certain characteristics in certain patterns. Refer to Erikson's and Piaget's stages for the age group (Chapters 17 to 23) being assessed to determine at what point a particular child should be relative to ego and cognitive development. Be aware that some cultures do not value the promotion of independence of the adolescent child.

IMMUNIZATIONS

The Centers for Disease Control and Prevention (see the Website at *www.cdc.gov*) makes recommendations about immunizations, and the state in which the child resides mandates the immunizations. All children should receive the appropriate immunizations to prevent disease. Evaluate the immunization status of the child at his or her first visit to determine which immunizations are current and which need to be given. When examining a new immigrant, you should be aware of immunizations that are commonly given in the child's country of origin (see Chapter 24).

 ## PHYSICAL EXAMINATION

Physical examination is based on the age of the child, not his or her cultural background. See the age-appropriate guidelines in Chapters 17 to 23.

Some common findings are that children with dark skin have a higher incidence of Mongolian spots (i.e., darker skin patches, usually located on the back and abdomen). Asian-Americans have smaller hip girdles, are generally smaller in stature, have higher palates, and rarely have facial hair. Chinese infants tend to have higher bilirubin levels at birth. African-American, Asian-American, and Hispanic children tend to be lactose intolerant. African-American, Native Americans, and Hispanic children are generally more obese than children of other cultures.

 ## ANTICIPATORY GUIDANCE

Anticipatory guidance should always include the same five areas: growth and development, safety issues, dental health, nutritional issues, and parenting. For adolescents, also include pubertal events, mortality and violence, sexuality issues (e.g., contraception, sexually transmitted diseases), and risk behaviors (e.g., bulimia and anorexia, drugs, depression). Although specific information should be given on these topics, cultural beliefs should be taken into account. Discuss with the parents their views on these issues to determine the type of care the child is receiving and what, if any, interventions need to be included.

TEST YOUR KNOWLEDGE OF CHAPTER 25

1. What are four basic characteristics of culture? Describe them.
2. Describe the differences in diverse populations concerning space, communication, relationships, health-related beliefs, and health-related customs and practices.

3. What are your responsibilities when interacting with children from diverse cultural backgrounds?
4. How do children adjust when they are growing up in a country different from their parental homeland?
5. What are some common physical complaints of children from culturally diverse backgrounds?
6. What is the approach to the examination of a child from a culturally differing background?
7. What concerns about immunizations should be considered with children from culturally diverse backgrounds? How about immigrants?
8. Describe some common physical findings in children from different races.
9. What components of anticipatory guidance should be discussed with parents of children from culturally diverse backgrounds?

BIBLIOGRAPHY

Geissler, E. M. (1998). *Mosby's pocket guide series: Cultural assessment.* St. Louis: Mosby.

Huff, R. M., & Kline, M. V. (1999). *Promoting health in multicultural populations: A handbook for practitioners.* London: Sage.

Jarvis, C. (2000). *Physical examination and health assessment.* Philadelphia: W. B. Saunders.

Purnell, L.D., & Paulanka, B. J. (1998). *Transcultural health care: A culturally competent approach.* Philadelphia: F. A. Davis.

Seidel, H. M., Ball, J. W., Dains, J. E., & Benedict, G.W. (1999). *Mosby's guide to physical examination.* St. Louis: Mosby.

Spector, R. E. (1996). *Guide to heritage assessment and health traditions.* Stamford, CT: Appleton & Lange.

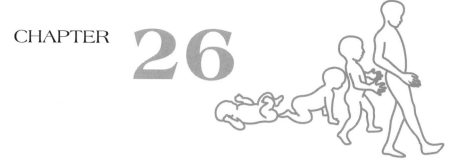

CHAPTER **26**

Sports Physical Examinations

MARGARET R. COLYAR AND
GEETA MAHARAJ

OBJECTIVES
• Describe the necessary components of sports physical examination.
• Determine what problems disqualify a child from contact, collision,
  and noncontact sports.

Most states require children to undergo preparticipation screening and medical clearance before they can take part in sports to ensure safe participation. The goal of sports physical examinations is to determine whether any health problems would affect a child's ability to play, worsen with participation, or increase the chance of injury or result in death. You may need to treat problems that pose a risk, defer permission to participate until problems are identified or treated, or disqualify children from activities when participation would pose risk of injury or illness.

HISTORY

Sports physical examinations must include a medical history that consists of a history of injuries, immunization status, current medications, and allergies. The review of systems should focus on the cardiorespiratory, neurological, visual, musculoskeletal, and genitourinary systems (Table 26–1). Also check the family history for cardiovascular problems (i.e., myocardial infarction, cerebrovascular accident, arrhythmias, sudden death, and hypertension), asthma, seizures, and musculoskeletal problems.

421

TABLE 26–1. REVIEW OF SYSTEMS FOR SPORTS PHYSICAL EXAMINATIONS	
System	Focus On
HEENT	Visual problems
Cardiovascular	Exertional syncope, dizziness, or chest pain with activity
	Murmurs
	Irregular heartbeats, palpitations
	Hypertension
	MVP
Respiratory	Active tuberculosis
	Asthma
	Pulmonary insufficiency
	Spontaneous pneumothorax
CNS	Seizure disorder
	Concussion
Abdominal	Hepatitis
	Diabetes
	Pancreatitis
Genitourinary	Single kidney
	Kidney problems
Musculoskeletal	Fractures
	Sprains
	Torn tendons or ligaments

CNS = central nervous system; HEENT = head, eyes, ears, nose, and throat; MVP = mitral valve prolapse.

APPROACH

Introduce yourself and demonstrate an interest in the sport in which the child is going to participate. Make the examination nonthreatening, and let the child know what to expect. Determine whether the sport is a contact, collision, or noncontact activity (Table 26–2).

TABLE 26–2. CATEGORIES OF SPORTS		
Contact	Collision	Noncontact
Field hockey	Soccer	Aerobics
Football	Wrestling	Track
Martial arts	Ice hockey	Fencing
Rodeo	Rugby	Swimming
Boxing	Baseball	Running
Lacrosse	Basketball	Weightlifting
		Archery
		Golf
		Tennis
		Crew
		Riflery

PHYSICAL EXAMINATION

A complete physical examination must be performed with increased emphasis on the cardiovascular, respiratory, neurological, vision, orthopedic, psychosocial, and genitourinary systems. The physical examination must include height, weight, blood pressure, heart rate and rhythm, pulses, visual acuity, auscultation for murmurs, palpation of the abdomen, a thorough orthopedic examination, and testicular and inguinal canal examination in boys.

OBSERVATION

Start the examination by observing the standing patient from the front for symmetry of all features, including shoulders, trunk, and extremities. Observe the patient's gait.

AUSCULTATION, PALPATION, PERCUSSION—BY SYSTEMS

Head, Eyes, Ears, Nose, and Throat

Perform a complete head, eyes, ears, nose, and throat (HEENT) examination (see Chapter 5) with emphasis on the visual examination (see Chapter 6). Determine whether there is decreased or absent vision in either eye or a detached retina, which would disqualify the child from contact and collision sports.

Cardiovascular System

Palpate all peripheral pulses, and auscultate the heart. Perform the scratch test to determine the size of the heart. If any irregular heart sounds are heard, an electrocardiogram (EKG) is indicated. If an EKG is performed, pay particular attention to the QT interval. A prolonged QT interval can be a cause of sudden death and often occurs among members of a family. Also, refer the child for an echocardiogram if a murmur is detected and has not been performed previously. Most serious arrhythmias (99%) are detectable when the child holds his or her breath.

Hypertension in a child requires a thorough workup. The condition must be under control before the child can be allowed to participate in sports. The most common cause of severe hypertension in a child is a renal problem. Participation cannot be granted until cardiovascular abnormalities have been resolved.

Respiratory System

Auscultate all lung fields, both anteriorly and posteriorly. Check the oxygen saturation, if equipment is available. Asthma that is well controlled is not a

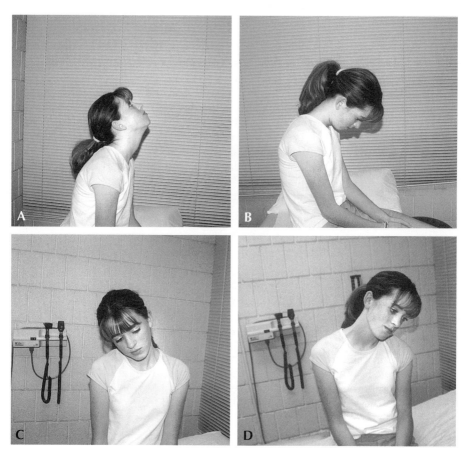

FIG. 26–1. Neck examination. *(A)* Hyperflexion. *(B)* Flexion. *(C)* Right lateral flexion. *(D)* Left lateral flexion.

reason to disqualify a child from sports participation. However, if a child has exercise-induced deoxygenation, contact and collision sports should be restricted.

Musculoskeletal System

The orthopedic examination must focus on looking for asymmetry in joints, muscles, range of motion (ROM), and strength. The examination is faster if you perform the maneuvers and then let the child imitate you.

Neck

To evaluate ROM in the cervical spine, ask the child to flex the neck forward and backward, to the right and left sides, and do a complete right-to-left rotation (Fig. 26–1).

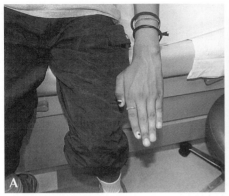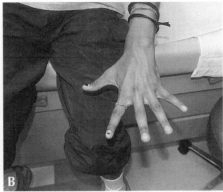

FIG. 26–2. Range of motion of fingers. *(A)* Together, *(B)* Spread.

Shoulders

To assess trapezius muscle strength, apply resistance as the child shrugs his or her shoulders. Next, assess deltoid muscle strength. Apply resistance as the child abducts his or her shoulders. Last, assess ROM of the glenohumeral joint. Observe the child as he or she performs external and internal rotation of his or her shoulder. Also, check the strength of the upper extremities by testing grip bilaterally.

Elbows

Assess ROM by observing the child extend the arms and flex the elbows. Assess ROM of the wrist and elbow by observing the child pronate and supinate the forearm.

Hands and Fingers

To evaluate ROM of the hand and fingers, observe the child clench the fist and then spread the fingers (Fig. 26–2).

Back

Observe the standing child to assess symmetry. Observe as the child stands with his or her knees straight and then flexes forward at the waist, first facing away from you and then facing toward you, to assess for ROM of the spine, hamstring flexibility, and scoliosis.

Legs

Observe for symmetry of the leg muscles as the child stands facing you with the quadriceps flexed. Instruct the child to duck-walk four steps (Fig. 26–3). Demonstrate if necessary. This position is used to assess strength, balance, and ROM of the hips, knees, and ankles. Have the child stand or walk on the

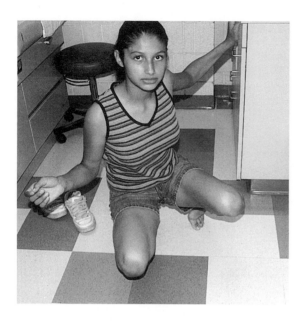

FIG. 26–3. Duck-walking. Assessment of strength, balance, and range of motions of the hip, knee, and ankle.

toes and then on the heels. This position is used to assess calf strength, symmetry, and balance.

Abdomen

Palpate the abdomen for pain or masses. Note liver and spleen size. Check for costoventebral vertebral angle tenderness. Perform a urinalysis and measure liver enzymes, if indicated.

Hernias

For boys, the presence of inguinal hernias must be ruled out (see Chapter 14—Assessment of the Genitourinary System). This is a good time to introduce the male athlete to testicular self-examination.

After the head-to-toe physical examination is completed, document findings on an approved sports physical examination form (Fig. 26–4). Use Table 26–3 as a guide to determine when to allow participation, refer for further workup, or disqualify the athlete from the proposed sport.

SPORTS PHYSICAL EXAMINATION

Health Record

Name_____ Age_____ (years) Grade_____Date_____

Address_____Phone_____

Sport(s)_____

PART I: HEALTH HISTORY

(To be completed by athlete and parent)

		YES	NO
1.	Have you ever had an illness that:		
	a. required you to stay in the hospital?	___	___
	b. caused you to miss 3 days of practice or a competition?	___	___
	c. is related to allergies?	___	___
	d. required an operation?	___	___
	e. is chronic (i.e., asthma, diabetes, etc.)?	___	___
2.	Have you ever had an injury that:		
	a. required you to go to an ER or see a doctor?	___	___
	b. required you to stay in the hospital?	___	___
	c. required x-rays?	___	___
	d. caused you to miss 3 days of practice or competition?	___	___
	e. required an operation?	___	___
3.	Do you take any medication or pills?	___	___
4.	Have any members of your family under age 50 had a heart attack, heart problems, or died unexpectedly?	___	___
5.	Have you ever:		
	a. been dizzy or passed out during or after exercise?	___	___
	b. been unconscious or had a concussion?	___	___
6.	Are you unable to run _ mile (2 times around the track) without stopping?	___	___
7.	Do you:		
	a. wear glasses or contacts?	___	___
	b. wear dental bridges, plates, or braces?	___	___
8.	Have you ever had a heart murmur, high blood pressure, or a heart abnormality?	___	___
9.	Do you have any allergies to any medicine?	___	___
10.	Are you missing a kidney?	___	___

11. When was your last tetanus booster? _____

For Females:

12. At what age did you experience your first menstrual period? _____

13. In the last year, what is the longest time you have gone between periods? _____

14. Explain any "yes" answers:

I hereby state that, to the best of my knowledge, my answers to the above questions are correct.

Signature of athlete_____

Signature of parent/guardian_____

FIG. 26–4. Sports physical examination form.

PART II: INTERIM HEALTH HISTORY

(Positive responses should trigger a medical evaluation)

Over the next 12 months, what sports do you wish to participate in?

_____

Have you missed more than 3 consecutive days of participation in usual activities because of an injury in the past year? _____Yes _____ No

If yes, please indicate:

Site of injury_____

Type of injury_____

Have you missed more than 5 consecutive days of participation in usual activities because of an illness, or have you had a medical illness diagnosed that has not been resolved in the past year? _____ Yes _____ No

If yes, please indicate type of illness _____

Have you had a seizure or concussion or been unconscious for any reason in the past year?

_____ Yes _____ No

Have you had surgery or been hospitalized in the past year? _____ Yes _____ No

If yes, please indicate:

Reason for hospitalization _____

Type of surgery _____

List all medications you are presently taking and what condition the medication is for:

Medication	Dose	Frequency	Condition

Are you worried about any problem or condition at this time?   _____Yes _____No

If yes, please explain: _____

I hereby state that, to the best of my knowledge, my answers to the above questions are correct.

Signature of athlete_____

Signature of parent/guardian_____

FIG. 26–4. Sports physical examination form (*continued*).

PART III: PHYSICAL EXAMINATION RECORD

Height_____Weight _____Pulse_____ BP_____

Vision: R_____/_____ Corrected_____ or uncorrected_____
         L_____/_____ Corrected_____ or uncorrected_____

System	Normal	Abnormal Findings	Initials
Eyes			
Ears, Nose, Throat			
Mouth and Teeth			
Neck			
Cardiovascular			
Chest and Lungs			
Abdomen			
Skin			
Genitalia/Hernia (males)			
M/S: ROM, strength			
Neck			
Spine			
Shoulders			
Arms/hands			
Hips			
Thighs			
Knees			
Ankles			
Feet			
Neuromuscular			

Physical Maturity   Tanner Stage 1 2 3 4 5 (circle one)

The following abnormalities were found and may require treatment:

PARTICIPATION RECOMMENDATIONS:

No participation in: _____

Limited participation in:_____

Full participation in: _____

Provider's signature _____

Address _____
_____

Telephone Number_____

FIG. 26–4. Sports physical examination form (*continued*).

429

TABLE 26–3. SPORTS PARTICIPATION DISQUALIFICATION TABLE

Problem	Contact	Collision	Noncontact
Acute infections: respiratory, genitourinary, mononucleosis, hepatitis, rheumatic fever, TB	X	X	X
Hemorrhagic disease: serious bleeding tendencies	X	X	X
Diabetes: Inadequately controlled	X	X	X
Diabetes: Controlled	O	O	O
Eyes			
Single eye or detached retina	X	X	O
Corrected visual acuity < 20/200	X	X	X
Glaucoma	X	X	O
Respiratory			
Severe pulmonary insufficiency*	X	X	X
Recurrent pneumothorax	X	X	O
Cardiovascular*			
Mitral or aortic valve stenosis or prolapse, aortic insufficiency, coarctation of aorta, cyanotic heart disease, recent carditis	X	X	X
Hypertension: Uncontrolled	X	X	X
Hypertension: Controlled	O	O	O
Previous heart surgery	J	J	J
Liver: Enlarged	X	X	O
Spleen: Enlarged	X	X	O
Skin: Boils, impetigo, herpes simplex	X	X	O
Hernia: Inguinal or femoral	X	X	X
Musculoskeletal			
Inflammatory	X	X	X
Congenital or acquired problems that are incompatible with skills required	X	X	X
CNS			
Previous serious head injury	X	J	O
Seizure disorder: Controlled	J	J	J
Seizure disorder: Uncontrolled	X	X	X
Previous head surgery	X	X	O
Kidneys			
One kidney present	X	X	O
Renal disease	X	X	X
Genitalia			
One testicle present	O	O	O
Undescended testes	O	O	O

*Refer and work up.
CNS = central nervous system; J = judge on individual basis with recommendations from cardiologist or surgeon; O = OK; TB = tuberculosis; X = exclusion.

430

TEST YOUR KNOWLEDGE OF CHAPTER 26

1. What type of physical examination is performed for sports physical examinations?
2. What review of systems must be covered in sports physical examinations?
3. What are the components of the history included in sports physical examinations?
4. Describe the different categories of sporting activities.
5. List five problems that would disqualify a child from contact, collision, and noncontact sports.

 ## BIBLIOGRAPHY

Greene, P. (2000). Recognizing young people at risk for sudden cardiac death in preparticipation sports physicals. *Journal of American Academy of Nurse Practitioners*, 12(1), 11–4.

Herbert, D. L. (1997). Preparticipation cardiovascular: Toward a national standard. *The Physician and Sports Medicine*, 25(3), 112–117.

Reich, J. D. (2000). It won't be me next time: An opinion on preparticipation sports physicals. *American Family Physician*, 61(6), 2618, 2620, 2625, 2629.

Yetter, J. T. (1990). Sports physicals. *American Family Physician*, 41(5), 1395, 1398.

SECTION III

Procedures and Diagnostic Testing

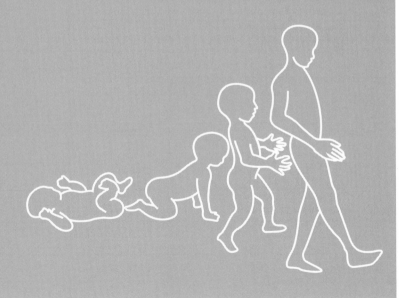

CHAPTER 27

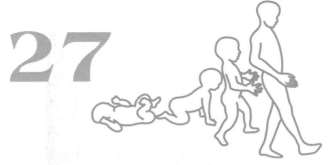

Assessment of Maturity

MARGARET R. COLYAR AND
GEETA MAHARAJ

OBJECTIVES
- *Understand the use of the Ballard (formerly Dubowitz) assessment tool for gestational age.*
- *Determine whether a newborn is large for gestational age or small for gestational age.*

A complicated pregnancy, maternal health problems, poor maternal health habits (e.g., abuse of alcohol and drugs, smoking), and poor prenatal care lead to many problems for newborns. Gestational age helps you understand what went on in utero. Gestational age and whether a child is larger or smaller than average for gestational age assist you in predicting problems the newborn may develop. Babies born before 36 weeks' gestation are considered premature, and babies born between 36 and 37 weeks' gestation are preterm. Term babies are born between 38 and 42 weeks' gestation. After 42 weeks' gestation, a baby is considered post-term. Because the placenta becomes less and less functional after 42 weeks, problems may occur with post-term newborns.

BALLARD GESTATIONAL AGE ASSESSMENT TOOL

To determine gestational age, seven external physical signs (Fig. 27–1) and six neuromuscular signs (Fig. 27–2) are used. This test should be completed within the first 5 days of extrauterine life. This standard scoring system is used to estimate actual gestational age within 2 weeks. Scoring is done on a

435

Physical maturity sign	Score							Record score here
	0	1	2	3	4	5	6	
Skin	Sticky, friable, transparent	Gelatinous, red, translucent	Smooth, pink, visible veins	Superficial peeling &/or rash, few veins	Cracking, pale areas, rare veins	Parchment, deep cracking, no vessels	Leathery, cracked, wrinkled	
Lanugo	None	Sparse	Abundant	Thinning	Bald areas	Mostly bald		
Plantar surface	Heel-toe 40-50 mm:-1 <40 mm:-2	>50 mm no crease	Faint red marks	Anterior transverse crease only	Creases ant. 2/3	Creases over entire sole		
Breast	Imperceptible	Barely perceptible	Flat areola, no bud	Stippled areola, 1-2 mm bud	Raised areola, 3-4 mm bud	Full areola, 5-10 mm bud		
Eye/Ear	Lids fused Loosely: -1 Tightly: -2	Lids open Pinna flat, stays folded	Sl. curved pinna; soft; slow recoil	Well-curved pinna; soft but ready recoil	Formed & firm instant recoil	Thick cartilage, ear stiff		
Genitals (Male)	Scrotum flat, smooth	Scrotum empty, faint rugae	Testes in upper canal, rare rugae	Testes descending, few rugae	Testes down, good rugae	Testes pendulous, deep rugae		
Genitals (Female)	Clitoris prominent, labia flat	Prominent clitoris, small labia minora	Prominent clitoris, enlarging minora	Majora & minora equally prominent	Majora large, minora small	Majora cover clitoris & minora		
						Total physical maturity score		

FIG. 27–1. Ballard scale—External physical maturity assessment scale.

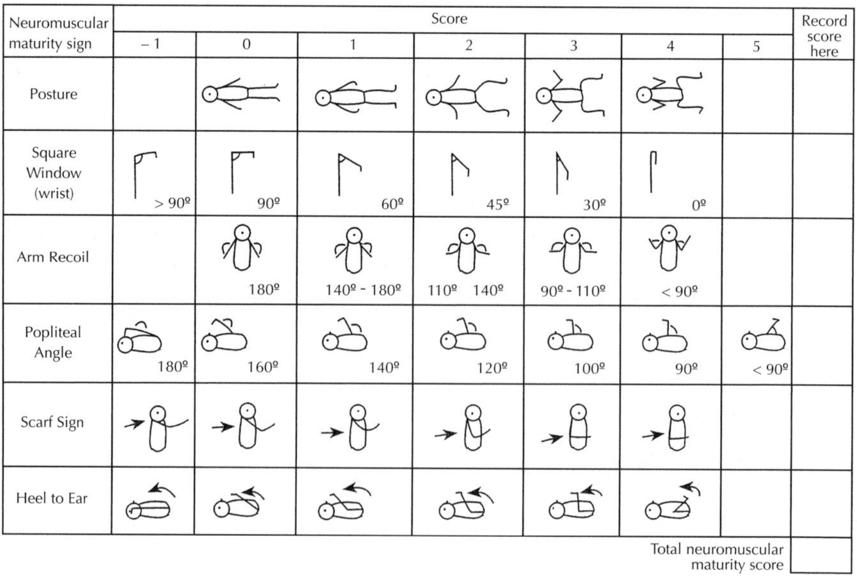

Neuromuscular maturity sign	Score							Record score here
	− 1	0	1	2	3	4	5	
Posture								
Square Window (wrist)	> 90º	90º	60º	45º	30º	0º		
Arm Recoil		180º	140º - 180º	110º 140º	90º - 110º	< 90º		
Popliteal Angle	180º	160º	140º	120º	100º	90º	< 90º	
Scarf Sign								
Heel to Ear								
						Total neuromuscular maturity score		

FIG. 27–2. Ballard scale—Neuromuscular scale.

436

SCORE

Neuromuscular ______

Physical ______

Total ______

MATURITY RATING

Total Maturity score	Gestational age (weeks)
5	26
10	28
15	30
20	32
25	34
30	36
35	38
40	40
45	42
50	44

GESTATIONAL AGE (weeks)

By dates ______

By ultrasound ______

By score ______

FIG. 27–3. Ballard scale—Maturity score sheet.

scale of −1 to 5. After assessing the physical or neuromuscular signs, circle the appropriate description under the correct column. Total the scores and plot them on the maturity score sheet (Fig. 27–3). If the score falls between a range, estimate the closest number and circle the score along with the gestational age.

EXTERNAL PHYSICAL MATURITY ASSESSMENT

The seven areas of the external physical maturity assessment (see Fig. 27–1) are:

1. Skin: The assessment of the skin ranges from sticky, friable, and transpar-

ent (score of 1) seen the in premature infants to leathery, cracked, and wrinkled (score of 5) seen in the overdue infant.
2. Lanugo: There is no lanugo in very premature infants. Whereas premature infants have abundant lanugo, mature infants are mostly without lanugo.
3. Plantar creases: Premature infants have faint creases, and mature infants have creases over the entire soles of the feet.
4. Breast: Immature infants have barely perceptible breast buds; mature infants have breast buds 5 to 10 mm in diameter.
5. Eyes and ears: Very immature infants have fused eyelids and pinna that are flat and stay folded. Mature infants have thick, stiff ear cartilage and well-formed eyes.
6. Genitals: Boys: As boys mature, the testes descend and rugae become evident.
7. Genitals: Girls: As the girls mature, the labia majora cover the clitoris and labia minora.

✹ NEUROMUSCULAR MATURITY ASSESSMENT

All six items of the neuromuscular maturity assessment (see Fig. 27–2) should be assessed with the child in the supine position.
1. Posture: As children mature, their arms and legs become more flexed. Observe children when they are quiet and in the supine position.
2. Square window: As children mature, their hand/wrist angle becomes more flexible. Flex the hand at the wrist gently but firmly to get as much flexion as possible. Score the angle between the anterior aspect of the forearm and the hypothenar eminence.
3. Arm recoil: Whereas immature infants have minimal flexion, mature infants have full flexion. Fully flex the forearm for 5 seconds, then extend the arms, and release. Note the amount of flexion.
4. Popliteal angle: The more flexion, the more mature the infant. Flex the leg and thigh fully, then extend. Release the leg and note the degree of flexion the infant assumes.
5. Scarf sign: As children mature, the scarf sign decreases. Extend the infant's hand and arm across the neck as far as possible to the opposite shoulder. Score according to the location of the elbow.
6. Heel to ear: The more immature the child, the easier it is to bring the heel to the ear. Keeping the pelvis flat, extend the foot to the head without forcing it.

✹ INTRAUTERINE GROWTH

SMALL FOR GESTATIONAL AGE

After determining maturity (gestational age) using the Ballard form, plot the length, weight, and head circumference on the intrauterine growth curve charts. Determine whether the child falls within the curve (normal) or is above or below the curve. A child who falls below the curve is considered small for gestational age (SGA). SGA children are shorter than normal, underweight, and have smaller heads than expected. This indicates that at some time, there was a problem in utero. SGA or growth-retarded babies have a higher incidence of problems, such as congenital viral infections, placental insufficiency, or fetal alcohol syndrome, during in utero development.

LARGE FOR GESTATIONAL AGE

A child who falls above the curve is considered large for gestational age (LGA). LGA children are longer and heavier, and have larger head circumferences than expected. LGA babies most commonly are associated with maternal diabetes. Refer to *www.cdc.gov* for intrauterine growth charts.

TEST YOUR KNOWLEDGE OF CHAPTER 27

1. Explain the concept of gestational age.
2. When should the Ballard Assessment Tool be used, and why?
3. What are the seven areas of external physical maturity assessed on the Ballard scale?
4. Describe how the six items of neuromuscular maturity are assessed on the Ballard scale.
5. Why is it important to determine if a child is large or small for gestational age?

BIBLIOGRAPHY

Algranati, P. S. (1992). *The pediatric patient: An approach to history and physical examination*. Baltimore: Williams & Wilkins.

Ballard, J. L., Khoury, J. C., Wedig, K., Wang, L., Eilers-Walsman, B. L., & Lipp, R. (1991). New Ballard score, expanded to include extremely premature infants. *Journal of Pediatrics*, (September), 417.

28

Mental Status Assessment

MARGARET R. COLYAR

OBJECTIVES
- Determine considerations for mental status assessment.
- Develop a list of areas of assessment for mental status in children.
- Become familiar with testing for attention-deficit disorder and attention-deficit hyperactivity disorder.
- Be able to identify the physical examination components of common mental status problems.
- Become familiar with manifestations of childhood depression.

Mental status is a child's cognitive and emotional functioning. Increased stress and traumatic events (e.g., death, serious illness) can tip the balance, leading to mental disorders. Children's behavior is the area of evaluation that leads providers to a diagnosis of mental disorder. A full mental status examination includes a systematic check of emotional and cognitive functioning.

 HISTORY

Most of mental status assessment is done through history taking. Determine the medical history of the child regarding neurological and psychiatric problems. Ask about brain injuries, brain surgeries, psychiatric counseling, and hospitalization. Note any family history of mental illness, alcoholism, addiction, retardation, learning disorders, and psychiatric disorders.

Conduct a thorough personal and social history, including emotional status, feelings about self, level of life stressors, anxiety, irritability, restlessness, weight changes (loss or gain), and appetite change. Also explore intellectual levels, sleeping patterns, and use of mood-altering drugs. Always check speech and language development. Note aberrations of behavior such as tantrums, holding breath, hyperactivity, impulsivity, decreased attention span, personality or behavior changes, and learning difficulties.

DEVELOPMENTAL CONSIDERATIONS

Language development occurs in a logical progression. Cooing begins at approximately 6 weeks of age. By age 1 year, children should be saying one-word sentences. Multiword sentences occur at age 2 years. A child's attention span gradually increases in through preschool age. By school age, children are able to sit and concentrate on their work for a long period. Thinking becomes more logical and systematic around age 7 years, with children being able to reason and understand. Abstract thinking develops between ages 12 and 15 years with the ability to consider a hypothetical situation (review Chapter 3). Then judgment begins to develop through experiences and education. Last, a set of values is developed and is reflected in children's thinking and actions.

MENTAL STATUS EXAMINATION

The mental status examination in children includes cognitive, behavior, and psychosocial development. For children up to 6 years old, use the Denver Development II scale to determine appropriate completion of milestones (see Chapter 3). For school-age children who are older than age 6 years, use a behavioral checklist that covers mood, play, school, friends, and family relations as a guide to determine need for referral for psychiatric evaluation (Table 28–1). For adolescents, use indicators of appearance, behavior, cognition, and thought process to evaluation mental status (Tables 28–2 to 28–4).

INDIVIDUAL AREAS OF ASSESSMENT

Evaluation of each area is dependent on the child's age and cognitive development.

Mood and Affect

Mood is the state of mind and expression of a child (Table 28–5). Affect is expressed by voice, demeanor, and facial expression.

Orientation

Orientation includes memory and attention. Orientation is the child's awareness of himself or herself relative to other people, time, and place. In general, younger children can focus attention for about 1 minute per year of age.

TABLE 28–1. SCHOOL-AGE CHILD BEHAVIORAL CHECKLIST OF INDICATIONS FOR PSYCHIATRIC REFERRAL*

1. Prefers to play alone
2. Gets hurt in minor accidents
3. Plays with fire
4. Has difficulties with teachers
5. Gets poor grades in school
6. Is frequently absent from school
7. Becomes angry easily
8. Seems to be daydreaming
9. Appears to be unhappy
10. Acts younger than other children his or her age
11. Does not listen to parents
12. Does not tell the truth
13. Unsure of himself or herself
14. Has trouble sleeping
15. Seems afraid of someone or something
16. Is nervous and jumpy
17. Has a nervous habit
18. Does not show feelings
19. Fights with other children
20. Is understanding of other people's feelings
21. Refuses to share
22. Shows jealousy
23. Takes things that are not his or hers
24. Blames others for his or her troubles
25. Prefers to play with children not his or her age
26. Gets along well with grown-ups
27. Teases others

*Scoring point system: 0 = never; 1 = sometimes; 2 = often. Scoring is reversed for items 20 and 26. Scores between 15 and 22 indicate closer following; scores above 22 warrant psychiatric evaluation.

Attention

Attention is the ability to focus and concentrate on one task. By school age, children should be able to focus on the task at hand for 15 to 30 minutes.

Memory

Memory is the retention of information. Beginning at preschool age, children should have recent memory. Remote memory is more developed in school-age children. Recent memory is the ability to recall information in the last minute, hour, and day. Remote memory is the ability to recall information in years.

Abstract Reasoning

Abstract reasoning is developed between ages 12 and 15 years. It is the ability to think in abstract terms and to grasp similarities and differences.

442

TABLE 28–2. ADOLESCENT MENTAL STATUS EVALUATION:
INDICATORS TO ASSESS

A = APPEARANCE

- Posture
- Body movements
- Dress
- Grooming and hygiene

B = BEHAVIOR

- Level of consciousness
- Facial expressions
- Speech
- Mood and affect

C = COGNITIVE FUNCTION

- Orientation
- Attention span
- Memory: Recent and remote
- Judgment

T = THOUGHT PROCESSES AND PERCEPTIONS

- Thought content (consistent and logical)
- Perceptions (visual, tactile, auditory, gustatory)
- Suicidal ideations

Judgment

Judgment is the ability to compare and evaluate alternatives, and decide on a course of action. Judgment is poorly developed in preschool-age children. Development of judgment improves progressively from school age to adolescence, depending on personal experiences.

Perception

Perception is the awareness of objects through any of the five senses. Depending on the cognitive stage the child is in his or her perceptions of the environmental qualities and relationships vary.

TABLE 28–3. ADOLESCENT MENTAL STATUS EVALUATION: THOUGHT CONTENT EVALUATION

Content	Description
Obsession	Persistent thoughts or impulses
Compulsion	Unwanted, repetitive acts
Delusion	False irrational beliefs
Hallucination	Altered sensory (visual, tactile, auditory, gustatory) perceptions
Illusion	Misperception of existing stimulus
Phobia	Irrational fear of a situation or object
Hypochondriasis	Morbid worry about personal health without actual reason

TABLE 28–4. ADOLESCENT MENTAL STATUS EVALUATION: THOUGHT PROCESS EVALUATION

Process	Description
Blocking	Interruption of train of thought; inability to complete sentences
Confabulation	Fabrication to fill memory gaps
Neologism	Invented words with no real meaning
Circumstantiality	Excessive and unnecessary detail in speech pattern
Loosening associations	Shifts topics quickly even though unrelated
Flight of ideas	Continuous rapid skipping from topic to topic; rapid speech
Word salad	Words, phrases, and sentences are mixed and are incoherent and illogical
Perseveration	Repetition of verbal or motor response
Echolalia	Mocking repetition of other people's words
Clanging	Choice of words based on sounds rather than meaning; rhyming

Appearance

Appearance includes dress, grooming, personal hygiene, posture, and body movements. Note the child's hair, teeth, nails, and skin. Compare one side of the body with the other. Excessive fastidiousness is seen in individuals with obsessive-compulsive disorders. Neglect or deterioration of personal hygiene may indicate depression. One-sided neglect usually occurs with lesions on the opposite side of the parietal cortex.

TABLE 28–5. MOOD AND AFFECT

Type of Expression	Description
Flat	Blunted expression of feelings; monotone voice
Depressed	Sad, gloomy, dejected
Ambivalent	Does not care about either side of an issue
Anxious	Apprehensive, worried, uneasy
Fearful	Apprehensive, worried, uneasy about identified danger
Irritable	Impatient, annoyed, or easily provoked
Elated	Increased motor activity, overconfident, optimistic
Euphoric	Excessively cheerful or highly elated
Rage	Furious; violent anger
Labile	Emotions shift quickly
Inappropriate	What the child does conflicts with what he or she is talking about (e.g., laughs when talking about his or her broken leg)
Depersonalized	Estranged, perplexed, loss of identity

Dress should be appropriate for the season, age, and gender. Although eccentric dress combinations occur in individuals with schizophrenia, school-age and adolescent children tend to follow dress fads. Keep up to date with the current trends.

Posture should be erect and relaxed. Anxiety can be seen in children who are tense, curled up, frowning, watchful, or crying. Depression is shown by a child's slumped posture, slow walk, dragging of the feet or pacing, hand wringing, and agitation.

Body movements should be deliberate, coordinated, smooth, and voluntary. Anxious children are restless and fidgety. Depressed children are apathetic and sluggish in movement. With schizophrenia, look for facial grimacing and abnormal posturing and gestures. Manic episodes present as singing, dancing, and expansive movements.

Speech

Note the quantity and quality of the child's speech. Is the child talkative or silent? Note the rate and rhythm. Is the speech rapid, slow, or hesitant? Note volume and loudness. Note quality by the fluency, inflection, and clarity.

COMMON MENTAL STATUS PROBLEMS IN CHILDREN

Attention-Deficit Disorder and Attention-Deficit Hyperactivity Disorder

Attention-deficit disorder (ADD) and attention-deficit hyperactivity disorder (ADHD) occur in 2% to 5% of all children. Also, these problems often run in families. Three components comprise the diagnosis of ADD and ADHD: inattention, hyperactivity, and impulsivity (Table 28–6). Inattention is difficulty concentrating on desired tasks when potentially distracting stimuli occur. Hyperactivity is an increase in the level of intensity of motor activity of a child. Impulsivity is a sudden inclination of urge that cannot be controlled.

Always assess the child at home and at school. Symptoms of ADD or ADHD must be present in all settings to complete the diagnosis. Questionnaires have been developed and tested to evaluate children who may be affected by ADHD (Fig. 28–1). Every adult member in the household and every teacher should fill out the questionnaire separately. Information from as many people as possible is helpful for baseline information and adequate scoring.

Scoring To score the questionnaire for ADD and ADHD, an inattention score and a hyperactivity/impulsivity score must be determined. To score inattention, add the odd-numbered item answers and determine a score. To score the hyperactivity/impulsivity section, add the even-numbered items and determine a score. Add both scores (inattention and hyperactivity/

TABLE 28–6. COMPONENTS OF THE DIAGNOSIS OF ATTENTION-DEFICIT HYPERACTIVITY DISORDER		
Inattention	**Hyperactivity**	**Impulsivity**
Easily distracted	Fidgets or squirms	Trouble taking turns
Fails to finish tasks	Cannot play quietly	Blurts out in class
Difficulty sustaining attention	Talks excessively	Fails to consider consequences
Does not listen	Loses things	Difficulty playing quietly
Difficulty following instructions	Difficulty remaining seated	Interrupts others
Does not seem to be listening	Shifts from one task to another	Engages in dangerous activities (not thrill seeking)

impulsivity) together to get a total score. Note where the child's score falls on the appropriate score chart by gender and age for all three areas. If the child is scored on inattention at the 93rd percentile or above but hyperactivity/impulsivity is below the 93rd percentile, the child is considered to have ADD. If the child is scored at the 93rd percentile or above on inattention and hyperactivity/ impulsivity, then the child is considered to have ADHD. If the scores are less than the 93rd percentile, then the child is not considered to have ADD or ADHD.

Anorexia Nervosa and Bulimia

Eating disorders can start as a temporary way to eliminate calories. It has been found that when the pattern of bingeing, purging, or dieting is established, it can be difficult to alter. Some adolescents become addicted to using the eating disorder as a coping mechanism to eat what they want but not alter their bodies. Common methods used to lose weight include dieting, fasting, vomiting, using laxatives, and taking diuretics.

Both anorexic and bulimic adolescents have the same negative self-image, which is influenced by weight and body shape. Teens with eating disorders may also be perfectionists who want a body that a American society believes is beautiful. Other reasons for eating disorders are a sense of personal ineffectiveness, and difficulties with communication and conflict resolution. Usually, teens with anorexia or bulimia are female, but boys do participate in this practice, especially if they are in a sport that has a weight requirement that is difficult to achieve. Examination questions to assess an eating disorder are provided in Table 28–7.

Childhood Depression

The incidence of childhood depression is estimated to be 2% in prepubertal children and approximately 5% in adolescents. Depression is more common in boys than in girls before puberty. During puberty, depression is common in both boys and girls.

ADHD RATING SCALE–IV—SCHOOL VERSION

Child's Name	Child's Age	Child's Grade
Completed by:	SEX: M F	Child's Race

Circle the number that best describes this student's behavior over the past 6 months (or since the beginning of the school year).	never or rarely	sometimes	often	very often
1. Fails to give close attention to details or makes careless mistakes in schoolwork.	0	1	2	3
2. Fidgets with hands or feet or squirms in seat.	0	1	2	3
3. Has difficulty sustaining attention in tasks or play activities.	0	1	2	3
4. Leaves seat in classroom or in other situations in which remaining seated is expected.	0	1	2	3
5. Does not seem to listen when spoken to directly.	0	1	2	3
6. Runs about or climbs excessively in situations in which it is inappropriate.	0	1	2	3
7. Does not follow through on instructions and fails to finish work.	0	1	2	3
8. Has difficulty playing or engaging in leisure activities quietly.	0	1	2	3
9. Has difficulty organizing tasks and activities.	0	1	2	3
10. Is "on the go" or acts as if "driven by a motor."	0	1	2	3
11. Avoids tasks (e.g., schoolwork, homework) that require sustained mental effort.	0	1	2	3
12. Talks excessively.	0	1	2	3
13. Loses things necessary for tasks or activities.	0	1	2	3
14. Blurts out answers before questions have been completed.	0	1	2	3
15. Is easily distracted.	0	1	2	3
16. Has difficulty awaiting turn.	0	1	2	3
17. Is forgetful in daily activities.	0	1	2	3
18. Interrupts or intrudes on others.	0	1	2	3

Questionnaire developed by DuPaul, Anastopoulos, Power, Murphy, and Barkley. Reprinted with permission. From: Gordon, M. & Irwin, M. (1997). *The diagnosis & treatment of ADD/ADHD: A no-nonsense guide for primary care physicians.* DeWitt, NY: GSI Publications.

FIG. 28–1. ADD/ADHD questionnaires: School and home versions and scoring.

ADHD RATING SCALE–IV—HOME VERSION

Child's Name		Child's Age	Child's Grade

Completed by: ❑ Mother ❑ Father ❑ Guardian ❑ Grandparent	Sex: M F	Child's Race

Circle the number that _best describes_ your child's home behavior over the past 6 months.	never or rarely	sometimes	often	very often
1. Fails to give close attention to details or makes careless mistakes in schoolwork.	0	1	2	3
2. Fidgets with hands or feet or squirms in seat.	0	1	2	3
3. Has difficulty sustaining attention in tasks or play activities.	0	1	2	3
4. Leaves seat in classroom or in other situations in which remaining seated is expected.	0	1	2	3
5. Does not seem to listen when spoken to directly.	0	1	2	3
6. Runs about or climbs excessively in situations in which it is inappropriate.	0	1	2	3
7. Does not follow through on instructions and fails to finish work.	0	1	2	3
8. Has difficulty playing or engaging in leisure activities quietly.	0	1	2	3
9. Has difficulty organizing tasks and activities.	0	1	2	3
10. Is "on the go" or acts as if "driven by a motor."	0	1	2	3
11. Avoids tasks (e.g., schoolwork, homework) that require sustained mental effort.	0	1	2	3
12. Talks excessively.	0	1	2	3
13. Loses things necessary for tasks or activities.	0	1	2	3
14. Blurts out answers before questions have been completed.	0	1	2	3
15. Is easily distracted.	0	1	2	3
16. Has difficulty awaiting turn.	0	1	2	3
17. Is forgetful in daily activities.	0	1	2	3
18. Interrupts or intrudes on others.	0	1	2	3

Questionnaire developed by DuPaul, Anastopoulos, Power, Murphy, and Barkley. Reprinted with permission. From: Gordon, M. & Irwin, M. (1997). _The diagnosis & treatment of ADD/ADHD: A no-nonsense guide for primary care physicians._ DeWitt, NY: GSI Publications.

FIG. 28–1. ADD/ADHD questionnaires: School and home versions and scoring (_continued_).

TABLE 28–7. EATING DISORDER EXAMINATION

1. Do you feel good about your body?
2. Do you think you eat too much?
3. What do you do when you are over your goal weight? When you have eaten too much? When you have eaten high-calorie foods?
4. Do you like to eat alone?
5. Do you need to take laxatives? How often?
6. Do you have a sore throat most of the time?
7. How often do you exercise?
8. Examination of these clients includes observation of:
   a. Height and weight
   b. Mouth and throat examination: Palatal trauma (from pharyngeal stimulation)
   c. Parotid gland examination (glands are usually inflamed if the client is constantly vomiting)
   d. Dental erosion because the enamel is chemically damaged by hydrochloric acid from the stomach
   e. Metacarpal-phalangeal bruises or calluses, which are constant abrasions, even scars, on the base of the index finger or finger used in purging
   f. Vital signs, bradycardia (a resting heart rate of $\leq$ 60 beats per minute is often found in anorexics), bradypnea, hypotension, hypothermia, and poor capillary refill
   g. Evaluate hydration state
   h. Scaphoid abdomen or organomegaly
   i. Skin edema of extremities (loss of protein)
9. Mental state, including apathy, psychomotor retardation, depression, anxiety, obsessive-compulsive traits

Clinical manifestations of major depression in children and adolescents are listed in Table 28–8. The etiology of depression is varied. Depression may have a biological origin or be secondary to parental depression, abuse, neglect, learned helplessness, cognitive distortion, social skills deficit, or family dysfunction. Childhood depression can be treated using a variety of modalities, including medication, play therapy, cognitive therapy, and group therapy.

TABLE 28–8. CLINICAL MANIFESTATIONS OF DEPRESSION IN CHILDREN

- Withdrawal from social activities
- Sleep disturbance (too much or too little)
- Appetite disturbance (too much or too little)
- Multiple somatic complaints
  - Headaches
  - Stomachaches
- Decreased energy
- Difficulty concentrating
- Difficulty making decisions
- Low self-esteem
- Feelings of hopelessness

TEST YOUR KNOWLEDGE OF CHAPTER 28

1. What information in a child's family history is needed with a mental status examination?
2. What are the developmental considerations with a mental status examination?
3. By age, what are the components of a mental status examination?
4. What are common mental status problems seen in children?
5. How are ADD and ADHD evaluated?
6. What are the components of an eating disorder examination?
7. What is the etiology of childhood depression?
8. What are the clinical manifestations of childhood depression?

 BIBLIOGRAPHY

Binder, R., & Ball, J. (1999). *Pediatric nursing: Caring for children*. Stamford, CT: Appleton & Lange.

Brantly, D. C., & Takacs, D. J. (1991). Anxiety and depression in preschool and school-aged children. In P. Clunn (Ed.), *Child psychiatric nursing*. St. Louis: Mosby; 351–365.

Goldbloom, R. B. (1997). *Pediatric clinical skills*. Philadelphia: Churchill Livingstone.

Jarvis, C. (1992). *Physical examination and health assessment*. Philadelphia: W. B. Saunders.

Kashani, J. H., & Eppright, T. D. (1997). Mood disorders in adolescents. In J. M. Weiner (Ed.), *Textbook of child and adolescent psychiatry*. Washington, DC: American Psychiatric Press; 248–260.

29

Eye Procedures

Margaret R. Colyar

> **Objectives**
> - *Determine when to treat an eye injury.*
> - *Understand the procedures of eyelid eversion and inspection for corneal abrasion.*
> - *Establish a safe method to quickly stabilize a child with a punctured globe and prepare for transfer.*

Children are prone to many eye problems, including conjunctivitis, superficial corneal abrasion, and puncture of the globe. Corneal abrasions can occur from simple rubbing of the eye to remove sand or dirt. In addition, children may sustain corneal abrasions by not wearing eye protection when watching someone weld. Laceration of the eyelid or sclera and puncture of the globe are both emergencies in which stabilization of the eye and transfer of the child to the appropriate emergency treatment facilities are necessary.

You should attempt to remove foreign bodies and treat corneal abrasions that are superficial. Corneal abrasions can be caused by trauma to the anterior globe of the eye, with or without penetration by a foreign object. Corneal foreign bodies result from superficial penetration by a foreign object to the anterior globe of the eye. Most injuries in children result from falls or sports injuries. However, rough play at school, tossing objects, or mass hysteria can also result in eye injuries. Assessment of the eye before performing procedures should include visual acuity, extraocular movement (EOM), palpation of the orbital bony structures, and fundoscopic examination (see Chapter 6).

EYELID EVERSION

CONTRAINDICATIONS

Do not evert the eyelid if the child is uncooperative, any foreign body is present, the eyelid is lacerated, or any of the conditions listed below are suspected. Stabilize the eye, and send the child to an emergency facility for any of the following:

- Ruptured globe
- Corneal or sclera lacerations
- Eyelid lacerations
- Conjunctival lacerations
- Corneal ulceration
- Any embedded foreign object
- Unsuccessful removal of foreign body
- Uncooperative child or infant who requires sedation

EQUIPMENT

- Nonsterile cotton-tipped applicator

PROCEDURE

- Instruct the child to look downward.
- Get the child to relax the eye. Explain the procedure to the child.
- Grasp the upper eyelashes between your thumb and forefinger. Pull down and forward gently.
- Using your other hand, place the tip of the cotton-tipped applicator on the upper eyelid approximately 1 cm above the eyelid margin.
- Push down with the cotton-tipped applicator and lift the eyelashes up gently. The eyelid will turn inside out. Do NOT put pressure on the eyeball (Fig. 29–1).
- After inspection, gently pull the eyelashes outward as the child looks up. The eyelid will return to normal position.

452

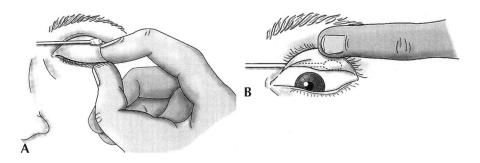

FIG. 29–1. Eversion of the eyelid. *(A)* Grasp the eyelid. Pull down and forward gently. *(B)* Push downward with the cotton-tipped applicator and lift the eyelid up.

CORNEAL ABRASION

CONTRAINDICATIONS

- Chemical acid or alkali exposure:
  - Apply ophthalmic anesthetic and begin vigorous irrigation with the use of standard intravenous (IV) tubing and 0.9% sodium chloride solution or lactated Ringer's solution for 15 minutes or 2 liters, whichever comes first.
- **Urgent (REFER within 48 hours to an ophthalmologist):**
  - Onset of corneal opacities
  - Presence of a "rust ring" at the former location of embedded foreign body
  - Increasing pain
  - Loss of vision
  - Nonresolution of corneal abrasion
  - Onset of preseptal cellulitis with periorbital cellulitis

EQUIPMENT

- Direct ophthalmoscope
- Nonsterile gloves
- Fluorescein strips (use individually packaged strips)
- Cobalt blue light (Wood's light or blue light on ophthalmoscope)
- Two eye patches if child is older than age 5 years
- Adhesive tape
- IV tubing with sterile 0.9% sodium chloride or lactated Ringer's solution
- Tissue or nonsterile 4 × 4 gauze
- Ophthalmic medication

PROCEDURE

- Cover the lateral corner of the face with a drape or facial tissue to prevent drainage of dye onto clothing because dye can cause permanent stain to clothing.

- Provide tissues for the child to wipe drips.
- Instill 1 to 2 drops of ophthalmic anesthetic if there are no contraindications.
- Moisten strips with 2 to 3 drops of sterile 0.9% sodium chloride.
- Touch the moistened strip to the base of the globe of lateral sclera until there is good fill.
- Instruct the child to blink several times to disperse the dye.
- Turn off the overhead light and turn on cobalt blue light.
  - Abrasions to the cornea are seen as bright yellow or yellow green.
- Note the size, shape, and location of the abrasion.
- **If abrasion is close to the central line of vision, consider REFERRING to an ophthalmologist because of a high incidence of permanent scarring in this area.**
- When inspection is completed, initiate a vigorous irrigation with 0.9% sodium chloride to remove all dye from the eye to lessen any further irritation. Always apply topical ophthalmic antibiotic of choice (e.g., tobramycin; hydrocortisone, bacitracin zinc, and polymyxin B sulfate [Cortisporin]; gentamicin; neomycin [Neosporin]) if an abrasion is found because of the avascular character of the cornea.
- Apply a single or double eye patch
  - Use of a patch should be considered in children older than 5 years of age.

DOCUMENTATION

Include when and how the abrasion occurred, assessment of vision, procedure performed, pictorial or written description of the location of the abrasion, and treatment administered. An example is as follows:

S (Subjective): Rubbed right eye after another child threw sand in face at noon today. Eye is painful. Denies visual difficulty

O (Objective): EYES: PERRLA (pupils equal, round, reactive to light and accommodation), EOMs intact.

Funduscopic: Vessels without nicking/twisting, disc edges smooth. Right eye: Reddened and tearing.

PROCEDURE: Cleansed right eye with sterile saline. Instilled ophthalmic anesthetic and fluorescein stain. Using Wood's lamp, visualized abrasion at 2:00 right eye. No rust ring. Tobramycin ophthalmic suspension applied. One eye patch applied and taped in place. Tolerated procedure well.

✪ SUPERFICIAL FOREIGN BODY REMOVAL

This is NOT a standard procedure because of the severity of risk if the child moves and the needle penetrates the eye. Use ONLY with very cooperative older adolescents. Do NOT attempt this procedure with uncooperative children.

CONTRAINDICATIONS

- History of high-velocity injury.
  - Apply a nonpressure eye shield. Transfer to an emergency room or ophthalmologist.
- **Urgent (REFER within 48 hours to an ophthalmologist):**
  - Onset of corneal opacities
  - Presence of a "rust ring" at the former location of embedded foreign body
  - Increasing pain
  - Loss of vision
  - Nonresolution of corneal abrasion
  - Onset of preseptal cellulitis with periorbital cellulitis

EQUIPMENT

- Sterile cotton-tipped applicators
- Sterile 25- or 27-gauge needle

PROCEDURE

- Position the child in a comfortable supine position
- Put on nonsterile gloves.
- Instill 1 to 2 drops of ophthalmic anesthetic. This will aid in performing the procedure.
- When the pain subsides, the child becomes more trusting.
- Spread the eyelids apart with the thumb and index finger.
- Have the child's head positioned so the foreign body is at the highest point on the eye globe.
- Instruct the child to fix his or her gaze toward a certain point.
- *If foreign body is not embedded,* use moistened sterile cotton-tipped applicator with gentle rolling motion to remove.
- *If foreign body is embedded superficially,* use 27- or 25-gauge needle bevel side up (Fig. 29–2).
- Rest the lateral side of your hand on the side of the client's cheek or forehead for more stability in movement.
- Approach the child's eye with the needle parallel to the eye globe.
- Gently apply pressure across the surface (bevel away from the eye) to dislodge the foreign body.
- After several unsuccessful attempts, apply antibiotic ointment and refer to an ophthalmologist.
- After removal of the foreign body, proceed to check for a corneal abrasion with fluorescein stain, followed by patching if indicated.

DOCUMENTATION

Include when and how the abrasion occurred, assessment of vision, procedure performed, pictorial or written description of the location of the abrasion, and treatment administered. An example is as follows:

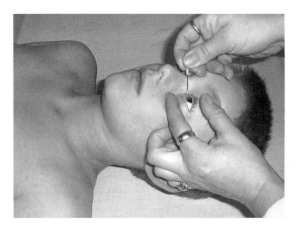

FIG. 29–2. Removal of foreign body from the eye using a 27-gauge needle.

S: Working in wood shop without safety glasses on. Thinks a splinter is in the left eye. Eye is painful. Denies visual difficulty.

O: EYES: PERRLA, EOMs intact.

Funduscopic: Vessels without nicking/twisting, disc edges smooth. Left eye: Reddened and tearing.

PROCEDURE: Cleansed right eye with sterile saline. Instilled ophthalmic anesthetic and fluorescein stain. Using Wood's lamp, visualized splinter at 1:00 left eye. Using sterile cotton-tipped applicator, gently removed splinter. No rust ring. Tobramycin ophthalmic suspension applied. Tolerated procedure well.

EYE TRAUMA STABILIZATION

Eye trauma includes blunt or penetration injuries to the globe of the eye. Complications include fractures of the facial bones and loss of sight in the affected eye. Thoroughly examine the region for anatomical defects:

- If possible, establish visual acuity.
- Avoid any pressure to the eyelid and the globe of the eye because pressure may precipitate a spontaneous and premature rupture and loss of the vitreous humor. Loss of vitreous humor results in permanent blindness.
- Inspect for disruption in the sclera. This includes rotating the globe in an upward and downward motion. (This is important because when the eyelid closes, the globe automatically rotates upward.)
- Fundoscopic examination:
  - Note any iritic infection.
  - Note the absence of the anterior chamber.
  - Note wrinkling of anterior chamber (represents rupture of the chamber).
  - Note the presence or absence of macular edema.
  - Check the vitreous humor for clouding (represents hemorrhage).
  - Note the presence or absence of retinal detachment (i.e., changes in the color and shape of the retinal eye background compared with the uninjured eye).
- Inspect the maxillary structures for loss of integrity.

456

- Inspect the orbit structures for loss of integrity.
- Perform a neurological examination to exclude accompanying head injury.

CONTRAINDICATIONS

- Do not perform the procedure for visualizing corneal abrasion (fluorescein staining) if a globe injury is suspected.

EQUIPMENT

- Ophthalmoscope
- Plastic or Styrofoam cup or large eye shield
- Two rolls of 4-inch gauze wrap
- Ophthalmic antibiotic ointment
- Eye patch
- Adhesive tape (1 or 2 inches wide)

PROCEDURE

- Position the child in a comfortable position with the eye easily accessible.
- Make a donut ring using the 4-inch gauze wrap (Fig. 29–3).
- Wrap loosely around the hand six to eight times in approximate diameter to encircle the eye.
- In a continuous motion, wrap the other 4-inch gauze in a circular fashion around the loose gauze until a firm donut forms.
- Anchor the end of the gauze with a piece of tape.
- Apply ophthalmic antibiotic ointment to the injured eye.
- Apply the gauze donut over the orbit of the eye without coming in contact with the globe.
- Place the plastic or Styrofoam cup or eye shield on the gauze donut.
- Anchor the cup or shield with 4-inch gauze around the head with several wraps.
- Apply an eye patch to the unaffected eye and continue wrapping the head to anchor both of the eye dressings (Fig. 29–4).
- Transport the client to the nearest emergency department via ambulance in a slightly upright position for further evaluation by an ophthalmologist.

DOCUMENTATION

Include when and how the abrasion occurred, assessment of vision, procedure performed, pictorial or written description of the location of the abrasion, and treatment administered. An example is as follows:

> S: Grinding metal without safety glasses on. Thinks metal is in the left eye. Eye is painful. Can't see well.

> O: EYES: Piece of metal visible in sclera of left eye at 5:00. PERRLA. EOMs intact.

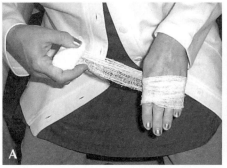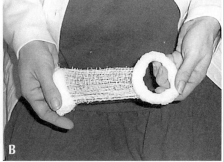

FIG. 29–3. *(A)* and *(B)* Preparation of the donut ring.

Fundoscopic: No wrinkling of anterior chamber. Disc, retina, and macula intact. No clouding or hemorrhage. Acuity not done. Left eyelid edematous without laceration. Orbits palpated; no crepitus or obvious fracture.

PROCEDURE: Shielded left eye with gauze ring and Styrofoam cup. Eye patch applied to right eye. Secured with 4-inch gauze. Transferred to emergency room via ambulance.

CLIENT INSTRUCTIONS

To prevent eye movement and further eye damage:

● It is necessary for both eyes to be covered.
● Try not to cough, sneeze, or breathe deeply.

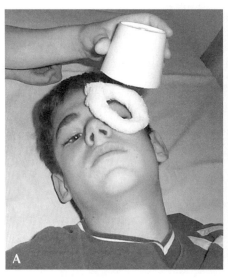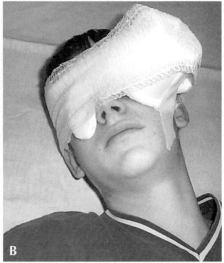

FIG. 29–4. *(A)* and *(B)* Completed stabilization of eye trauma.

🌀 HEALTH PROMOTION AND PREVENTION

- People of all ages should wear protective eyewear while participating in sports.
- People of all ages should wear protective eyewear when working around any machinery.
- Lessen the risk of BB gun injury through proper gun handling education classes.
- Lessen the risk of falling accidents with the use of good safety habits.
- People of all ages should wear protective eyewear against excessive and prolonged light exposure.

GENERAL PRINCIPLES

- Use of an eye patch for more than 48 hours increases the risk of amblyopia (especially for children who are younger than age 5 years).
- Tetanus booster: Needed if child was not immunized within past 5 years.

TEST YOUR KNOWLEDGE OF CHAPTER 29

1. Why is an eye examination necessary when an eye injury occurs?
2. What components of an eye examination are necessary when an eye injury occurs?
3. When are eyelid eversion and foreign body removal contraindicated?
4. Describe the procedure for eyelid eversion. When should the procedure be performed?
5. Describe the procedure for corneal abrasion treatment. When should the treatment be given?
6. How do you stabilize a child with a penetrating eye injury?
7. What types of eye injuries should be referred to the emergency room?
8. What types of eye injuries should be referred to the ophthalmologist?

🌀 BIBLIOGRAPHY

Colyar, M. R., & Ehrhardt, C. (1999). *Ambulatory care procedures for the nurse practitioner.* Philadelphia: F. A. Davis.

Goldbloom, R. B. (1997). *Pediatric clinical skills.* Philadelphia: Churchill Livingstone.

Pfenninger, J. L., & Fowler, G. C. (1994). *Procedures of primary care physicians.* St. Louis: Mosby.

CHAPTER 30

Respiratory Procedures

MARGARET R. COLYAR

OBJECTIVES
- *Become proficient in aerosol inhalation treatment.*
- *Become proficient in peak flow testing.*
- *Determine when to seek emergency assistance.*
- *Competently document respiratory procedures.*

Inhalation through aerosol administration of medication is commonly used in medical conditions of airflow obstruction such as bronchospasm and airway hyperresponsiveness. This method is considered an effective method of medication administration for the treatment of bronchiole pathway disorders, and it has few side effects. It is extremely effective in the administration of medication in children younger than 5 years of age. Fewer drug interactions and side effects have been associated with aerosol administration. Intervention for episodic or chronic therapy may be used.

Peak flow monitoring is particularly beneficial in asthmatic patients. It has been demonstrated that regular monitoring has reduced the frequency, duration, and severity of attacks. A peak flow meter is a hand-held device that provides an objective assessment of dynamic pulmonary function and response to clinical therapy of pulmonary diseases. It allows asthmatics to objectively self-monitor their respiratory status, permits clinicians of asthmatics to intervene early in therapy, and reduces the frequency of emergency room visits and hospitalizations. The result of the peak flow meter evaluation is expressed as the peak flow rate (PFR). Limitations of the peak flow meter include poor user skills, lack of motivation and individual effort, and the fact that children younger than age 5 years cannot use it properly.

460

CPT Codes

- 94642: Aerosol inhalation
- A7003: Aerosol administration set (tubing)
- J7619: Albuterol inhalation solution
- J7051: Sterile saline 5 mL
- J7644: Atrovent inhalation solution
- 94160: Vital capacity screening tests; total capacity, with timed forced expiratory volume (state duration), and peak flow rate
- 94360: Peak flow

 # CONTRAINDICATIONS

There are no contraindications to aerosal treatments and peak flow monitoring.

AEROSOL AND INHALATION ADMINISTRATION

EQUIPMENT

- Pulse oximeter
- Peak flow meter
- Oxygen with tubing and nebulizer mask
- Aerosol administration kit
- Air compressor (such as Pulmo-aide or Invacare Passport)
- 3 mL 0.9% sodium chloride
- Medication (commonly used) (Table 30–1)

PROCEDURE

- Have the child sit up or lie down.
- If the child is cooperative, apply the pulse oximeter and monitor continuously throughout the procedure. Otherwise, check pre- and post-procedure oxygen saturation.
- If the child is older than age 5 years and is cooperative, perform a peak flow reading and record it.
- Plug the air compressor in and open the aerosol administration kit.
- Insert the aerosol medication into the aerosol administration kit at an appropriate dosage and mixture.
- Determine the best method of administration. A mask is best for infants, and a mouthpiece is best for older children. This is dependent on the age of the child and his or her ability to handle the mouthpiece versus the mask. If using a mouthpiece, cover one end with tape and position the end with aerosol mist close to the child's mouth and nose.

461

Drug	Dosage	Comments
BETA-2 AGONIST: SHORT-ACTING BRONCHODILATOR		
Albuterol	By weight: • Age <12 years: 0.15–0.25 mg/kg (maximum: 5 mg) in 3 mL 0.9% sodium chloride every 4–6 hours • Age >12 years: 2.5 mg Using 0.5% solution: • Age <12 years: 0.01–0.05 mL/kg (maximum: 1 mL) in 3 mL 0.9% sodium chloride every 4 to 6 hours. • Age >12 years: 0.5 mL Using 0.083% solution: • Age <12 years: 0.06–0.03 mL/kg (maximum: 6 mL); no dilution required; treatment should be performed every 4–6 hours • Age >12 years: 3 mL	May repeat every 20 minutes if necessary Use with caution in children younger than age 2 years and in those with pre-existing cardiac conditions
ANTI-INFLAMMATORY AGENTS (CORTICOSTEROIDS)		
Decadron (methylprednisone) 0.5 mg	0.5 mg mixed in 3 mL 0.9% sodium chloride with or without administration of albuterol	One-time dosage administration Rapid and direct administration of corticosteroids to the lining of the bronchioles Not for use in emergency situations
CROMOGLYCATE		
Cromolyn sodium: 20-mg/2-mL ampule	1 ampule every 6 hours Children age >2 years: 20 mg four times per day	May be mixed with albuterol and administered simultaneously Slow onset of action, may be several days before significant reduction of airway obstruction occurs

(continued)

TABLE 30–1. MEDICATIONS COMMONLY USED IN AEROSOL INHALATION ADMINISTRATION

Drug	Dosage	Comments
ANTICHOLINERGICS		
Atropine 0.1 mg/mL	Children: 0.03–0.05 mg/kg/dose three to four times per day; maximum 2.5 mg/dose	Rarely used because of potential side effects Use only when reduction in bronchospasm has not occurred with conventional therapy and potential life-threatening situation is occurring
Ipratropium	Neonates: 25 μg/kg/dose three times per day Infants and children: 125–250 μg three times per day Children age >12 years: 500 μg three to four times per day	Can be diluted with saline but not required Poorly absorbed from the lung, so systemic effects are rare Not indicated for initial treatment of acute episodes of bronchospasm

- Turn on the machine; a fine mist should form.
- Instruct the child to breath normally until the mist disappears (Fig. 30–1).
- When the aerosol mist stops, the medication is depleted. Stop the machine.
- Perform post-treatment peak flow and oxygen saturation measurement Record.

PATIENT TEACHING

- Perform home treatments every 6 hours using the medications ordered. Do not perform treatments more often than every 6 hours unless instructed to by a healthcare provider.

FIG. 30–1. Child receiving an aerosol inhalation treatment.

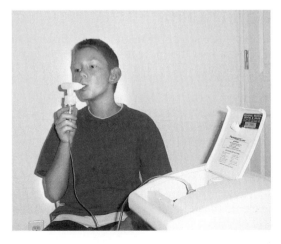

- Breathe slowly in and out to maximize the effectiveness of the medication.
- Side effect of the medications may include:
  - Nervousness or a jittery feeling
  - Fast heart rate or palpitations
- Seek emergency treatment if any of the following occur:
  - Nasal flaring
  - Intercostal retractions
  - Blueness of the fingertips or nail beds, or around the mouth

DOCUMENTATION

Document the type of treatment, and amount and type of medication used; peak flow meter results, both before and after the treatment; status of the child's respiratory system, both before and after the treatment; and how the child tolerated the procedure. An example is as follows:

> Procedure: Nebulizer treatment with 0.5% albuterol in 3 mL of normal saline.
>
> Pretreatment: Peak flow: 250. Lungs: Inspiratory and expiratory wheezes throughout.
>
> Posttreatment: Peak flow: 400. Lungs: clear bilaterally to auscultation anterior and posterior.
>
> Tolerated procedure well.

PEAK FLOW METER

EQUIPMENT

- Peak flow meter (Fig. 30–2)
- Mouthpiece

PROCEDURE

- Place the appropriate-size mouthpiece over the peak flow meter.
- Check that the indicator is at the bottom of the chamber.
- Hold the peak flow meter in the proper direction (as recommended by the manufacturer).
- Take a breath as deep as possible.
- Seal lips over the mouthpiece and blow out as quickly as possible (like blowing out candles) (Fig. 30–3).
- Note the reading on the dial.
- Repeat the above procedure a total of three times and record the highest reading.

The normal predicted average peak expiratory flow for children and adolescents (based on height) is shown in Table 30–2.

FIG. 30–2. Peak flow meter.

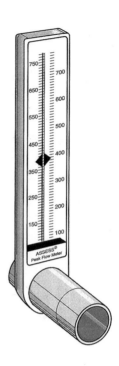

FIG. 30–3. Seal lips over the mouthpiece and blow out as quickly as possible.

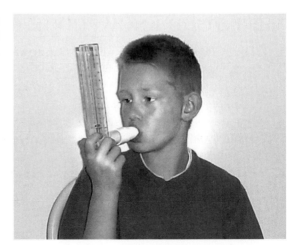

TABLE 30–2. NORMAL PREDICTED AVERAGE PEAK EXPIRATORY FLOW (CHILDREN AND ADOLESCENTS)*

Height, Inches	PFR
43	147
44	160
45	173
46	187
47	200
48	214
49	227
50	240
51	254
52	267
53	280
54	293
55	307
56	320
57	334
58	347
59	360
60	373
61	387
62	400
63	413
64	427
65	440
66	454

*Testing for this table was performed at sea level. These values are considered averages and may vary widely from individual to individual.
PFR = peak flow rate.

TEST YOUR KNOWLEDGE OF CHAPTER 30

1. What is the procedure for administering an aerosol inhalation treatment?
2. Which medications are commonly used in aerosol inhalation treatments?
3. How do the dosages of medications commonly used in aerosol inhalation treatments differ by age of child?
4. What are common side effects of aerosol inhalation medications?
5. When should parents seek emergency treatment for a child with respiratory problems?
6. What are the necessary components of respiratory treatment documentation?
7. How is "normal" peak flow determined?

BIBLIOGRAPHY

American Medical Association. (1996). *Physicians' current procedural terminology.* Chicago: American Medical Association.

Busse, W., & Holgate, S. (Eds.). (1995). *Asthma and rhinitis.* Cambridge, MA: Blackwell.

Fisons Pharmaceuticals. (1995). *Using a peak flow meter* [handout].

National Asthma Education and Prevention Program. (Feb. 1997). *Expert panel report II: Guidelines for the diagnosis and management of asthma.* Bethesda, MD: National Heart, Lung, and Blood Institute.

Pfenninger, J. L., & Fowler, G. C. (1994). *Procedures of primary care physicians.* St. Louis: Mosby.

Siberry, G. K., & Iannone, R. (Eds.). (2000). *The Johns Hopkins Hospital: The Harriet Lane handbook.* St. Louis: Mosby.

Summer, W., Elston, R., Tharpe, L., Nelson, S., & Haponik, E. (1989). Aerosol bronchodilator delivery methods. *Archives of Internal Medicine, 149,* 618–623.

Takotomo, C. K., Hodding, J. H., & Kraus, D. M. (2000). *Pediatric dosage handbook.* Cleveland: Lexi-Comp Inc.

CHAPTER 31

Interpretation of Radiographs

M<small>ARGARET</small> R. C<small>OLYAR</small>

O<small>BJECTIVES</small>
- *Review the basic rules of interpreting radiographs.*
- *Improve appreciation of the normal radiographic appearance of the pediatric chest, abdomen, and bones.*
- *Determine abnormalities and when to refer.*

An adequate knowledge base of anatomy and physiology is necessary for the proper interpretation of radiographs. Use an orderly and systematic approach to interpret chest, abdominal, and bone radiographs. A chest radiograph is considered the best radiological screening and diagnostic tool for most lung diseases because of its ability to generate high spatial resolution and to visualize various densities within the thoracic cavity. Radiographs of the musculoskeletal system are taken to determine the presence of disease, such as arthritis, spondylitis, bone lesions, and fractures.

An abdominal radiograph is considered a basic radiological screening tool for evaluating abdominal disorders. Abdominal radiographs give a visual overview of the basic pathophysiology of gastrointestinal, vascular, renal, and skeletal systems. Radiographs should not be the sole criterion of diagnosis; rather, radiographs should be correlated with clinical history, physical examination, and results obtained from additional diagnostic tools.

HISTORY

Obtain a thorough history of present illness from the primary caregiver and child, if possible. Include information on when the problem started or

CPT Codes

- 74000: Abdomen: One view
- 74010: Abdomen: Two views
- 74020: Abdomen: Three views
- 74022: Abdomen Acute
- 73600: Ankle: Two views
- 73610: Ankle: Three views
- 73000: Clavicle
- 73080: Elbow: Three views
- 70200: Eye: Orbits
- 70150: Facial bones
- 73550: Femur: Two views
- 73140: Fingers
- 73620: Foot: Two views
- 73630: Foot: Three views
- 73090: Forearm
- 73120: Hand: Two views
- 73130: Hand: Three views
- 73120A: Hand bilateral
- 73520: Hip bilateral
- 73510: Hip unilateral
- 73060: Humerus
- 73562: Knee: Three views
- 73592: Leg: Infant
- 73590: Leg: Lower
- 70160: Nasal bones
- 70360: Neck soft tissue
- 73540: Pelvis: Infant/child
- 73010: Scapula
- 73030: Shoulder: Two+ views
- 70222: Sinus
- 70260: Skull: Four views with Waters view
- 72050: Spine: Cervical: Four views
- 72100: Spine: Lumbar
- 72221: Spine: Sacrococcyx: Two+ views
- 72074: Spine: Thoracic
- 72069: Spine, Trunk, Scoliosis
- 70330: Temporomandibular joint
- 73660: Toe(s)
- 73110: Wrist

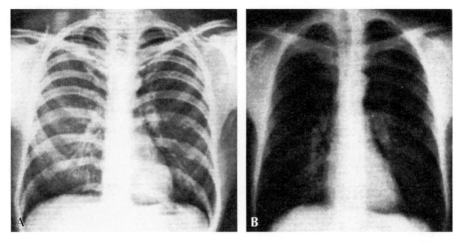

FIG. 31–1. (A) Chest radiograph, correct exposure. (B) Chest radiograph, overexposure.

occurred, what the child was doing at the time, how the condition has progressed, and what has been done to correct the problem.

✸ BASIC INFORMATION ABOUT RADIOGRAPHS

SHADES OF GRAY

An x-ray beam is a large amount of photons that travel through the body. They produce an x-ray shadow on film. The x-rays are absorbed in varying amounts, depending on the tissue through which they pass. There are five basic shades (Table 31–1) visible on plain radiographs: air, fat, water, soft tissue, and bone. Because air does not absorb much radiation, the photons pass through the body and expose the film more. This causes a dark area to be produced. On radiograph films, fat is generally a shade of gray that is darker than soft tissue, and bone is almost white.

EXPOSURE

Exposure is the measure of the ionization of air produced by a beam of radiation (Fig. 31–1). A correctly exposed film should have enough contrast for identification of structures and abnormalities. A correctly exposed chest radiograph should allow visualization of vessels to the peripheral one third of the lung and allow visualization of the left hemidiaphragm behind the heart. Overexposed films are dark. Overexposure makes it easier to see behind the heart and regions of the clavicle and thoracic spine. The lungs appear very dark, and the esophagus is visible. Underexposed films are very light. Underexposure accentuates the pulmonary vasculature but occludes the structures behind the heart and edges of the ribs.

470

TABLE 31–1. SHADOW COLOR OF TISSUE ON RADIOGRAPH

Tissue	Shadow Color
Air	Dark
Fat	Dark gray
Water (blood and muscle)	Lighter gray
Soft tissue	Light gray
Bone and calcium	Almost white

VIEWING

When putting radiographs on the view box, always remember to place them so that you view the chest radiograph as if you are facing the client. Thus, the client's right will be on your left. The technician usually marks the radiograph to indicate which is the client's right side or, in the case of radiographs of the extremities, whether it is the right or left arm or leg. After ordering the radiograph, a logical approach to the examination of the radiograph should be used (Table 31–2). After the radiograph has been reviewed and a diagnosis made, treatment and follow-up can be determined.

NORMAL CHEST RADIOGRAPHS

Always order an upright posteroanterior (PA) and a left lateral (LAT) view. These radiographs should be taken with the child in full inspiration. This may be difficult to accomplish with children. For more definitive evaluation of pleural opacity (which shows up as unexpected white area) noted on the conventional PA and LAT views, a decubitus view should be ordered. A decubitus view is taken using a sidelying position with the suspicious side of the patient's thoracic cavity dependent. This position allows the cause of the pleural opacity (usually a pleural effusion) to be free moving and results in layering along the lateral chest wall. When a portable chest radiograph is taken, you get an anteroposterior (AP) view, which makes the heart look artificially larger. Order an expiratory view if a pneumothorax is suspected.

TABLE 31–2. LOGICAL APPROACH TO RADIOGRAPH EXAMINATION

- Orient yourself to the radiograph ordered.
- Look at the name and age on the radiograph label (make sure you have the correct patient).
- Review normal and expected anatomy, and refer to an anatomy and physiology book, if needed.
- Decide if there are any abnormal findings.
- Describe the abnormal findings using correct anatomical descriptors.
- Complete a differential diagnosis.
- Order an overread by a radiologist if you are unsure.

TABLE 31–3. SYSTEMATIC EVALUATION OF A CHEST FILM

- Determine the age, gender, and history of the patient.
- Identify the projection and technique used (i.e., AP, PA, LAT, decubitus).
- Identify the position of the patient (i.e., adequate, hypoinflated, hyperinflated)
  - (Count the number of ribs (nine or 10 is adequate).
  - Identify the clavicles and spineous processes.
  - Identify the diaphragm.
- Identify the obvious and common abnormalities.
  - Heart size
  - Heart shape
  - Upper mediastinal countours
  - Airway or tracheal deviation
  - Lung symmetry
    - Mediastinal shift
    - Hilar position
  - Lung infiltrates, masses, or nodules
  - Pulmonary vasculature (increased, decreased, or normal)
  - Blind spots
    - Behind the heart
    - Behind the hemidiaphragms
    - In the lung apices
    - Chest wall
    - Lytic rib lesions
    - Shoulders
- Decide what the findings are and their locations.
- Correlate findings with clinical history.

AP = anteroposterior; LAT = lateral; PA = posterior-anterior.

Pleural density that migrates away from the lateral chest wall indicates free fluid. This view is most useful in children with pleural pulmonary infection. Indistinct lung markings usually indicate motion during the filming process. Look at inspiratory effort. Adequate inspiratory effort is shown as 9 or 10 ribs visible. Evaluate the radiographs in an organized manner (Table 31–3).

Inspect for the presence of any foreign bodies in the thoracic cavity. Systematically inspect the thoracic region skeletal system. Identify the anatomical skeletal landmarks within the thoracic cavity and occurrence of any aberration (Figs. 31–2 and 31–3).

COUNT THE RIBS

There should be 9 to 10 posterior ribs or five to six anterior ribs. Note the appearance of the ribs, beginning with identification of the posterior segments of the first rib on the right and proceeding through the twelfth rib. Repeat this process on the opposite side of the thoracic cavity. Note any widening of the rib spaces. Identify any demineralization (which shows up as darker area on the bone) in the skeletal structure. Determine any lack of continuity and symmetry of skeletal structure (including the clavicles, scapulae, humeri, and sternum).

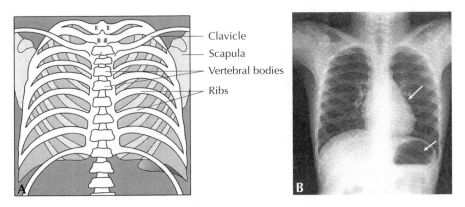

FIG. 31–2. *(A)* Anatomical skeletal landmarks as seen on the posteroanterior (PA) view of the chest. *(B)* Normal PA chest radiograph of a 7-year-old child. *Top arrow* shows the heart, and *bottom arrow* shows the gas bubble.

SOFT TISSUE MASSES

Systematically inspect for the presence of soft tissue masses. Note the contour of the neck. Look for asymmetry and shadow density changes in breast shadows or hepatic and splenic shadows. Check for the presence of a gas bubble in the stomach shadow. Note any evidence of changes in or shifting of the mediastinal shadows.

CARDIAC SYSTEM

Systematically inspect the cardiac system. Evaluate the contour of the heart, mediastinum, and great vessels. Begin at the upper right side of the medi-

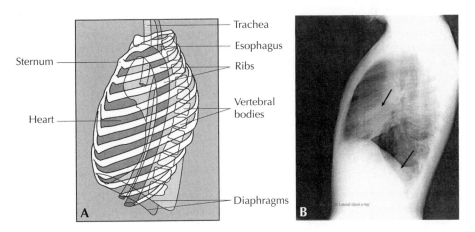

FIG. 31–3. *(A)* Anatomical skeletal landmarks as seen on the lateral view of the chest. *(B)* Normal lateral chest radiograph of 7-year-old child. *Top arrow* shows the heart, and the *bottom arrow* shows the diaphragms.

473

PA view

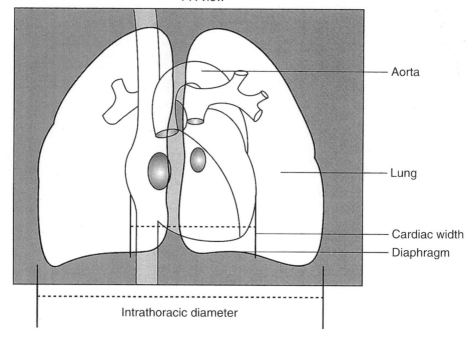

FIG.31–4. Inspect the cardiac system. Measure the intrathoracic diameter. Divide the intrathoracic diameter by 2. Measure the cardiac width. Normal cardiac size is less than half the intrathoracic diameter.

astinum and slowly progress to the apex. Evaluate the size of the heart. Note the shape of the cardiac silhouette, which is easily visible. Measure the intrathoracic diameter (Fig. 31–4). Note the width of inside of the rib cage at the level of the diaphragm on the right side plus the rib cage width on the left side. Divide the intrathoracic diameter by one-half. This should equal the cardiac size. Normal cardiac size is less than one-half the width of the thoracic diameter. Note the clarity of the cardiac borders, which should be well defined. Note increased calcification of the heart silhouette. Calcifications within the silhouette represent the valvular structures of the heart.

VASCULAR SYSTEM

Systematically inspect the presentation of vascular system. Evaluate the peripheral vessels. Correct exposure of the radiograph shows the peripheral vessels to at least the peripheral one third of the lung; you should also be able to see the left hemidiaphragm behind the heart. If the exposure is too dark, the vessels may not be seen. Underexposed films are extremely white, which makes small pulmonary vessels extremely prominent. Note any

474

anatomical shift or calcifications in the pulmonary arteries and aorta. The main pulmonary arterial branches should be equal in size, shape, and contour. Inspect the size and shape of the thoracic aorta. Locate the base of the aorta as it extends from the cardiac silhouette. Note the presence of aortic dilatation, straightening or coarctation of the aortic arch, or calcifications of the aorta.

LUNG SILHOUETTE

Systematically inspect the lung silhouette. Check for cohesiveness to the pleural borders, lucency of air within the lungs, presence of pleural lines within the confines of the ribs, and calcifications or densities within the lung field. Accentuated areas of white within the pulmonary black background represent pleural thickening or pleural fluid and can prevent clear demarcation of the anatomical borders. Note the presence of blunting of the costophrenic borders. Bronchovascular markings are normally symmetrical side to side and should be sharply marginated.

HEMIDIAPHRAGMS (DIAPHRAGM)

Systematically inspect the diaphragm. Note the presence or absence of flattening. Note the integrity and symmetry of the anatomical location. Note the absence or presence of the contralateral hemidiaphragm. The right hemidiaphragm is higher than the left. Both should be dome shaped. Costophrenic angles should be acute and well defined. With hyperinflation or air trapping, the diaphragm may appear more flat than dome shaped. When diaphragms are flat, the costophrenic angles may be obliterated.

THYMUS

Evaluate the thymus. In babies and young children, the normal thymus appears on radiographs as a triangular sail-shaped structure with well-defined borders projecting from the right or both sides of the mediastinum. In older adolescents, the thymus is not visible.

NORMAL VARIANTS

Normal variants may simulate disease. These include:

- Trachea buckling to the right at the thoracic inlet is common in infants and young children.
- The thymus can mimic mediastinal mass or lung consolidation.
- Suboptimal chest radiographs may lead to misinterpretation such as asymmetrical appearance of the lungs. Check for rotation by comparing anterior rib–spine and anterior rib–lateral chest distances.
- Check for asymmetrical positioning of the upper extremities. Table 31–4 provides common chest radiograph abnormalities.

TABLE 31–4. COMMON ABNORMAL CHEST RADIOGRAPH FINDINGS

Abnormality	Description
Pneumothorax	More lucent (blacker than the adjacent lung)
Pleural fluid	Always more opaque (whiter) than the adjacent lung
Viral infection	Generalized involvement
Aspiration, asthma, BPD, CF	Interstitial infiltrates seen as increased prominence and decreased sharpness of the lung markings
Bacterial infection	Diffuse, focal consolidation: Single focal area of opacity
Free fluid	Pleural opacification: Obtain an ultrasound infection or decubitus view
Mycoplasma infection	Bibasilar interstitial-nodular densities
Foreign bodies	Frontal radiographs ● Inspiratory: Usually normal ● Expiratory: Mediastinal shift away from the object Fluoroscopy (most accurate) Decubitus radiographs
Abscesses, fungus, and lymphomas	Appearance of "balls" in the chest; diaphragm may be pulled up
CF	Low, flat diaphragm; small heart; large lungs
Pneumonia	More white and less black in whichever lobe is affected
Pneumothorax	Lobe of lung is decreased in size or absent
Sarcoidosis	Masses in hylar area
Tuberculosis	Infiltrates and ball-like scarring in apices

BPD = bronchial pulmonary disease, CF = cystic fibrosis.

NORMAL BONE RADIOGRAPHS

Evaluating skeletal trauma is one of the most important aspects of pediatric radiology. The pediatric skeleton has increased potential for growth and greater elasticity of bone, cartilage, and soft tissue. Because of developmental changes in bone anatomy and physiology, fractures that occur in children differ from those that occur in adults. An injury that would produce a sprain or dislocation in an adult can cause a fracture or growth plate injury in the child.

Always obtain both an AP and a LAT view. Other views may also be appropriate. It is important to compare one side with the other. Therefore, if the injury is to one knee, also obtain a radiograph of the other knee to get a comparison. The long bones should not be radiographed without the joint. Describe fractures in terms of location, direction of the fracture line, type of fracture, and degree of angulation or displacement.

Describe the type of fracture (i.e., open or closed). An open fracture is one in which the bone has penetrated the skin. With open fractures, there is a greater risk of infection. With a closed fracture, the bone does not penetrate the skin.

Describe the nature of the fracture line (i.e., complete or incomplete). The three types of incomplete fractures are plastic, buckle, and greenstick (Table 31–5). Also note whether the fracture is transverse, oblique, spiral, comminuted, impacted, or avulsed (Fig. 31–5).

TABLE 31–5. TYPES OF INCOMPLETE FRACTURES	
Type	**Radiographic Presentation**
Plastic	Bending of the bone without cortical disruption or angulation
Buckle (torus)	Fracture on the compressed side of bone with an intact cortex on the tension side
Greenstick	Bone is bent but fractured on only one side of the cortex

The systematic approach to the interpretation of bone radiographs includes inspection of anatomical alignment and position. Check the epiphyseal growth plates (Fig. 31–6). Growth of the epiphyses begins to appear at birth and is completed at puberty. Ossification is usually completed by age 20 years in women, and age 23 years in men. Examine the bone density, which should be consistent over the entire bone. Changes in bone density indicate fractures, tumors, or sclerosis. Note spotted lucency and dense sclerosis. These may indicate bone metastases or congenital, infectious, neoplastic, or metabolic diseases. Periosteum thickening indicates stress fractures or inflammation. Check for abnormalities in contour or excess calcification. Last, check for soft tissue inflammation, which may indicate osteomyelitis.

COMMON FRACTURES IN CHILDREN

GROWTH PLATE FRACTURES

Common fractures in children include injuries of the epiphyseal plates, the epiphysis, and the metaphysis. Growth plate cartilaginous tissue in children

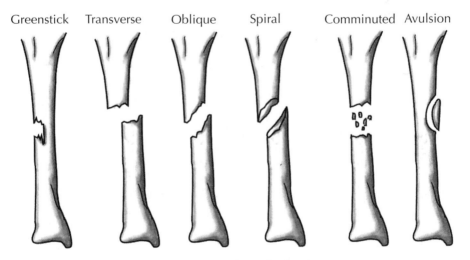

Greenstick   Transverse   Oblique   Spiral   Comminuted Avulsion

FIG. 31–5. Inspect bone for fractures.

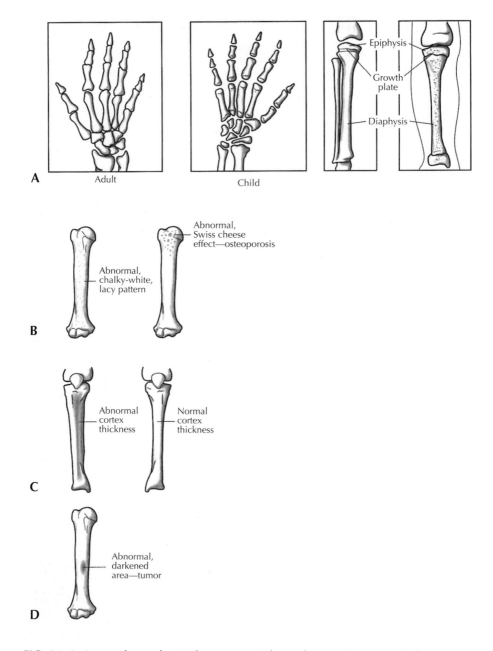

FIG. 31–6. Inspect bones for *(A)* bone age, *(B)* bone density, *(C)* cortex thickness, and *(D)* lucency.

478

TABLE 31–6. GROWTH PLATE FRACTURES: SALTER-HARRIS CLASSIFICATION

Type	Description
I	Caused by shearing or avulsion forces parallel to the growth plate
II	Extends through part of the metaphysis
III	Results from vertical shearing force; extends vertically through the epiphysis and horizontally through the growth plate; typically occurs in the knee and ankle
IV	Crosses the epiphysis, growth plate, and metaphysis; usually requires open reduction and internal fixation; associated with limb shortening deformities
V	Produces a crush fracture at the epiphyseal plate that is caused by a compressive injury; usually involves the ankle and knee; many times, the initial radiograph is normal; obtain additional radiographs if the child continues to experience pain and point tenderness 5 to 7 days after the initial evaluation

is much weaker than the adjacent joint capsule and ligamentous structures. The growth plate is also weaker than surrounding bone. The Salter-Harris classification system is used to describe growth plate injuries (Table 31–6).

AVULSION FRACTURES

An avulsion fracture occurs when bone fragments are torn away at the site of ligamentous or tendinous attachments. Osgood-Schlatter disease occurs when fragments of the tibial tubercle are separated from the underlying bone (Fig. 31–7).

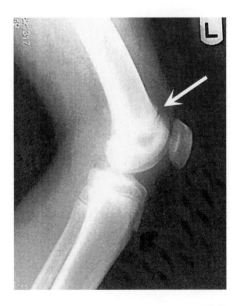

FIG. 31–7. Avulsion fracture of proximal tibial tuberosity, which is a feature of Osgood-Schlatter disease.

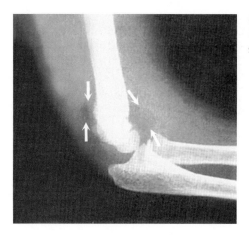

FIG. 31–8. Supracondylar fracture of the humerus. *Arrows* denote the fat pad signs.

SUPRACONDYLAR FRACTURE OF THE DISTAL HUMERUS

A supracondylar fracture extends across the distal aspect of the humerus. The radiograph will show marked anterior displacement of the anterior fat pad and visualization of the posterior fat pad (Fig. 31–8), which are usually not visualized. Extend a line down the anterior humerus. It should normally extend down through the middle third of the capitellum, which is the round end of the humerus. If a supracondylar fracture has occurred, there will be displacement of the capitellum from the anterior humeral line.

PHALANGEAL FRACTURES

These fractures are usually caused by crush injuries. Examples include fingers caught in a door or dropping something on a hand or foot. Always check the neurovascular status and tendon function when an injury occurs to an extremity. These fractures usually are associated with shortening, angulation, or rotational deformity of the digit (Fig. 31–9).

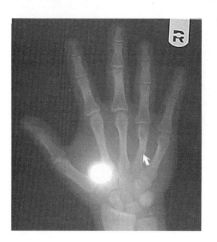

FIG. 31–9. Fracture of the fourth metacarpal.

FIG. 31–10. Clavicle fracture.

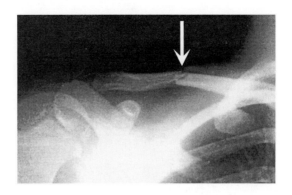

ACROMIOCLAVICULAR SHOULDER JOINT SEPARATION

This process may be caused by falling on the shoulder. Look at the child in the upright position. The top of the shoulder will look deformed, with upward displacement of the clavicle. Bring the arm across the body, approximating the elbow to the contralateral shoulder. Pain will localize in the acromioclavicular (AC) joint. Always radiograph both shoulders because AC joint separation may be missed without a comparison view.

SHOULDER DISLOCATIONS

In anterior shoulder dislocations, the mechanism of injury is abduction accompanied by external rotation of the arm. The arm will usually be held abducted and externally rotated. The acromium will be prominent. On radiographs, the humeral head is displaced anteriorly and is displaced out of the glenoid fossa.

Although posterior is rarer than anterior dislocation, the cardinal sign of a posterior dislocation is an arm held in adduction and internally rotated. The mechanism of injury is violent internal rotational force. This could occur with a fall with the arm flexed forward and internally rotated. This type of dislocation is often seen with seizures. On radiograph, the greater tuberosity of the humeral head is internally rotated, and the normal elliptical pattern produced by overlap of the humeral head and the posterior glenoid rim is lost.

CLAVICLE FRACTURES

Most clavicular fractures (Fig. 31–10) occur in either the middle or the distal third of the clavicle. They are usually caused by direct impact on the clavicle or a fall on the shoulder, causing the clavicle to buckle. Clavicle fractures are usually obvious on observation. A lump will be obvious over the fracture.

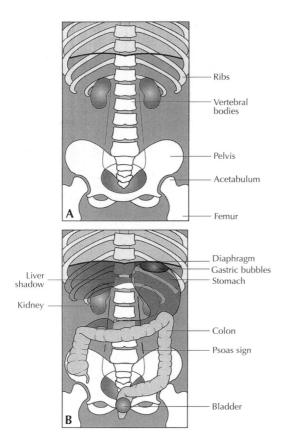

FIG. 31–11. Anatomical skeletal landmarks within the abdominal cavity. *(A)* Identify anatomical skeletal landmarks of the abdomen. *(B)* Inspect the soft tissues of the abdomen.

Ribs

Vertebral bodies

Pelvis

Acetabulum

Femur

Diaphragm
Gastric bubbles
Stomach

Liver shadow

Kidney

Colon

Psoas sign

Bladder

HEALING OF BONE FRACTURES

On radiographs, new bone formation is typically visible within 4 to 6 weeks. Children's bones have a great capacity for remodeling. Granulation tissue forms between the fracture fragments, and immature osteoid tissue is laid down on the injured bone. The granulation tissue becomes calcified and then woven bone is laid down, creating a new bone union. The healing process is generally complete in 4 to 6 months.

NORMAL ABDOMINAL RADIOGRAPHS

For problems with the abdomen, order flat plate and upright views (Fig. 31–11). If free air is suspected, order a left lateral decubitus view and a PA view of the chest. Place the flat and upright radiographs as well as left lateral decubitus and chest radiographs (if ordered) on the view box with adequate illumination. Systematically evaluate the abdominal radiographs (Table 31–7). Remember that gas is dark and stool is light gray. Also become familiar with the patterns of the small and large bowels (Table 31–8 and Fig. 31–12) to make it easier to identify structures.

TABLE 31–7. FEATURES ON NORMAL ABDOMINAL RADIOGRAPHS

GAS PATTERNS
- Stomach
- Small bowel
- Rectosigmoid

ORGAN SHAPES AND SIZES
- Liver
- Spleen
- Kidneys
- Soft tissue pelvic masses

CALCIFICATION
- Asymmetrical psoas margins
- Skeleton
- Basilar lung abnormalities

Inspect for the presence of any foreign bodies in the abdominal cavity. Systematically inspect the abdominal region skeletal system. Identify anatomical skeletal landmarks (e.g., lumbar, sacrum, and pelvis) within the abdominal cavity. Determine any aberration. Note the absence or presence of demineralization. Note the lack of continuity or symmetry of skeletal structures, which may represent fracture, dislocation, metastases (lytic means low density; sclerotic means high density; and mixed), and calcifications of the lumbar-sacral spine, iliosacral region, pelvis, acetabulum, and femur region. Note the presence of pathological calcifications.

Systematically inspect the soft tissues. Note the presence or absence of the psoas sign (see Fig. 31–11). Note the presence or absence of an air-fluid pattern under the diaphragm. Note the homogeneous uniform density of the hepatic shadow and the presence or absence of full visualization of hepatic edge. In young children, the tip of the liver can be seen at the right costal margin. The splenic shadow is generally hidden by the gastric bubble and splenic flexure of the colon unless splenomegaly is present. The pancreas is not usually visible. The entire renal shadow outlines are generally not clear-

TABLE 31–8. ABDOMINAL RADIOGRAPHS: EVALUATION OF GAS PATTERNS

Normal Findings
- Dilatation of structure and assessment of wall or mucosal thickness in stomach, small bowel, colon, and rectosigmoid

Abnormal Findings
- Free air under diaphragm on upright film
- Free air on supine films (double bowel wall sign)
- Right upper quadrant
  - Portal vein
  - Biliary system
- Small bubbles in an abscess

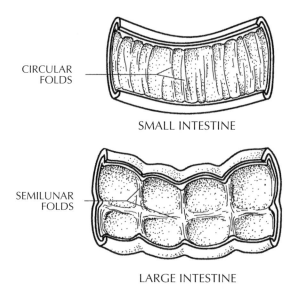

FIG. 31–12. Bowel patterns.

CIRCULAR
FOLDS

SMALL INTESTINE

SEMILUNAR
FOLDS

LARGE INTESTINE

ly demarcated. It may be difficult to estimate the overall size of the organs. If the bladder is filled, it appears as a round, homogeneous mass. The uterus is usually not visible; however, it can present as an irregular mass if fibroids are present. Note the presence of any calcifications, widening, or tortuosity of the aorta or renal arteries.

GASTROINTESTINAL EVALUATION

Stomach

Note the gastric shadow with presence of gastric bubble usually located in the midline to the left upper quadrant region.

Intestines

Note the patterns made by the small and large intestines. Air shadow location is scattered in a random and nonspecific pattern throughout the abdominal cavity. Variables, such as age, amount of air ingested, length of small or large intestine, stool concentration, and pathology, can cause normal presentations to appear abnormal and vice versa.

Abdominal Gas Pattern

The location is generally nonspecific. Abnormal concentration of abdominal gas in one location or unilateral appearance of the air gas pattern on one side with the absence of any air on the opposite side may suggest bowel displacement. The location and concentration of air with accompanying dilated bowel proximally and decreased air shadows distally are suggestive of paralytic ileus. Localization with the presence of dilated bowel with or without

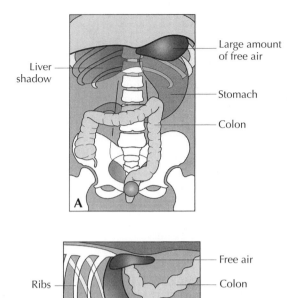

Liver shadow

Large amount of free air

Stomach

Colon

A

FIG. 31–13. Pneumoperitoneum. *(A)* Upright view. *(B)* Left lateral decubitus view.

Ribs

Free air

Colon

B

Liver

air or fluid levels proximally and absence of air shadows distally is suggestive of local obstruction.

PERITONEUM

Note free air in the peritoneal cavity (pneumoperitoneum) (Fig. 31–13). This is usually caused by the disruption of the abdominal wall. Usually seen with left lateral decubitus and chest PA views, dark air shadows can be visualized in the diaphragm and against the inferior hepatic margin. Inspect for intraperitoneal fluid, which usually obscures the hepatic edges and displaces the abdominal gas pattern.

TEST YOUR KNOWLEDGE OF CHAPTER 31

1. What questions should be included in determining the history of a fracture?
2. How are air, fat, water, soft tissue, and bone exhibited on radiographs?
3. How do you determine if a radiograph is underexposed, overexposed, or correctly exposed?
4. How are radiographs correctly placed on the view box?
5. What views should be ordered for chest radiographs?
6. What are the steps in evaluating a chest radiograph?
7. How can you determine if the heart is large or small?
8. Describe the common types of bone fractures.

485

9. How are abnormal bone structures revealed on bone radiographs?
10. What are common fractures seen with children?
11. What views should be ordered for abdominal radiographs?
12. What structures can be visualized on abdominal radiographs?
13. How can a blockage of the bowel be determined from abdominal radiographs?
14. How can the small bowel be differentiated from the large bowel?

 BIBLIOGRAPHY

Amorosa, J. K., Novelline, R. A., & Squire, L. F. (1993). *Chest, abdomen, bone and clinical skills: A problem-based text.* Philadelphia: W. B. Saunders.

Barloon, T., & Weissman, A. (1996). Diagnostic imaging in the evaluation of blunt abdominal trauma. *American Family Physician, 54*(1), 205–211.

Brown, J. H., & Salvatore, D. A. (1992). Growth plate injuries: Salter-Harris classification, *American Family Physician, 46*, 1180–1184.

Chen, M., Pope, R. L., & Ott, D. J. (1996). *Basic radiology.* New York: McGraw-Hill.

Caffner, R. H. (1993). *Clinical radiology: The essentials.* Philadelphia: Williams & Wilkins.

Edmunds, M. W., & Mayhew, M. S. (1996). *Procedures for primary care practice.* St. Louis: Mosby.

Hurst, W. (1995). *Cardiac puzzles.* St. Louis: Mosby.

Merier, L. R. (1991). *Practical orthopedics.* St. Louis: Mosby.

Mettler, F. A., Guiberteau, M. J., Voss, C. M., & Urbina, C. E. (2000). *Primary care radiology.* Philadelphia: W. B. Saunders.

Pierro, J. A., Berens, B. M., & Crawford, W. L. (1989). *Manual of diagnostic radiology.* Philadelphia: Lee & Febiger.

Scialabba, F., & Salvatore, D. (1990). Saccular aneurysms of thoracic aorta. *American Family Physician, 42*(5), 1475–1478.

Simon, R. R., & Koenigsknecht, S. J. (1995). *Emergency orthopedics: The extremities.* Stamford, CT: Appleton & Lange.

Spilane, R., Shepard, J., & Salvatore, D. (1994). Radiographic aspects of pneumothorax. *American Family Physician, 51*(2), 459–464.

Stimac, G. (1992). *Introduction to diagnostic imaging.* Philadelphia: W. B. Saunders.

Sutton, D. (1998). *Textbook of radiology & imaging* (6th ed.). Hong Kong: Longman Asia Ltd.

Vine, D. (1990). Congestive heart failure. *American Family Physician, 42*(3), 739.

Wilson, J. (Ed.). (2000). *Harrison's principles of internal medicine.* New York: McGraw-Hill.

Zitelli, B. J., & Davis, H. W. (1997). *Atlas of pediatric physical diagnosis.* St. Louis: Mosby.

32

Cardiac Procedures

MARGARET R. COLYAR

OBJECTIVES
- *Become proficient in placing electrocardiograph (ECG) leads appropriately on a child.*
- *Determine when an ECG is needed.*
- *Understand components of an ECG.*
- *Differentiate between normal and abnormal ECG results.*
- *Ascertain venipuncture techniques for children of different ages.*

CPT Codes

- 93000: ECG complete
- 93005: ECG technical component
- 36415: Venipuncture: Finger, heel, or ear

The ECG is a unique tool used to assist clinicians in diagnosing or ruling out myocardial infarction (MI); potentially life-threatening arrhythmias; and many heart problems caused by medications, electrolyte imbalance, or disease processes. Interpreting an ECG is not difficult. After learning the basic rules, understanding and application are easier. The ECG is performed on almost every child presenting to the emergency department or ambulatory healthcare facility with chest pain that is not obviously lung related. It is indicated to assist in differential diagnosis of cardiac problems and for baseline data if the child is at risk for cardiac problems.

TABLE 32–1. COMMON ERRORS IN ELECTROCARDIOGRAPH LEAD PLACEMENT

Error in Placement	Result
Inaccurate precordial positioning	Creates the impression of mirror-image dextrocardia or possible lateral MI
Exchange of two or more precordial leads	Produces misleading patterns
Exchange of right and left leg leads	No significant change
Exchange of left leg and left arm leads	Insignificant Q wave in lead III
Exchange of left arm and right leg leads	Low voltage in lead III
Leg leads placed on abdomen or arm leads placed on upper chest	Distortion of pattern
Exchange of right and left arm leads	Misinterpretation of pattern: Lateral MI
Exchange of right arm and right or left leg leads	Misinterpretation of pattern: Inferior wall MI or previous MI, pericardial effusion, emphysema, or thyroid problem

MI = myocardial infarction.

⬥ ELECTROCARDIOGRAPH LEAD PLACEMENT

To ensure an accurate ECG, correct lead placement is vitally necessary. Misplaced leads can cause potentially dangerous interpretation errors. Common errors are shown in Table 32–1.

CONTRAINDICATIONS

There are no contraindications.

EQUIPMENT

- ECG machine with limb leads, chest leads, and cable
- ECG paper
- Electrodes
- Grounded safe electrical outlet

PROCEDURE

- Position the child in the supine position.
- Plug in the machine.
- Enter child's identification data into the machine, if required.
- Set speed at 25 mm per second and size sensitivity at 10 mm per second.
- If the child's skin is dirty or oily, cleanse it.

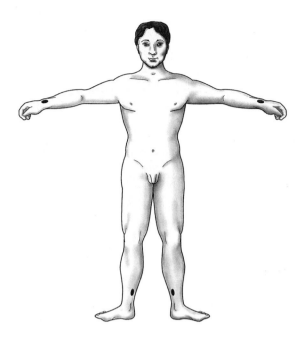

FIG. 32–1. Limb leads.

- Apply the electrodes in the proper configuration.
- Limb leads (Fig. 32–1) are as follows:
  - Legs: Distal third of the lower leg on the anterior medial surface
  - Arms: Volar surface of the distal third of the forearm
- Chest leads (Fig. 32–2) are as follows:
  - V_1: Fourth intercostal space (ICS), right sternal border
  - V_2: Fourth ICS, left sternal border
  - V_3: Halfway between V_2 and V_4
  - V_4: Fifth ICS, midclavicular line
  - V_5: Anterior axillary line lateral to V_4
  - V_6: Midaxillary line lateral to V_5
- Attach the cable to the electrodes.
- Push the record button.
- If an arrhythmia is seen, obtain a rhythm strip (long lead II).
- Remove the electrodes and cleanse the skin if needed.

⬮ ELECTROCARDIOGRAPH INTERPRETATION

BASIC CARDIAC INFORMATION

- Depolarization: Electrical stimulation of the heart muscle causing the heart cells to contract
- Repolarization: Resting or relaxation phase of the heart muscle
- ECG components (Fig. 32–3)

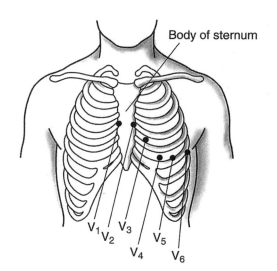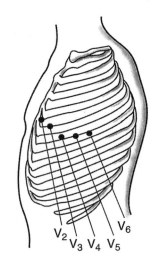

FIG. 32–2. Chest leads.

- P wave: Depicts atrial stimulation or depolarization.
- PR interval: Depicts the time it takes atrial stimulation to reach the atrioventricular (AV) node; during this time, blood flows from the atria through the AV valves into the ventricles; normal time is less than 0.20 second.
- QRS complex: Depicts the beginning of ventricular contraction or depolarization; normal time is less than 0.12 second.
- Q wave: The first downward deflection of the QRS complex; notice that sometimes the Q wave is absent from the QRS complex; do not be alarmed because this is a physiologic variation that happens occasionally.
- R wave: The first upward deflection of the QRS complex.
- S wave: Any downward deflection that is first preceded by an upward deflection of the QRS complex.
- ST segment: The pause after the QRS complex; the line should be flat; if it is *elevated* or *depressed*, there is a major problem.
- T wave: Depicts ventricular repolarization or relaxation.
- ECG paper
  - One small square is 1 mm long and wide (0.04 second).
  - One large square (from one heavy line to the next heavy line) is 5 mm long and wide (0.020 second).
  - Limb leads are measured in the frontal plane (Table 32–2); a pair of electrodes (one is + and one is −) forms a limb lead.
  - Chest leads are measured in the horizontal plane (Fig. 32–4); the chest leads normally produce a *positive* deflection in a progressive manner.
  - The placement of the chest leads correlates with the area of the heart that is being measured (Table 32–3).

490

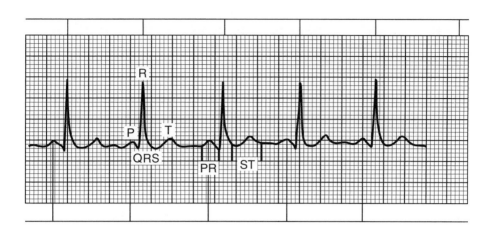

FIG. 32–3. ECG components.

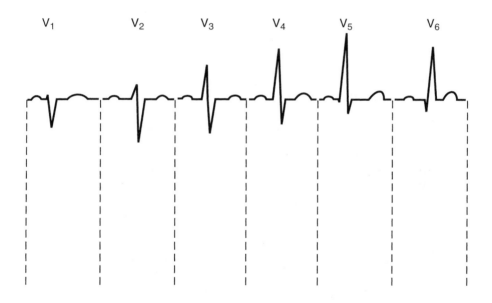

Progressively positive deflection

FIG. 32–4. Normal chest leads.

491

TABLE 32–2. 12-LEAD ECG TRACING: LIMB LEADS, LOCATIONS, AND NORMAL CONFIGURATIONS

Limb Lead	Placement	Normal Configuration
I	Left arm + → right arm −	Lead I
II	Left leg + → left arm −	Lead II
III	Left arm + → right arm −	Lead III
aV<u>R</u>	<u>R</u>ight arm +; left arm and left leg −	AV<u>R</u>
aV<u>L</u>	<u>L</u>eft arm +; right arm and left leg −	AV<u>L</u>
AV<u>F</u>	Left <u>f</u>oot +; right and left arms −	AV<u>F</u>

TABLE 32–3. ECG CHEST LEADS AND WHAT THEY MEASURE

Lead	Placement	What Is Measured
V_1	4th intercostal space (ICS), right sternal border (RSB)	Right side of the heart
V_2	4th ICS, left sternal border (LSB)	Right side of the heart
V_3	Halfway between V_2 and V_4	Intraventricular septum
V_4	5th ICS, midclavicular line	Intraventricular septum
V_5	Anterior axillary line lateral to V_4	Left side of the heart
V_6	Midaxillary line lateral to V_5	Left side of the heart

✍ METHODOLOGICAL INTERPRETATION

The five general areas of interpretation are rate, rhythm, axis, hypertrophy, and infarction.

RATE

The following is the best method for measuring rate or beats per minute (bpm) on the 12-lead ECG because it is based on 3 seconds of tracing. Other methods are easier for measuring rate on a rhythm strip. Look at the ECG paper and measure from one R wave to the next one.

- First heavy black line to the next heavy black line (1/300 minute) = 300 bpm
- Then = 150 bpm (2 heavy lines = 2/300 or 1/150)
- Then = 100 bpm (3 heavy lines = 3/300 or 1/100)
- Then = 75 bpm (4 heavy lines = 4/300 or 1/75)
- Then = 60 bpm (5 heavy lines = 5/300 or 1/60)
- Then = 50 bpm (6 heavy lines = 6/300 or 1/50)

Within a 6-second strip, count the cycles from R wave to R wave and multiply by 10 (number of 6-second intervals in 1 minute = cycles/minute). (See Chapter 3 for a discussion of the normal heart rates in children.)

RHYTHM

The rhythm is the pattern of electrical conduction phenomena of the heart observed as the electrical current passes from the sinoatrial node (SA) through the AV node through the bundle of His, bundle branches, and Purkinje fibers. The rhythm can be regular or irregular. With a regular rhythm, the distance between R waves is always equal. With an irregular rhythm, the distance between R waves is *not* always equal. Examples of irregular rhythms are shown in Figures 32–5 and 32–6.

The presence of ectopic foci (Figs. 32–7 and 32–8) is another reason for irregular rhythms. Included are paroxysmal atrial tachycardia, supraventricular tachycardia, ventricular tachycardia, premature atrial contractions,

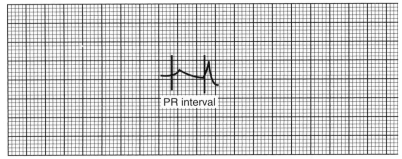

A

PR interval greater than 0.20 mm (5 small blocks)

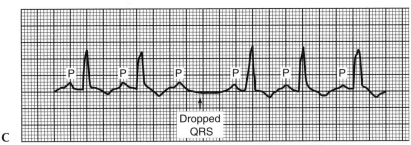

B

PR interval elongates and a QRS complex is dropped.

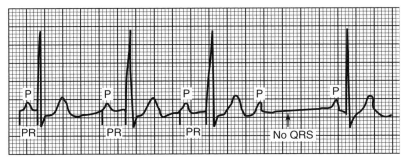

C

A QRS segment is dropped with no lengthening of PR intervals.

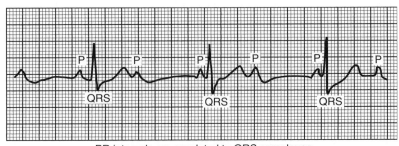

D

PR intervals are unrelated to QRS complexes.

FIG. 32–5. AV blocks. *(A)* First-degree AV block. *(B)* Second-degree Wenckebach (type I) block. *(C)* Second-degree Mobitz II (type II) block. *(D)* Third-degree block (complete heart block).

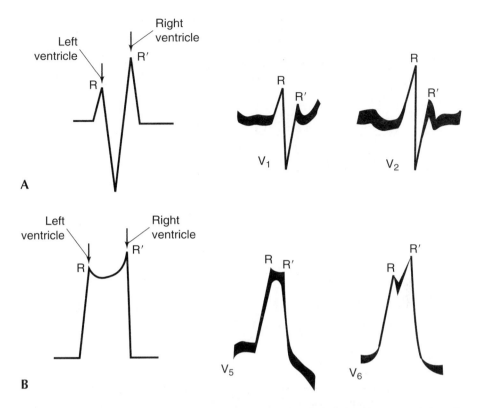

FIG. 32–6. Bundle branch blocks. *(A)* Right bundle branch block. *(B)* Left bundle branch block.

early SA node contraction, flutter, fibrillation, and premature ventricular contractions (PVCs; i.e., early ventricular firing). PVCs can be *unifocal* or *multifocal*. A unifocal PVC comes from an abnormal focus in the *same place* in the ventricle *every* time and looks the same each time. A multifocal PVC comes from *several* abnormal foci in the ventricles and looks different each time. A multifocal PVC is an indicator of more serious heart disease is than a unifocal PVC. Flutter can be atrial or ventricular in origin. A flutter has a regular, single ectopic foci, and it appears sawtoothed on ECGs. Fibrillation can also be atrial or ventricular in origin. A fibrillatory beat is irregular and comes from multiple foci. It is irregular in appearance and is a indicator of much worse heart disease.

AXIS (VECTOR)

The axis means the direction and magnitude of the electrical stimulus of depolarization, starting at the AV node and continuing through the ventricles. It is measured in degrees. With a normal axis, the mean QRS (+0 to +90 degrees) vector points downward and toward the client's left side because that is the way the normal heart lies in the chest (Fig. 32–9). To measure the axis, do the following:

495

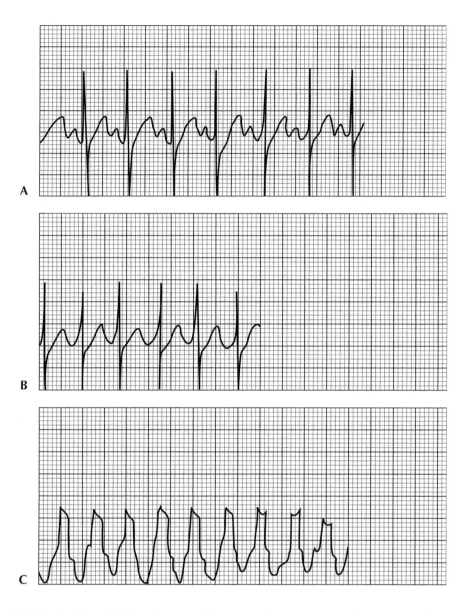

FIG. 32–7. *(A)* to *(C)* Ectopic foci. *(A)* Paroxysmal atrial tachycardia, 150 to 200 beats per minute. *(B)* Supraventricular tachycardia. *(C)* Paroxysmal ventricular tachycardia.

496

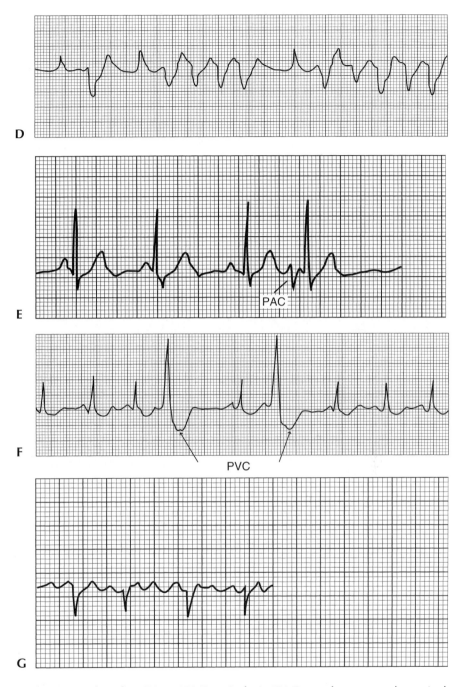

FIG. 32–7 (continued). *(D)* to *(G)* Ectopic foci. *(D)* Runs of paroxysmal ventricular tachycardia. *(E)* Premature atrial contraction (PAC). *(F)* Premature ventricular contractions. *(G)* Atrial flutter.

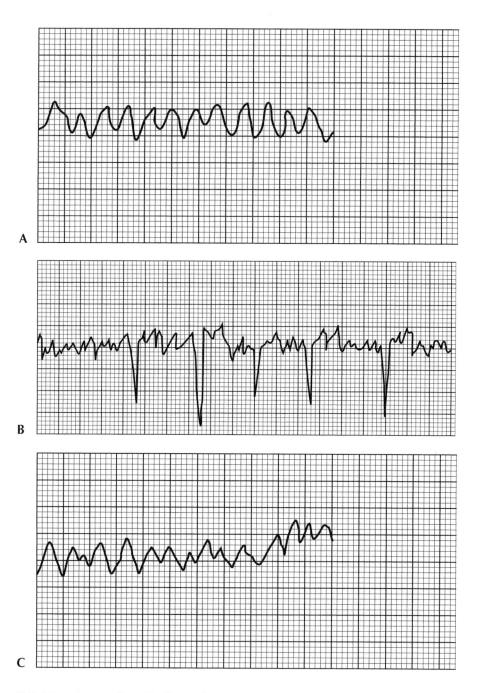

FIG. 32–8. Ectopic foci: fibrillation/flutter. *(A)* Ventricular flutter. *(B)* Atrial fibrillation. *(C)* Ventricular fibrillation.

- With the AV node as the center, imagine a circle around the heart measured in degrees both positive (+) and negative (−). Positive degrees are measured in the lower half of the heart, and negative degrees are measured in the top the half of the heart.
- In lead I, measure the right and left spheres (halves) of the axis (left is +; right is −). Thus, a + deflection occurs when the stimulus is moving toward the left (i.e., left axis deviation). A − deflection occurs when the electrical stimulus is moving toward the right (i.e., right axis deviation).
- AVF measures the upper and lower spheres (halves) of the axis (upper is −; lower is +). If the deflection is mainly +, then the mean QRS vector is downward. If the deflection is mainly −, then the mean QRS vector is upward.
- Chest leads record the axis on a horizontal plane. They should be − in V_1 and V_2 and + in leads V_5 and V_6. A progression from − in V_1 to + in V_6 is normal.
- Because of its position, lead V_2 projects through the anterior wall of the heart to the posterior wall of the heart, giving the best information on anterior and posterior wall MIs.

Problems That Affect the Axis

- Obesity: Pushes the heart up. Thus, the mean QRS vector is directed to the left of +0 degrees.
- Infarction: No electrical stimulus will go through dead tissue, and the mean QRS vector *turns away* from the infarcted area of tissue.
- Atrial hypertrophy (Fig. 32–10). Hypertrophy is an increase in heart size or wall thickness caused by an increased volume in the chambers of the heart.
  - P wave depicts contraction of the atria.
  - Lead V_1 is placed directly over the atria (4th intercostal space [ICS]), right sternal border [RSB]).
  - Hypertrophy of the atria is shown as a *diphasic* wave (+ or − deflection) P wave in lead V_1.
  - If right atrial hypertrophy is present, the *beginning* portion of the diphasic wave is larger.
  - If left atrial hypertrophy is present, the *end* portion of the diphasic wave is larger.
- Ventricular hypertrophy (Fig. 32–11): Ventricle has electrical activity, and the mean QRS vector deviates *toward* the enlarged ventricle. QRS wave depicts the contraction of the ventricles. Lead V_1 tracing is usually negative (small R wave and large S wave) because depolarization is *away* from the right side of the heart toward the thicker left side of the heart. Hypertrophy of the ventricles is shown by the deflection of the QRS in lead V_1 (+ or −).
  - Right ventricular hypertrophy (RVH): V_1 has a + deflected QRS. This means that the electrical stimulus is away from the left side toward the thicker right side. Progression of V_1: V_6 starts with large R waves in V_1 and ends with a small R wave in V_6. V_2 is directly over the right ventricle and is the best place to look for right ventricular *strain*.

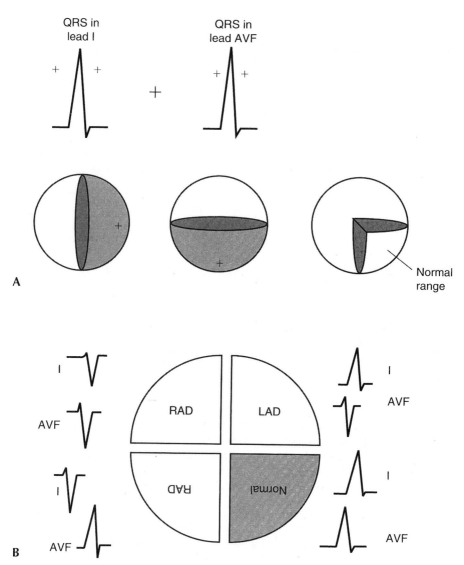

FIG. 32–9. Check leads I and aVF to determine *(A)* normal axis or *(B)* axis deviation.

- Left ventricular hypertrophy (LVH): More depolarization toward the left than usual. Thus, there is a *very small R wave* and *very deep S wave* in V_1. Lead V_5 is directly over the left ventricle, so if the left ventricle is enlarged, V_5 will have a more + deflection, resulting in a *very tall R wave*. (You must *add* the S wave in V_1 and the R wave in V_5 together in millimeters. If these add up to more than 35 mm, LVH is present.)
- T waves also indicate ventricular hypertrophy. V_5 and V_6 are directly over the left ventricle and are the best place to look for left ventricular *strain*. The wave will be *inverted* and *asymmetrical*.

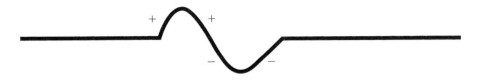

Diphasic P wave

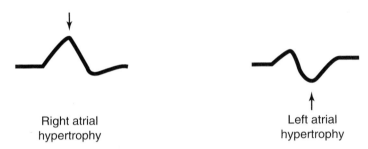

Right atrial
hypertrophy

Left atrial
hypertrophy

FIG. 32–10. Atrial hypertrophy.

HYPOXIA

Hypoxia is the occlusion of a coronary artery (by thrombus or arteriosclerotic plaques), producing lack of blood supply to the heart that results in decreased oxygenation to the cells. Usually only the left ventricle suffers an MI. On the ECG, you can determine whether the heart has suffered *ischemia, injury,* or *infarction.*

- *Ischemia* (decreased blood supply): "Smiley face" configuration (Fig. 32–12)
  - Shown as a T wave inversion and symmetry. In V_2–V_6, this indicates pathology. In limb leads, this is a normal variation.
- *Injury* (acuteness of infarct): "Frowny face" configuration (Fig. 32–13)
  - Shown as elevated ST segment. Elevation of ST segment *only* indicates a small acute infarct, pericarditis, or ventricular aneurysm (T does *not* return to baseline).
  - Depressed ST segment may indicate a partial-thickness (subendocardial) infarct or digitalis effect.
- *Infarction* (Fig. 32–14): Not diagnosable if left bundle branch block (LBBB) is present. Check all leads for *significant Q waves.* Q waves that are significant are 0.04 second (1 small square) wide OR one third the amplitude of the entire QRS. Q waves (first downward deflection of the QRS) are usually absent in normal individuals. *Tiny Q waves are insignificant* in leads I, II, V_5, and V_6.

501

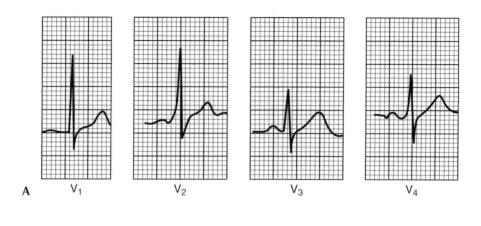

A   V₁   V₂   V₃   V₄

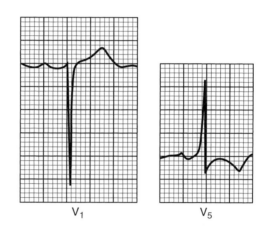

B   V₁   V₅

FIG. 32–11. Ventricular hypertrophy. *(A)* Right ventricular hypertrophy. *(B)* Left ventricular hypertrophy.

- *Anterior infarction* (V_1–V_4): Check all chest leads (V_1–V_4) for the presence of significant Q waves (0.04 second) and for elevated ST segment. Because all chest leads are anteriorly placed, it makes sense to check these leads.
- *Lateral infarction*: Check aVL and lead I for significant Q waves and elevated ST segment.
- *Inferior infarction*: Check aVF and leads II and II for significant Q waves or elevated or depressed ST segments.
- *Posterior infarction*: V_1 to V_2. Opposite picture from anterior MI. There is a larger R wave and an obviously depressed ST segment.
- Do the mirror test. Turn the ECG upside down and look at it in a mirror. It should look like the classic acute infarct.

502

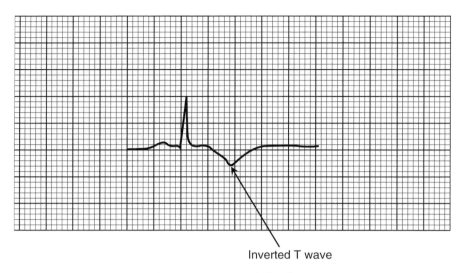

Inverted T wave

FIG. 32–12. Myocardial ischemia.

⊕ QUICK AND EASY INTERPRETATION

1. Rate: 300, 150, 100, 75, 60, 50. With bradycardia, check 6-second strip and multiply by 10.
2. Rhythm: Regular or irregular? Atrioventricular (AV) block or bundle branch block (BBB)?

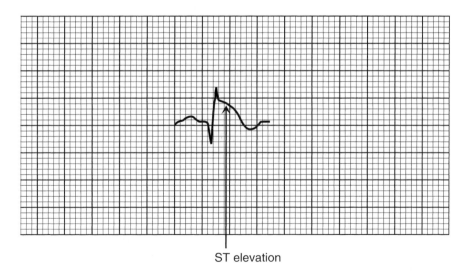

ST elevation

FIG. 32–13. Myocardial injury.

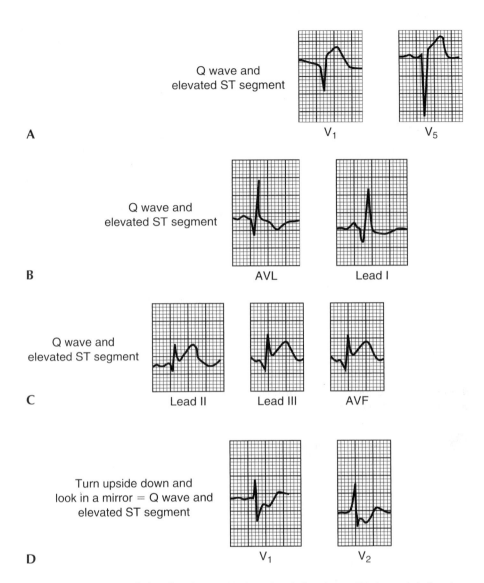

FIG. 32–14. Myocardial infarction. *(A)* Anterior infarction. *(B)* Lateral infarction. *(C)* Inferior infarction. *(D)* Posterior infarction.

3. Axis: Right or left? Positive or negative? If abnormality is present, consider hypertrophy and infarction.
4. Hypertrophy
- Atrial V_1: Diphasic P wave
  - Large *initial* positive deflection = right atrial hypertrophy
  - Large *ending* negative deflection = left atrial hypertrophy

504

- Ventricular
  - V_1: Positive deflection of QRS = RVH
  - V2: Inverted and asymmetrical T wave = RVH
  - Check V_1: If deep S wave, measure
  - Check V_5: If large R wave, measure
  - Add V_1 and V_5 together; if greater than 35 mm = LVH
  - Check V_5 and V_6: If inverted and asymmetrical T wave = LVH
5. Hypoxia
- Ischemia: Smilelike configuration: T wave inverted and symmetrical in V1–V6 only
- Injury: Frownlike configuration: ST segment elevation = acute full-thickness MI
  - Depressed ST segment = partial-thickness MI
- Infarction: Q wave present, ST elevation
  - Anterior MI: Q in V_1 to V_4 and ST wave elevation
  - Lateral MI: Leads aVL and I = Q and ST wave elevation
  - Inferior MI: Leads aVF, II, and III = Q wave and ST wave elevation
  - Posterior MI: Opposite of anterior MI; larger R wave with ST wave depression

CLIENT INSTRUCTIONS

- Lie still while the ECG machine is running.
- There will be *no* electrical shock.

VENIPUNCTURE

CONTRAINDICATIONS

- Inability to stabilize the vein site as required for successful blood drawing

EQUIPMENT

- Blood specimen tube
- Plastic needle holder
- Needles for plastic needle holder (16, 18, and 21 gauge)
- Vacuum butterfly adapters
- Alcohol swabs
- Povidone-iodine (Betadine) swabs
- Cotton balls
- Adhesive tape
- Plastic adhesive bandages
- Nonsterile gloves
- 2 × 2 gauze
- Indelible marking pen
- Tourniquets

- Puncture-resistant sharps box container with biohazard approval and markings

PROCEDURE

- Prepare the equipment.
- Determine the type of needle or butterfly infusion needle needed.
- Attach the unused needle to the plastic needle holder.
- Select the appropriate blood specimen tube for the test.
- Position the child in a comfortable position.
- Talk with the child. Let the child know what he or she should do and what you are going to do.
- Palpate the vein. The median vein of the antecubital space of the arms is usually the best site in children older than age 1 year (Fig. 32–15).
  - Avoid thrombosed veins.
  - If there are no viable antecubital veins, inspect the sites distally.
  - Choose a distal site before a proximal site.
- Put on your gloves.
- Cleanse the site with an antiseptic agent (Betadine or alcohol preps) in a circular pattern beginning at the center and expanding outward.
- Apply a tourniquet approximately 4 to 6 inches above the vein that has been selected, firmly enough to obstruct venous flow without obstructing arterial flow. For infants and toddlers, use a rubber band as the tourniquet.
- Do not leave the tourniquet on longer than 1 minute.
- After a suitable vein is located, have the child make a fist.
- Palpate the vein. It should be an elastic sensation without pulsation.
- Uncap the needle.
- Stabilize the site. Have someone assist by holding the child's arm still because children have a tendency to jerk away when stuck with a needle. Try distraction techniques if the child is fearful.
- Insert the needle bevel side up at a 15-degree angle in line with the vein in a smooth, clean motion.
- When the needle penetrates the vein, decreased resistance will be felt.
- Decrease the angle and slowly insert the needle approximately an eighth of an inch or more or until the blood flow is adequate.
- Push the blood specimen tube onto the distal end of the needle.
- Allow the blood to flow until the tube is filled.
- Pull back on the blood specimen tube to dislodge it from the needle in the plastic needle holder. This will release the pressure.
- Release the tourniquet.
- Remove the needle.
- Apply pressure to the puncture site with a cotton ball in a smooth motion.
- Have the child apply pressure to the site if he or she is old enough to assist.
- Keep pressure on the site for 1 minute (unless the child is taking anticoagulant therapy; then apply pressure for 3 to 5 minutes).

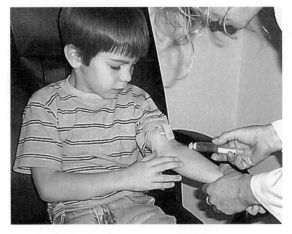

FIG. 32–15. Drawing blood from the median vein in a child.

- Deposit the needle in a puncture-proof container.
- Apply a plastic adhesive bandage or cover the cotton ball with tape at the venipuncture site.
- Reward the child with a sticker and praise.

CLIENT INSTRUCTIONS

- You may remove the adhesive bandage in 15 minutes.
- Do not rub the puncture site because that will increase risk of oozing and result in a bruised appearance.

⦿ HEEL AND FINGER STICK FOR CAPILLARY BLOOD

EQUIPMENT

- Capillary specimen tube or filter paper for required test (Fig. 32–16)
- Lancet
- Alcohol swabs
- Povidone-iodine (Betadine) swabs
- Cotton balls or 2 × 2 gauze
- Plastic adhesive bandages
- Nonsterile gloves
- Puncture-resistant sharps box container with biohazard approval and markings

PROCEDURE

- Warm the heel or finger to increase blood flow.
- Cleanse the area with alcohol.
- Dry the area with sterile gauze or a cotton ball.
- Use a lancet that is 2.4 mm in length or less.

507

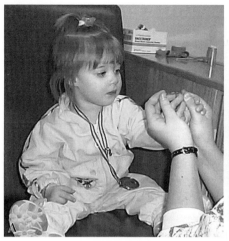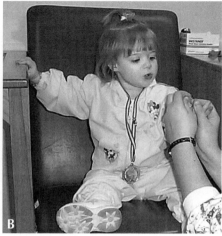

FIG. 32–16. Using finger stick for capillary blood.

- Use a swift, clean puncture on the plantar surface.
- Wipe away the first drop of blood.
- Allow a large blood drop to form.
- Using filter paper of test strip, gently touch the blood drop to the filter paper and completely saturate it. The entire circle must be filled. Avoid squeezing the puncture site.
- Using a capillary tube, fill the tube to the specified line. Milk the heel or finger to produce enough blood for the test.
- Cover the puncture site.
- Send the specimen to the laboratory for evaluation.
- For the filter paper test strip:
  - Dry the specimen in a horizontal position and mail it within 24 hours.
  - Do not transport the sample in a plastic bag because condensation may occur.

TEST YOUR KNOWLEDGE OF CHAPTER 32

1. When is an ECG necessary?
2. Describe ECG lead placement.
3. What are the components of methodological ECG interpretation?
4. How is rate measured on an ECG?
5. Describe irregular rhythms.
6. Why is axis information important?
7. Differentiate among ischemia, injury, and infarction.
8. What are the differences on ECG leads with anterior, inferior, posterior, and lateral infarctions?
9. Describe the quick ECG interpretation method.

10. Describe how to perform a venipuncture.
11. Describe how to perform a heel/capillary blood draw.

 BIBLIOGRAPHY

College of American Pathologists. (1992). *So you're going to collect a blood specimen: An introduction to phlebotomy* (5th ed.). Washington, DC: College of American Pathologists.

Dubin, D. (2000). *Rapid interpretation of ECGs* (4th ed.). Tampa, FL: Cover Publishing Co.

Edmunds, M. W., & Mayhew, M. S. (1996). *Procedures for primary care practitioners*. St. Louis: Mosby.

Gray, H., Pick, T., & Howden, R. (1977). *Anatomy, descriptive and surgical*. Philadelphia: Running Press; 539–540.

Grauer, K. (1998). *A practical guide to ECG interpretation*. St. Louis: Mosby.

McCall, R. E., & Tankersley, C. M. (1997). *Phlebotomy essentials*. Philadelphia: J. B. Lippincott.

Peberdy, M. A., & Ornato, J. P. (1994). ECG leads: Misplacement and misdiagnosis. *Emergency Medicine*, (October), 37–38.

Thaler, M. S. (1999). *The only ECG book you'll ever need* (2nd ed.). Philadelphia: J. B. Lippincott.

33

Circumcision and Dorsal Penile Nerve Block

MARGARET R. COLYAR

OBJECTIVES
- *Determine contraindications to circumcision.*
- *Describe dorsal penile nerve block (DPNB).*
- *Differentiate between two types of circumcision procedures.*

 CPT Codes

- 54150: Circumcision (clamp): Newborn
- 54152: Circumcision (clamp): Child
- 54160: Circumcision, other (Plastibell): Newborn
- 54161: Circumcision, other (Plastibell): Child

The American Academy of Pediatrics (AAP) has recently formulated a new policy on circumcision. The AAP does not recommend circumcision as a routine procedure because it believes that the benefits of circumcision are not significant enough, but notes that the provider should take into account the cultural, religious, and ethnic traditions of the parents and allow them to make an informed choice. Additionally, the AAP feels that it is essential that pain relief be provided to the infant before the circumcision procedure. The new policy is based on evaluation of research published in the past 10 years on urinary tract infections, penile cancer, sexually transmitted diseases, analgesia, and complications of circumcision.

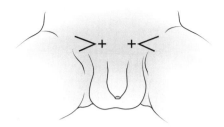

FIG. 33–1. Dorsal penile nerve block injection sites.

The three most commonly used methods used to circumcise the penis are the Gomco clamp, Plastibell, and Mogen clamp techniques. There is no significant advantage of one method over the others. Both the Gomco and Mogen clamps protect the glans while producing crushing of the nerve endings and blood vessels to promote hemostasis. The Plastibell causes necrosis of the remaining foreskin by strangulation. The Gomco clamp and Plastibell techniques are outlined in this chapter. The child to be circumcised should be at least 1 hour postprandial because of the risk of regurgitation. The child should have had at least one documented void.

Many providers are concerned about the amount of pain neonates experience during the procedure. Research has indicated that neonates who receive DPNB or local anesthesia cry less, have less tachycardia, are less irritable, and have fewer behavioral changes in the 24 hours after the circumcision procedure.

 CONTRAINDICATIONS

Contraindications for circumcision and DPNB include:
- Hypospadias
- Unusual-appearing genitalia (e.g., chordee, hypospadias, epispadias, ambiguous genitalia)
- Severe illness
- Infant younger than 12 hours old
- Prematurity

 DORSAL PENILE NERVE BLOCK

The sites for DPNB are shown in Figure 33–1.

EQUIPMENT
- Restrainer board with padding
- 1% lidocaine without epinephrine
- 1-mL tuberculin syringe
- 26-gauge needle
- Nonsterile gloves
- Alcohol

PROCEDURE

- Restrain the child.
- Inspect the genitalia.
- Cleanse with antiseptic solution.
- Insert needle at the 2 o'clock position 0.3 to 0.5 cm at the base of the penis beneath the skin surface.
- Aspirate. If there is no blood return, inject 0.2 to 0.4 mL of lidocaine.
- Repeat at the 10 o'clock position.
- Wait 4 minutes.
- Proceed with the circumcision.

CIRCUMCISION

Two commonly used methods of circumcision, the Gomco clamp and the Plastibell methods, are described.

EQUIPMENT

- Restrainer board with padding
- Sterile gloves
- Fenestrated drape
- Povidone-iodine (Betadine)
- Gauze pads
- Hemostats (two curved and one straight)
- Scissors
- Gomco clamp or Plastibell
- #10 scalpel
- Petroleum jelly

GOMCO CLAMP METHOD

This method is shown in Figure 33–2.

Procedure

- Restrain the child.
- Inspect the genitalia.
- Cleanse with antiseptic solution.
- Grasp the foreskin with the two hemostats at the 10 o'clock and 2 o'clock positions.
- Gently probe and lyse adhesions underneath the foreskin with the curved hemostat. Do not extend beyond the corona.
- Place the straight hemostat approximately two-thirds of the distance from the foreskin to the opening of the corona. Keep in place for 1 minute. This crushes the skin and marks the area for placing the dorsal slit.

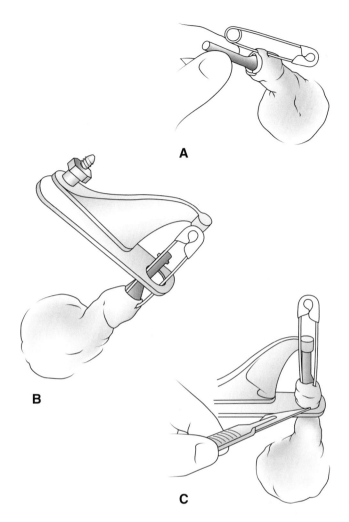

FIG. 33–2. Steps of Gomco clamp method of circumcision. (*A*) After incising the dorsal slit, retract the foreskin, and place the Gomco bell. (*B*) Bring the bell, safety pin, and foreskin through the Gomco ring. Tighten the screw. (*C*) Trim the excess foreskin with a #11 scalpel.

- Remove the hemostat.
- Cut through the middle of the crushed area.
- Peel back the foreskin with gauze and remove any additional adhesions.
- Place the Gomco bell over the penis with the dorsal slit secured over the bell.
- Pull the foreskin over the bell.
- Bring the bell and foreskin through the Gomco clamp ring.

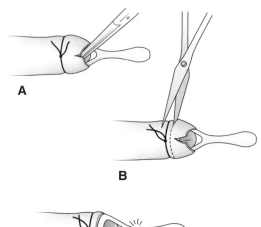

A

B

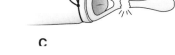

C

FIG. 33–3. Steps of Plastibell method of circumcision. (*A*) Place the Plastibell over the glans and place the string over the Plastibell indentation. (*B*) Trim the foreskin. (*C*) Break off the Plastibell shaft, leaving the bell in place.

- Tighten the thumbscrew until it is snug.
- Remove visible foreskin with a #10 scalpel distal to the junction of the bell and clamp device.
- Keep the Gomco clamp in place for 5 minutes to allow for hemostasis, which decreases the incidence of bleeding.
- Loosen the thumbscrew and gently loosen the foreskin.
- Wrap the penis in gauze with petroleum jelly.
- The first void after the procedure should be documented.

PLASTIBELL METHOD

This method is shown in Figure 33–3.

- Restrain the child.
- Inspect the genitalia.
- Cleanse with antiseptic solution.
- Grasp the foreskin with the two hemostats at the 10 o'clock and 2 o'clock positions.
- Gently probe and lyse adhesions underneath the foreskin with the curved hemostat. Do not extend beyond the corona.
- Place the straight hemostat approximately two-thirds of the distance from the foreskin to the opening of the corona. Keep in place for 1 minute. This crushes the skin and marks the area for placing the dorsal slit.
- Remove the hemostat.
- Cut through the middle of the crushed area.
- Peel back the foreskin with gauze and remove any additional adhesions.
- Place the Plastibell over the glans.
- Pull the foreskin over the Plastibell.

514

- Place the Plastibell so that the indentation is below the apex of the incision.
- Place a 2-inch string over the indentation of the Plastibell and tighten it until it is in place but not firm.
- Check the placement of the string and bell. Make sure that the Plastibell moves freely over the glans.
- Tighten the string and hold the tension for 30 seconds.
- Tie a square knot (right over left; left over right).
- Remove hemostats.
- Cut the foreskin with scissors, 1/8 inch to 3/16 inch distal to the string.
- Hold the Plastibell and gently snap off the shaft.
- Wrap the penis in gauze with petroleum jelly.
- The first void after the procedure should be documented.

INSTRUCTIONS TO PARENTS

- Yellow film will develop on the glans in the next few days. This is normal granulation tissue and will disappear in the next few days.
- Keep the penis clean and dry.
- Apply petroleum jelly on the circumcised area after each diaper change until the wound is healed.
- The Plastibell should fall off in 10 to 14 days. If it does not, call the health-care provider.

TEST YOUR KNOWLEDGE OF CHAPTER 33

1. What is the placement of anesthetic for the dorsal penile nerve block?
2. What are the two most commonly used methods of circumcision?
3. Why is circumcision performed?
4. Describe the steps of the Gomco clamp method of circumcision.
5. Describe the steps of the Plastibell method of circumcision.

 ## BIBLIOGRAPHY

American Academy of Pediatrics. (2001). *Policy statement: Circumcision. www.aap.org*
Hashmat, A. I., & Das, S. (1993). *The penis.* Philadelphia: Lea & Febiger.
Holman, J. R., Lewis, E. L., & Ringler, R. L. (1995). Neonatal circumcision techniques. *American Family Physician, 52,* 511–517.
McMillian, J. A., DeAngelis, D. C., Feigin, R. D., & Warshaw, J. B. (1999). *Oski's pediatrics: Principles and practice.* Philadelphia: Lippincott Williams & Wilkins.
Pfenninger, J. L., & Fowler, G. C. (1994). *Procedures for primary care physicians.* St. Louis: Mosby.

CHAPTER **34**

Lumbar Puncture

MARGARET R. COLYAR

OBJECTIVES
- *Determine the contraindications of lumbar puncture.*
- *Determine the indications for lumbar puncture.*
- *Ascertain a safe method of lumbar puncture.*
- *Ascertain appropriate laboratory testing of cerebrospinal fluid (CSF).*

 CPT Codes

- 62270: Spinal puncture, lumbar, diagnostic

In the ambulatory care setting, lumbar puncture is indicated for patients with suspected infection. Lumbar puncture is the most direct and accurate method of determining central nervous system (CNS) infection. CSF is completely replaced about three times a day. There is about 120 to 150 mL of CSF in the system at a time. Although about 500 mL of CSF is formed every day, much of it is reabsorbed into the blood.

 PURPOSE

- Diagnosis
  - To rule out CNS infection
  - To determine the level of pressure in the spinal column
  - To determine CNS infection

516

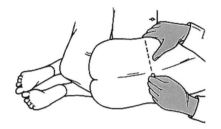

FIG. 34–1. Lateral recumbent position for lumbar puncture.

Symptoms of CNS infection include:
- Fever
- Malaise
- Irritability

 CONTRAINDICATIONS

- Lumbar skin infection
- Platelet count less than 50,000/mm^3

 EQUIPMENT

- Spinal tap tray
- Sterile gloves
- Fenestrated drape
- 1% lidocaine
- Povidine-iodine
- 2 × 2 gauze
- Tape

 PROCEDURE

- Position the child in the tripod or lateral recumbent (fetal) position (Fig. 34–1).
- Draw a line across the back between the tops of the iliac crests. Locate the interspace between either L3 and L4 or L4 and L5.
- Open the spinal tray.
- Apply sterile gloves.
- Cleanse the skin 6 inches around the interspace with povidone-iodine in a circular motion.
- Cleanse the same area with 70% alcohol.
- Draw up 3 mL of 1% lidocaine.
- Assemble the manometer with the three-way stopcock.
- Inject the lidocaine at the site, raising a wheal in the skin. Inject 0.5 mL of lidocaine into the posterior spinous region.

517

- Insert the spinal needle with the stylet in place through the skin just below the palpated spinous process. Angle the needle about 15 degrees cephalad.
  - If you hit bone or the needle meets with resistance, withdraw the needle slightly and redirect it.
- Advance the needle slowly.
- After the needle is inserted a few millimeters, withdraw the stylet to see if CSF is present. You may hear a popping sound when the needle penetrates the dura.
- Advance the needle 1 to 2 mm farther.
- Remove the stylet.
- Attach the manometer to the hub of the inserted needle. Note the level of pressure on the manometer.
- Open the stopcock to allow the CSF to flow into the test tubes.
- Label the tubes (Table 34–1).
- When enough CSF has been obtained, replace the stylet and remove the needle.
- Cover the insertion site with a 2 × 2-inch pressure dressing and leave it in place for 2 hours.
- Send the tubes to the laboratory for analysis within 2 hours. Do NOT refrigerate the tubes.
- To prevent headache:
  - Have the patient lie still for 4 to 8 hours after the procedure.
  - Encourage fluids by offering at least one to two 8-ounce glasses of water. Popsicles are often a great substitute.
  - Ask the caregiver to assist the patient with activities and rest while he or she is lying down over the next 4 to 8 hours.

TABLE 34–1. LABELING TUBES	
Tube Number	**Purpose of Test**
1: Biochemistry	Glucose, protein
2: Bacteriology	Gram's stain, culture (bacterial)
	Indicate if the following are needed:
	• Fungal culture
	• TB culture
	• Viral culture
3: Hematology	Cell count, differential
4: Optional	VDRL
	India ink (fungal)
	Cytology
	Myelin basic protein
	Oligoglional bands

TB = tuberculosis; VDRL = Venereal Disease Research Laboratory.

TABLE 34–2. NORMAL CEREBROSPINAL FLUID VALUES		
Test	**Value**	**Indication**
Opening pressure	50–200 mm H$_2$O	No intracranial pressure
		No obstruction
WBC count	<5/mm^3	No infection
Glucose	50%–80% of serum glucose	No hypo- or hyperglycemia
Protein	15–45 mg/dL	No hemorrhage
		No tumors
		No traumatic tap

WBC = white blood cell.

CEREBROSPINAL FLUID TESTS

WHAT TEST RESULTS INDICATE

- Normal result: No infection; no intracranial pressure (Table 34–2)
- Abnormal result: See Table 34–3

PROCEDURE

- 2 mL of CSF in each tube
- Nonfasting
- Color of tube: Clear plastic tubes that come in the spinal tray
- Special treatment of sample
  - Do not refrigerate
  - Storage: Send to laboratory within 2 hours.

INTERFERING FACTORS

- Medications: None
- Food: None

TEST YOUR KNOWLEDGE OF CHAPTER 34

1. What are the reasons for lumbar puncture?
2. What are the contraindications for lumbar puncture?
3. What is the correct positioning of the child for lumbar puncture?
4. Where is the appropriate placement of the stylus for lumbar puncture?
5. Describe the lumbar puncture procedure.
6. What testing of the CSF is done?
7. What are the normal and abnormal results of CSF testing?

TABLE 34–3. ABNORMAL CEREBROSPINAL FLUID VALUES

Test	Normal	Abnormal	Indication
Appearance	Clear	Cloudy	Infection
		Bloody	Hemorrhage, obstruction, or traumatic tap
		Brown	Elevated protein, RBCs
		Yellow-orange	Hemolysis present for 3 days or more
Protein	15–45 mg/dL	Increased	Tumors, trauma, hemorrhage, diabetes mellitus, polyneuritis, blood in CSF
		Decreased	Rapid CSF production
Gamma globulin	3%–12%	Increased	Multiple sclerosis, neurosyphilis, Guillain-Barré syndrome
Glucose	50%–80%	Increased	Systemic hyperglycemia
		Decreased	Systemic hypoglycemia, bacterial or fungal infection, meningitis, mumps
Cell count	0–5 WBCs as per mm^3	Increased	Active disease Meningitis, tumor, abscess, infarction, multiple sclerosis,
	No RBCs per mm^3	RBCs present	Hemorrhage, traumatic tap
VDRL	Nonreactive	Positive	Neurosyphilis
Chloride	118–130 mEqL	Decreased	Meningitis, TB
Gram stain	Negative	Gram-positive or gram-negative organisms	Bacterial meningitis

CSF = cerebrospinal fluid; RBC = red blood cell; TB = tuberculosis; VDRL = Venereal Disease Research Laboratory; WBC = white blood cell.

 BIBLIOGRAPHY

Diagnostics. An A-Z guide to laboratory tests. (2000). Springhouse, PA: Springhouse.

Ewald, G. A., & McKenzie, C. R. (Eds.). (1999). *Manual of medical therapeutics* (32nd ed.). Boston: Little, Brown, & Co.

Fischbach, F. (1999). *A manual of laboratory & diagnostic tests* (6th ed.). New York: J. B. Lippincott.

Siberry, G. K., & Iannone, R. (2000). *Johns Hopkins Hospital: The Harriet Lane handbook* (15th ed.). St. Louis: Mosby.

CHAPTER **35**

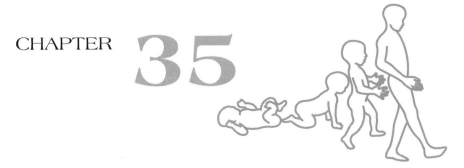

Serum Diagnostic Testing

MARGARET R. COLYAR

OBJECTIVES
- *Become familiar with serum diagnostic tests that are common for children.*
- *Ascertain the correct procedure and storage for common serum diagnostic tests.*
- *Identify interfering factors for common serum diagnostic tests.*

 CPT Codes

- 36415: Venipuncture: Finger/heel/ear
- 8502: CBC/platelet/full auto differential
- 8502: CBC/platelet/manual differential
- 8272: Ferritin
- 8296: Fingerstick glucose
- 82947: Fasting serum glucose
- 8302: Hemoglobin electrophoresis
- 8365: Lead level
- 8007: Liver enzymes (hepatic function panel)
- 8403: PKU
- 8630: Mononucleosis
- 8444: TSH
- 8443: Free T_4
- 8470: hCG: Serum quantitative
- 84703: hCG: Serum qualitative
- 86318: *H. pylori*

Several serum diagnostic tests are performed in pediatric patients. Tests included are specific for infection, inflammation, anemia, liver disease, thyroid disease, pregnancy, and amino acids.

COMPLETE BLOOD COUNT

PURPOSE

● Diagnosis: To determine infection, inflammation, anemia, coagulation problems, morphology of white blood cells, and hydration

NORMAL VALUES BASED ON AGE

Table 35–1 lists the normal values based on age.

WHAT TEST RESULTS INDICATE

Each part of the complete blood count (CBC) indicates different disease processes (Table 35–2).

PROCEDURE

● 3 to 7 mL preferred; 0.5 mL Microtainer; 0.25 mL for newborns and infants
● Whole blood
● Nonfasting
● Lavender-top capillary tube
● Special treatment of sample: May be stored at ambient temperature for 8 hours or refrigerated for 24 hours

INTERFERING FACTORS

● Medications
  ● Antineoplastic agents may cause leukopenia.
  ● Antibiotics may alter white blood cell (WBC) count.
● Food: None.
● Rough handling: May cause hemolysis.
● Frozen or clotted specimen.
● Exercise and stress: May increase WBC count.

CORTISOL

Abnormal changes in cortisol levels are caused by hypothalamus, pituitary, or adrenal malfunction. Peak levels are in the morning (6:00 AM) and lowest levels are in the evening (10:00 PM).

TABLE 35–1. VALUES FOR COMPLETE BLOOD COUNT COMPONENTS FOR CHILDREN

Component	Premature Infants	Newborns	Age 1 Month	Age 2 Months	Age 6 Months	Ages 6 Months to 2 Years	Ages 2 to 6 Years	Ages 6 to 12 Years	Ages 12 to 18 Years
WBC	4.4	9.0–30.0	5.0–19.5	—	6.0–17.5	6.0–17.0	5.0–15.5	4.5–13.5	4.5–13.5
Hgb	11.0	16.5	13.9	11.2	12.6	12.0	13.5	14.5	14.5
HCT	35.0–41.5	42.0–51.0	33.0–44.0	28.0–35.0	31.0–36.0	33.0–36.0	34.0–37.0	35.0–40.0	46.0–43.0
MCV	106.0–118.0	98.0–108.0	91.0–111.0	84.0–106.0	68.0–85.0	70.0–84.0	75.0–87.0	77.0–95.0	80.0–100.0
Platelets	180.0–317.0	290.0	250.0	—	—	150.0–350.0	—	—	—

HCT = hematocrit; Hgb = hemoglobin; MCV = mean corpuscular volume; WBC = white blood cell.

523

TABLE 35–2. COMPLETE BLOOD COUNT

Component	Indication
WBC COUNT	
Increased	Bacterial infection, inflammation
Decreased	Viral infection, bone marrow failure
Neutrophils	Bands: Acute infection (increased, or shift to the left): Elevated bands and decreased total WBCs indicate bone marrow depression
	Segmented neutrophils (increased, or shift to the right): Elevated segments indicate long-term infection
Basophils	Increased with allergic reactions and anaphylaxis
Granulocytes	Increased with stress
Monocytes	Second line of defense; increased with long-term infections, collagen vascular disease, carcinoma, leukemia, or lymphoma
Lymphocytes	Increased: Infection, mononucleosis, other viral infections
	Decreased: Debilitating illness, increased adrenocorticosteroids, immunodeficiency
Eosinophils	Increased with allergic reactions and parasitic infections
RBC COUNT, Hgb, Hct	
Increased	Dehydration, polycythemia
Decreased	Anemia, fluid overload, recent hemorrhage
MCV	Increased: Macrocytic anemia: vitamin B_{12} or folate deficiency
	Decreased: Microcytic anemia: iron deficiency, thalassemia
MCHC	Decreased: Iron deficiency, thalassemia
Platelets	Increased: Hemorrhage, infection, malignancy, recent surgery, stress, inflammatory disorder, collagen vascular disorder
	Decreased: Bone marrow disease, macrocytic anemia, pooling of platelets in spleen, DIC

DIC = disseminated intravascular coagulation; Hct = hematocrit; Hgb = hemoglobin; MCHC = mean corpuscular hemoglobin concentration; MCV = mean corpuscular volume; RBC = red blood cell.

PURPOSE

- Diagnosis of Cushing's syndrome, renal disease, diabetes mellitus, Addison's disease, or adrenal insufficiency

NORMAL VALUES FOR ANY AGE

Normal values are 6 to 18 µg/dL in the morning and 0 to 9 µg/dL in the evening.

WHAT TEST RESULTS INDICATE

Increases indicate:

- Cushing's syndrome
- Renal disease
- Diabetes mellitus

524

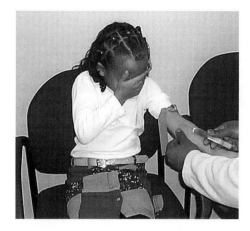

FIG. 35–1. Blood being drawn in a school-age child.

Decreases indicate:

- Primary adrenal insufficiency: Addison's disease
- Secondary adrenal insufficiency: Tuberculosis (TB), fungal infection, hemorrhage

Absence of diurnal variation indicates Cushing's syndrome or stress.

PROCEDURE

- 7 mL needed
- Serum
- Nonfasting
- Color of tube: Green heparin, lavender-top, or tiger-top tube
- Special treatment of sample: Storage at room temperature
- Other: Collection should be early, between 6:00 and 8:00 AM

INTERFERING FACTORS

- Medications
  - Oral contraceptives
  - Estrogen replacement
  - Androgens
  - Phenytoin
- Food: No extra salt for 3 days before test
- Exercise: Limit physical activity 10 to 12 hours before test
- Rough handling: May cause hemolysis

FERRITIN

Ferritin is a protein stored in the bone marrow. Only small amounts show up in serum. The serum ferritin level is determined to screen for iron-deficiency anemia and iron overload.

PURPOSE

- Diagnosis: To rule out anemia and iron overload
  - Symptoms: Pallor, shortness of breath, weakness, dizziness
- Follow-up: To determine effectiveness of treatment

NORMAL VALUES BASED ON AGE

- Newborn: 25 to 200 ng/mL
- Infant (age ≤ 1 month): 200 to 600 ng/mL
- Infant (age 2 to 5 months): 50 to 200 ng/mL
- Infant (age 6 months to 15 years): 7 to 140 ng/mL

WHAT TEST RESULTS INDICATE

- Increases indicate acute or chronic hepatic disease, iron overload, leukemia, Hodgkin's disease, chronic hemolytic anemias.
- Decreases indicate chronic iron-deficiency anemia.

PROCEDURE

- 1 mL needed
- Serum
- Nonfasting
- Red-top or lavender-top tube or heparin tube

INTERFERING FACTORS

- Medications: None
- Food: None
- Improper storage: None
- Recent blood transfusion: Will cause an increase

GLUCOSE

Plasma glucose is less accurate than a 2-hour postprandial plasma glucose test. This test cannot be used to diagnose diabetes mellitus.

PURPOSE

- To screen for diabetes mellitus
  - Symptoms
    - Polyuria
    - Polydipsia
    - Polyphagia
    - Blurred vision
    - Tiredness

NORMAL VALUES BASED ON AGE

- Premature infants: 20 to 65 mg/dL
- Newborn (age ≤ 1 day): 40 to 60 mg/dL
- Infant (age > 1 week): 50 to 90 mg/dL
- Child: 60 to 100 mg/dL
- Adolescents and young adults: 70 to 110 mg/dL

WHAT TEST RESULTS INDICATE

- Increases: Two elevated blood glucose results strongly suggest diabetes mellitus or may also indicate pancreatitis, acute illness, Cushing's syndrome, acromegaly, pheochromocytoma, chronic hepatic disease, nephrotic syndrome, brain tumor, sepsis, anoxia, or convulsive disorder.
- Decreases: Hyperinsulinism, hypoglycemia, myxedema, adrenal problems, hypopituitarism, or malabsorption.

PROCEDURE

- 5 mL needed
- Whole blood
- Fasting
- Gray-top tube
- Special treatment of sample: Store in refrigerator

INTERFERING FACTORS

- Medications
  - False-positive: Acetaminophen (Tylenol), diuretics, oral contraceptives, benzodiazepines, phenytoin, lithium, corticosteroids
  - False-negative: Propranolol, ethanol, insulin, oral hypoglycemic agents, monoamine oxidase inhibitors (MAOIs)
- Food: Fasting required
- Improper storage: Must refrigerate or glycolysis will occur, leading to a false-negative result
- Other
  - False-positive: Nonfasting, recent illness, infection, pregnancy

✇ *HELICOBACTER PYLORI* ANTIBODY: IgG AB

Persons with *Helicobacter pylori* develop serum antibodies. Three serum antibody tests are available: IgG, IgA, and IgM. These tests match antibody production against certain antigen bands specific to *H. pylori*. IgG is matched against more bands (98%), then IgA (30%), and last, IgM (3 %). Circulating antibodies for *H. pylori* are predominantly of the IgG class. Therefore, choose the IgG serum antibody test. *Do not* use the serum antibody tests to check for effectiveness of treatment because the patient will continue to have antibodies.

PURPOSE

- To detect the presence of *H. pylori*
  - Symptoms
    - Epigastric abdominal pain
    - Gastric reflux
    - Bloating

NORMAL VALUES FOR ANY AGE

The finding of no *H. pylori* present is normal for any age.

WHAT TEST RESULTS INDICATE

A positive result indicates presence of *H. pylori.*

PROCEDURE

- 5 mL needed
- Serum: 0.1 mL needed to place on test slide
- Nonfasting
- Heparin, lavender-top, or tiger-top tube
- Test slide
- Special treatment of sample: Handle gently to prevent hemolysis
- Temperature: May store at room temperature for 2 days or refrigerate up to 2 weeks

INTERFERING FACTORS

- Medications: None
- Food: None
- Improper storage
  - Hemolysis
  - Freezing and thawing
- Other: Severely lipemic blood sample

 # HEMOGLOBIN ELECTROPHORESIS

Hemoglobin electrophoresis evaluates the type and distribution of hemoglobin (Hgb) in the blood. It is the most useful test to measure abnormal Hgb levels.

PURPOSE

- Diagnosis: To detect:
  - Abnormal Hgb levels
  - Thalassemia
  - Sickle cell disease and trait
  - Hereditary or acquired methemoglobinemia

NORMAL VALUES BASED ON AGE

- Newborns: Hgb F: 50% of Hgb and Hgb S and C are absent.
- Infants: Hgb F replaced by Hgb A_1
- Toddlers: Hgb A_1 predominates
- Preschoolers: Hgb A_1 predominates
- School-age children: Hgb A_1 predominates
- Adolescents: Hgb A_1 predominates
- Young adults: Hgb A_1 predominates

WHAT TEST RESULTS INDICATE

Abnormal results indicate:
- Thalassemia: Hgb F greater than 5% after 6 months
- Sickle cell trait: A/S pattern: A = 60% to 80%; S = 20% to 40%; F = small amount
- Sickle cell anemia: S/S pattern: S = 80% to 100%; F = rest of sample; A = 0%
- Methemoglobinemia: M = ≤ 40% of total Hgb

PROCEDURE

- 3 to 7 mL needed
- Whole blood
- Nonfasting
- Lavender-top tube
- Special treatment of sample
  - Fill tube completely and rotate gently
  - Storage: *Do not* store at ambient temperature; must be refrigerated

INTERFERING FACTORS

- Medications: None.
- Food: None.
- Improper storage: *Do not* leave at room temperature.
- Other: Blood transfusion within the past 4 months.
- Rough handling.

⟡ HUMAN CHORIONIC GONADOTROPIN: SERUM PREGNANCY QUANTITATIVE

The two types of tests that can be ordered to detect pregnancy are urine qualitative and serum quantitative. The serum quantitative test is more sensitive than the urine qualitative test for human chorionic gonadotropin (hCG). Glycoprotein is released after conception, and it may be detected 9 days after ovulation and implantation of the ovum in the uterine wall. Levels of hCG increase steadily in the first trimester, peaking at the tenth week. The levels may vary during pregnancy.

PURPOSE

- Diagnosis: To detect pregnancy
  - Symptom: Missed menstrual period

NORMAL VALUES

The normal value is < 3 mIU/mL.

WHAT TEST RESULTS INDICATE

- Increases:
  - hCG increases steadily in the first trimester; peaks at the tenth week.
  - Significantly higher levels indicate multiple pregnancy or hydatidiform mole carcinomas that secrete hCG (gastric, pancreatic, ovarian).
- Decreases: Ectopic pregnancy, or pregnancy less than 9 days.

PROCEDURE

- 2 to 5 mL needed
- Serum
- Nonfasting
- Tiger-top tube
- Special treatment of sample: handle gently to prevent hemolysis.
- May keep at ambient temperature for 48 hours, refrigerated for 7 days, and frozen for 3 months

INTERFERING FACTORS

- Medications: None
- Food: None
- Improper storage: Hemolysis
- Diseases: Hepatitis: Decreased hCG

LEAD LEVELS

PURPOSE

- Diagnosis: To rule out lead poisoning
- Symptoms
  - Anemia
  - Blue line at gum margin
  - Colic
  - Coma
  - Constipation
  - Convulsions
  - Delirium
  - Headache
  - Metallic taste
  - Lethargy
  - Abdominal pain
  - Weight loss
  - Irritable
  - Anorexia

NORMAL VALUES

Normal value is < 30 µg/dL in children.

TOXIC VALUES

Toxic value is > 40 µg/dL.

WHAT TEST RESULTS INDICATE

Table 35–3 lists the results and what they indicate.

TABLE 35–3. LEAD LEVEL RESULTS	
Blood Level (µg/dL)	**Indication or Action**
< 9	No lead poisoning
10–14	Evaluate environment; decrease exposure to lead; follow up in 3 months
15–19	Decrease lead exposure
	Dietary interventions:
	• Increase iron
	• Increase calcium
	• Eat regular meals (lead absorbs more on empty stomach)
20–40	Decrease lead exposure
	Continue dietary interventions
20–41	Consider pharmacologic interventions
> 40	Chelation therapy within 48 hours

PROCEDURE

- 7 mL; 0.5 mL for newborns, infants, toddlers, and preschoolers
- Whole blood
- Nonfasting
- Heparin tube
- Special treatment of sample
  - Storage: Room temperature

INTERFERING FACTORS

- Medications: None
- Food: None
- Improper storage: Do not freeze

🌀 LIVER ENZYMES (HEPATIC FUNCTION TESTS)

Liver enzyme tests are usually not routinely ordered. However, they are indicated if liver or biliary tract disease is in your differential diagnosis list. Alanine aminotransferase and aspartate aminotransferase are indicators of liver cell damage. Alkaline phosphatase, bilirubin, and gamma-glutamyl transpeptidase are very sensitive to mild biliary system obstruction.

PURPOSE

- Diagnosis: To detect liver cell damage or biliary system obstruction
  - Symptoms
    - Jaundice
    - Right upper quadrant pain
    - Nausea, vomiting, diarrhea

NORMAL VALUES BASED ON AGE

Table 35–4 lists normal values based on age.

TABLE 35–4. NORMAL VALUES: LIVER ENZYMES

Age Group	ALT, U/L	AST, U/dL	Bilirubin, mg/dL	ALP, IU/L	GGT, U/L
Newborns		25–75	1.5 – 12		All ages
Infants	< 54	25–75	0.2–1	150–400	Boys: 6–28
					Girls: 4–18
Children ages					
2 to 10 years	1–30	0–40	0.2–1	100–300	
Adolescents	1–30		0.2–1	Boys: 50–375	
				Girls: 30–300	

ALP = alkaline phosphatase; ALT = alanine aminotransferase; AST = aspartate aminotransferase; GGT = gamma-glutamyl transpeptidase.

TABLE 35–5. LIVER ENZYMES: ABNORMAL RESULTS

Enzyme	Increased Levels	Indications
ALT	50× normal	Viral or severe drug-induced hepatitis
	Moderate	Mononucleosis, chronic hepatitis, cholecystitis, hepatic congestion
	Slight to moderate	Acute liver injury: Active cirrhosis, drug-induced or alcoholic hepatitis
AST	20× normal	Viral hepatitis, severe skeletal muscle trauma, extensive surgery
	10 to 20× normal	MI, mononucleosis, alcoholic cirrhosis
	5 to 10× normal	Duchenne muscular dystrophy, dermatomyositis, chronic hepatitis
	2 to 5× normal	Hemolytic anemia, metastatic hepatic tumors, acute pancreatitis, pulmonary emboli, delirium tremens, fatty liver
Bilirubin	Elevated	Hepatic damage, hemolytic anemia, congenital enzyme deficiencies, biliary obstruction
ALP	Sharp	Biliary obstruction
	Moderate	Biliary obstruction, cirrhosis, mononucleosis, viral hepatitis
	<20 IU/L	Hypophosphatasia, protein or magnesium deficiency
GGT	Sharp	Obstructive jaundice, hepatic metastases
	Moderate	Acute pancreatitis, renal disease, prostatic metastases, brain tumors

ALP = alkaline phosphatase; ALT = alanine aminotransferase; AST = aspartate aminotransferase; GGT = gamma-glutamyl transpeptidase; MI = myocardial infarction.

WHAT TEST RESULTS INDICATE

Table 35–5 lists the abnormal results indicated by increases. Decreases are not applicable.

PROCEDURE

- 1 mL needed
- Serum
- Nonfasting
- Color of tube: Tiger-top or green heparin tube
- Special treatment of sample: *Do not* freeze; keeps well at ambient temperature for 24 hours; can be refrigerated for 7 days.

533

INTERFERING FACTORS

- Medications: None.
- Food: None.
- Improper storage: Serum must be separated from cells before storage.

MONOSPOT

Infectious mononucleosis is a self-limiting disease caused by the Epstein-Barr virus. It peaks between the ages of 4 and 8 years. Detection can occur after 1 week of infection. It peaks at 2 to 4 weeks and declines by 12 weeks.

PURPOSE

- Diagnosis: To detect infectious mononucleosis
  - Symptoms
    - Fatigue
    - Pharyngitis
    - Fever
    - Lymphadenopathy
    - Splenomegaly
    - Hepatitis

NORMAL VALUES

- 1:56 is suspicious.
- $\geq$ 1:224 indicates infectious mononucleosis.

WHAT TEST RESULTS INDICATE

- Increases: False-positive results with lymphoma, hepatitis A and B, leukemia, and pancreatic cancer
- Decreases: Not applicable

PROCEDURE

- Amount needed: One capillary tube full.
- Whole blood: Finger or heel stick.
- Nonfasting.
- Capillary tube.
- Special treatment of sample: Store at $\geq$ 72°F or 2 to 8°C or use immediately.

INTERFERING FACTORS

- Medications: None
- Food: None

TABLE 35–6. PERIPHERAL BLOOD SMEAR	
RBC Shape	**Indications**
Elliptical (pencil shaped)	Iron deficiency; thalassemia, possibly hereditary
Spherocytes (small, spherical)	Hemolysis
Target cells (shooting target)	Iron deficiency, thalassemia, abnormal hemoglobin, liver disease
Blue stippling	Thalassemia, hemolysis, lead poisoning
Schistocytes (fragmented RBCs)	Seen with artificial heart valves, severe atherosclerosis, thrombocytopenic purpura

RBC = red blood cell.

- Improper storage: None
- Rough handling: Can depress titer

PERIPHERAL BLOOD SMEAR

Peripheral blood smears provide information on size and shape of red blood cells (RBCs). This information is important in determining response or lack of response to treatment for anemia.

PURPOSE

- Diagnosis: To determine response or lack of response to treatment for anemia
  - Symptoms
    - Pallor
    - Shortness of breath
    - Weakness
    - Dizziness

NORMAL VALUES

Biconcave disk-shaped RBCs are normal.

WHAT TEST RESULTS INDICATE

Table 35–6 lists abnormally shaped RBCs and the information they provide on disease processes.

PROCEDURE

- Amount needed: 0.1 mL
- Whole blood
- Nonfasting
- Color of tube: Tiger-top or capillary tube
- Special treatment of sample: Place on plate immediately

INTERFERING FACTORS

- Medications: None.
- Food: None.
- Improper storage: Place on plate immediately.

 # PHENYLKETONURIA

All states screen for phenylketonuria (PKU). The incidence of PKU is 1:10 per 15,000 white children born in the United States. It occurs infrequently in individuals of other ethnicities. Treatment for a positive PKU result must start as soon as possible after birth. The best time to maximize detection is 72 hours after birth. Because of early hospital discharge, newborns must be checked at their 10-day visit. Check your state regulations for other testing of newborns. Most states screen for congenital hypothyroidism, PKU, and galactosemia.

PURPOSE

- Diagnosis: To screen for phenylalanine
  - To prevent severe mental retardation

NORMAL VALUES BASED ON AGE

- Premature infants: 2.0 to 7.5 mg/dL
- Newborns: 1.2 to 3.4 mg/dL
- Young adults: 0.8 to 1.8 mg/dL

WHAT TEST RESULTS INDICATE

Increases may indicate hepatic disease, galactosemia, or delayed development of certain enzyme systems. Decreases are not applicable.

PROCEDURE

- Few drops needed.
- Capillary blood from a heel stick.
- Nonfasting.
- Special filter card provided by the state; must completely fill three of the four circles on the card.
- Special treatment of sample: Air dry flat and mail.

INTERFERING FACTORS

- Medications: None.
- Food: None.
- Other: Infant must receive 3 full days of breast milk or formula before test; otherwise, the test will have a false-negative result.

TABLE 35–7. THYROID TEST RESULTS

Test	Result	Indication
TSH	Elevated	Primary hypothyroidism
	Decreased	Hyperthyroidism, secondary or tertiary hypothyroidism
Free T$_4$	Elevated	Thyrotoxicosis, Graves' disease
	Decreased	Hypothyroidism

Free T$_4$ = free thyroxine.

THYROID TESTS

The two main tests used to screen for thyroid disorders are thyroid-stimulating hormone (TSH) and free thyroxine (free T$_4$) levels. TSH is used to detect primary hypothyroidism. Free T$_4$ is used to exclude hyperthyroidism and determine if replacement medication is needed.

PURPOSE

- Diagnosis: To screen for thyroid disorders and pituitary problems
  - Symptom: Fatigue in older children

NORMAL VALUES: TSH

- Newborns
  - Age 1 to 3 days: < 13.3
  - Age 2 to 4 weeks: < 10
  - Age > 4 weeks: < 5.5

NORMAL VALUES: FREE T$_4$

- Newborns
  - Age 1 to 10 days: 0.6 to 2.0
  - Age greater than 10 days: 0.7 to 1.7

WHAT TEST RESULTS INDICATE

Both TSH and free T$_4$ levels must be evaluated together (Tables 35–7 and 35–8).

TABLE 35–8. EVALUATION OF THYROID-STIMULATING HORMONE AND FREE THYROXINE TOGETHER

	Hypothyroidism	Hyperthyroidism
TSH	Elevated	Decreased
Free T$_4$	Decreased	Elevated

Free T$_4$ = free thyroxine; TSH = thyroid-stimulating hormone.

PROCEDURE

- 0.5 mL in neonates and infants; otherwise, 7 mL; can also do heel stick for infants and use filter card
- Serum
- Nonfasting
- Tiger-top tube
- Special treatment of sample: Send to laboratory immediately; may keep at ambient temperature for 8 hours, refrigerated for 48 hours, and frozen for 3 months

INTERFERING FACTORS

- Medications
  - Aspirin, corticosteroids, and heparin lower levels
  - Potassium iodide raises levels
- Food: None
- Improper storage: None
- Rough handling: May interfere with accurate determination of results

TEST YOUR KNOWLEDGE OF CHAPTER 35

1. What do the components of the CBC indicate?
2. Which tests assist in evaluation of hormone function?
3. Which tests assist in evaluation of anemia? What information does each of the tests contribute?
4. To evaluate for sickle cell trait versus anemia, which test should be ordered? How would trait versus anemia be determined?
5. Which serum tests are also used as screening tests, and why?
6. What do the components of the hepatic function tests indicate?
7. What tests might be ordered for a child with abdominal pain and bloating?
8. Which test is best to evaluate pregnancy, and why?

BIBLIOGRAPHY

Diagnostics. An A-Z guide to laboratory tests. (2000). Springhouse, PA: Springhouse.

Ewald, G. A., & McKenzie, C. R. (Eds.). (1999). *Manual of medical therapeutics* (32nd ed.). Boston, MA: Little, Brown & Co.

Fischbach, F. (1999). *A manual of laboratory and diagnostic tests* (6th ed.). New York: J. B. Lippincott.

Siberry, G. K., & Iannone, R. (2000). *Johns Hopkins Hospital: The Harriet Lane handbook* (15th ed.). St. Louis: Mosby.

36

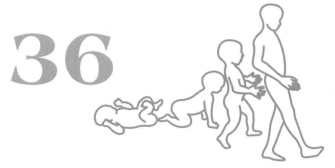

Urine Diagnostic Testing

Margaret R. Colyar

 ## CPT Codes

- 81003: Urinalysis
- 81015: Microscopic
- 87086: Urine culture
- 81025: Urine pregnancy: hCG

Understanding when and why to perform a urinalysis, microscopic analysis of urine sediment, urine culture and sensitivity, and urine pregnancy test is necessary for providing comprehensive care to the pediatric client.

 ## URINALYSIS

The routine urinalysis (UA) is an easy test that gives the provider much valuable information. It can be performed easily and quickly in any office setting. The elements of evaluating a UA include color, odor, opacity, specific gravity, and pH, as well as rough measurement of protein, glucose,

TABLE 36–1. URINALYSIS RESULTS AND WHEN TO ORDER OTHER TESTS

Urinalysis Component	Normal Value	Abnormal Value	Other Tests to Order
pH	4.5–8.0		
Specific gravity	1.025–1.030	1.001–1.003	BUN, creatinine
		1.10	BUN, creatinine
		1.030	Consider BUN, creatinine, or liver function tests
Leukocytes	Negative	0–Trace	Microscopic analysis Urine C & S
Nitrites	Negative	Positive	Urine C & S
Glucose	Negative	Positive	Serum glucose
Ketones	Negative	Positive	Consider serum glucose
Protein	Negative	Positive	BUN, creatinine
Blood	Negative	Positive	BUN, creatinine
Urobilinogen	0.2	> 0.2	Liver function tests

BUN = blood urea nitrogen; C & S = culture and sensitivity.

ketones, red blood cells (RBCs) and white blood cells (WBCs), casts, crystals, nitrates, and albumin. Based on the results of the UA, a microscopic analysis of the urine sediment can be done to determine etiology of the cells, casts, and crystals.

Abnormal findings suggest the presence of disease and mandate further urine or blood tests. Knowing when to order a microscopic analysis of urine sediment, a urine culture and sensitivity, a vaginal examination, kidney function tests, or other laboratory tests is crucial in the ambulatory care setting (Table 36–1).

PURPOSE

- Diagnoses: In well-child examinations for screening urinary pathology; to diagnose urinary tract infections, cystitis, and pyelonephritis
  - Symptoms children present with include:
    - Back or low abdominal pain, unexplained fever, unexplained irritability, holding urine, crying when urinating, frequency, burning, and urgency
- Follow-up: To determine effectiveness of treatment

WHAT TEST RESULTS INDICATE

Table 36–2 lists possible results and what they indicate.

PROCEDURE

- 1 to 3 mL of urine is needed.
- The first voided specimen in the morning is best because there is a greater amount of sediment in the urine.

540

TABLE 36–2. URINALYSIS RESULTS

Test	Range	Indications
pH	4.5–8.0	Alkaline urine (pH < 7.0) indicates a diet high in vegetables, citrus fruits, and dairy products but low in meat. Acid urine (below 7.0) indicates a high-protein diet.
Specific gravity	1.025–1.030	Elevated specific gravity (closer to 1.030) most often indicates dehydration but can also be present with hepatic disorders, congestive heart failure, and nephrosis. Depressed specific gravity (1.001–1.003) indicates renal disorders or diabetes insipidus. Fixed specific gravity (1.010) indicates severe renal damage.
Leukocytes (leukocyte esterase)	Negative	Positive indicates infection or inflammation. If no leukocytes are present but symptoms of urinary frequency, burning, urgency or suprapubic pain are present in a girl, suspect a vaginal infection and perform a vaginal examination.
Nitrites	None	Nitrites with flank pain indicate pyeleonephritis. If the test result is positive, culture the urine.
Glucose	None	A positive test result indicates > 180 mg/dL of glucose in the blood. If the test result is positive, order a fasting serum glucose.
Ketones	None	Positive ketones indicate fat metabolism, which may be caused by weight loss, dieting, starvation, or exercise. School-age children and adolescents have positive ketones because of their higher metabolic rate. Ketones are often present with diarrhea and vomiting.
Protein	None	Positive protein indicates leakage of proteins through the kidneys caused by kidney disease or damage.
Blood	None	Positive blood may indicate infection (cystitis), passage of a kidney stone, kidney disease or damage, strenuous exercise, and menses in women.
Urobilinogen	< 0.2 EU/dL	0.2 EU/dL may indicate hepatic problems. Also, drugs that acidify the urine can cause a higher than normal urobilinogen level. This test should be performed on first morning clean-catch midstream specimens.

- Type of collection container: Sterile collection cup is best.
- Special treatment of sample: Perform the test immediately if possible. If not possible, store in refrigerated area at 39° to 41°F. Refrigeration will make the urine become cloudy. This is normal and does not indicate infection.

INTERFERING FACTORS

- Medications: Be aware of medications the child is currently taking; some medications may falsely indicate an abnormal value on the UA.
- Food: None.
- Improper storage: If the urine is not refrigerated, bacteria will grow.

⊗ MICROSCOPIC ANALYSIS OF URINE SEDIMENT

Microscopic analysis of urine sediment is performed only when infection or renal disease is suspected. Microscopic examination of urinary sediments provides many valuable clues in the detection and evaluation of urinary tract disorders. If infection is suspected but the UA leukocytes are 0 to trace, a microscopic analysis should be conducted. Finding WBCs helps to determine the presence of infection. Analysis of casts and crystals can also help identify pathology.

PURPOSE

- Diagnosis To determine the extent of infection or if renal tubular problems exist
  - Symptoms children present with include:
    - Back pain
    - Low abdominal pain
    - Unexplained fever
    - Unexplained irritability
    - Holding in urine
    - Crying when urinating
    - Frequency
    - Burning
    - Urgency
- Follow-up: To determine the effectiveness of treatment

WHAT TEST RESULTS INDICATE

Table 36–3 lists possible results and what they indicate.

PROCEDURE

- 10 mL of urine is needed.

TABLE 36–3. RESULTS OF MICROSCOPIC ANALYSIS OF URINE SEDIMENT

Sediment	Implications
CELLS	
Numerous WBCs	Indicates urinary tract inflammation
WBCs and white cell casts	Strongly suggests renal infection
Increased numbers of epithelial cells	Suggests renal tubular degeneration
Yeasts*	Yeast infection
CASTS	
Increased numbers of casts	Suggests renal disease
Hyaline	Renal disease, febrile illness, strenuous exercise, CHF
Epithelial	Inflammation of the kidney
Granular	Strenuous exercise, diuretic phase of acute renal disease
Fatty	Nephrotic syndrome, diabetic nephropathy
Waxy	Urinary stasis within kidney, chronic renal disease
RBC	Renal parenchymal disease, especially glomerulonephritis
WBC	Infection, usually pyelonephritis
CRYSTALS	
Some crystals present	May be normal or indicate hypercalcemia
Leucine (polyhedral with radial or concentric striations)	Leucine crystals indicate liver disease
Tyrosine (sheaves of needles)	Tyrosine crystals indicate liver disease
Cystine (hexagonal)	Cystinosis
Sulfonamide (dumbbells, stalks of wheat, hexagonal plates)	
OTHER	
Parasites	Most common is *Trichomonas vaginalis*

* Appear as pale, ovoid red blood cells that are variable in size and sometimes budding.
CHF = congestive heart failure.

- The first voided specimen in the morning is best because there is a greater amount of sediment in the urine. Both cells and casts are destroyed in later, more diluted specimens, particularly if pH is above 7.
  - Centrifuge for 5 minutes.
  - Pour off 9 mL and get specimen from the remaining 1 mL.
  - Use a pipette to collect the sediment.
  - Place 2 drops on a slide, add 1 drop of Sedi-Stain, and examine under the microscope.
- Type of collection container: Sterile collection cup is best.
- Special treatment of sample: Perform the test immediately if possible. If not possible, store in refrigerated area at 39° to 41°F. Refrigeration will make the urine become cloudy. This is normal and does not indicate infection.
- Change in acidity and alkalinity will alter results.

INTERFERING FACTORS

- Food: None
- Improper storage: If urine is not refrigerated, bacteria will grow

 # URINE CULTURE AND SENSITIVITY

Urine culture and sensitivity (C & S) studies should be ordered only if leukocytes or nitrites are reported on the UA. The urine C & S identifies the causative organism of the infection and specifies which antibiotic is most effective. Accurate diagnosis results from the presence of a single type of bacteria. More than two organisms in the urine strongly suggest contamination during collection. There is no need to do a culture if the child is taking antibiotics.

PURPOSE

- Diagnosis: To determine the etiology of an infecting organism; to detect true infection versus contamination
    - Symptoms children present with include:
        - Back or low abdominal pain, unexplained fever, unexplained irritability, holding urine, crying when urinating, frequency, burning, and urgency
- Follow-up: To determine effectiveness of treatment

NORMAL VALUES

Normally, urine is sterile; no organisms should grow.

WHAT TEST RESULTS INDICATE

Table 36–4 lists possible results and what they indicate.

PROCEDURE

- Clean-catch or midstream urine specimen.
- 10 mL of urine is needed.
- The first voided specimen in the morning is best because there is a greater amount of sediment in the urine. Both cells and casts are destroyed in later, more diluted specimens, particularly if pH is above 7.
    - Centrifuge for 5 minutes.
    - Pour off 9 mL of urine and get specimen from the remaining 1 mL of sediment.
    - Dip a cotton swab into the sediment to collect the specimen.
    - Swab onto Thayer-Martin agar plate. Roll swab in Z pattern. Then cross-streak with sterile wire loop.

TABLE 36–4. ABNORMAL RESULTS OF URINE CULTURE

- *Escherichia coli*
- Coliform bacilli
- Enterococci
- Gonococci
- *Klebsiella*
- *Mycobacterium tuberculosis*
- *Proteus*
- *Pseudomonas aeruginosa*
- *Staphylococcus*: coagulase positive or negative
- *Streptococcus*: Beta-hemolytic groups B and D
- *Trichomonas vaginalis*
- *Candida albicans*
- Other yeasts

- Type of collection container: Sterile collection cup is best.
- Special treatment of sample: Within 30 minutes, store at 39.4°F (4°C). Store for only 2 hours before plating.

INTERFERING FACTORS

- Medications: Diuretics and antibiotics
- Food: None
- Improper storage: Failure to use within 30 minutes of refrigeration

✿ HUMAN CHORIONIC GONADATROPIN: URINE PREGNANCY TEST

Human chorionic gonadotropin (hCG) is a glycoprotein produced after conception and implantation in the uterus that prevents degeneration of the corpus luteum. It can be detected in urine 10 days after conception. There are two types of urine hCG testing: qualitative and quantitative. Qualitative hCG urine pregnancy testing should be done using the first early morning urine when it is most concentrated. Urine testing to detect pregnancy done on subsequent urine specimens is not reliable, and serum hCG testing should be done. Quantitative urine hCG testing is indicated if there is a question of the viability of the pregnancy or presence of an hCG-excreting tumor.

PURPOSE

- Diagnosis
  - Qualitative analysis
    - To detect the presence or absence of pregnancy
    - As a basis for starting oral and injectable contraception methods

- Quantitative analysis
  - To determine whether a pregnancy is viable or nonviable
  - To detect the presence of hydatidiform mole and hCG-excreting tumor

WHAT TEST RESULTS INDICATE

- Qualitative
  - Positive test result indicates pregnancy.
  - Negative test result indicates no pregnancy, urine too dilute, or too soon to detect agglutinins.
- Quantitative: Positive if agglutinins fail to appear
  - First trimester: 500,000 IU/24 hours
  - Second trimester: 10,000 to 25,000 IU/24 hours
  - Third trimester: 5000 to 15,000 IU/24 hours
  - A very high level may indicate multiple pregnancies or erythroblastosis fetalis.
  - A depressed level usually indicates threatened abortion or ectopic pregnancy.
  - Undetectable within a few days after delivery.
- Increases
  - During the first trimester of pregnancy, hCG levels rise steadily and rapidly.
  - The level peaks around the tenth week of gestation.
  - Tapers off to less than 10% of peak levels during gestation.
- Decreases: Initial increase followed by decreasing values indicates loss of tissues of pregnancy.

PROCEDURE

- How much urine is needed:
  - Qualitative: A few drops
  - Quantitative: 24-hour urine specimen
- Nonfasting
- The first voided specimen is best because it has an increased concentration of hCG. If the test is done on a specimen later in the day and pregnancy is strongly suspected, do a serum hCG.
- Type of collection container: Clean urine cup
- Special treatment of sample: Refrigerate 24-hour urine specimen and keep on ice during collection.

INTERFERING FACTORS

- Medications: Phenothiazines and anticonvulsants cause both false-positive and false-negative results.
- Food: None.

- Improper storage.
- Proteinuria, hematuria, and elevated sedimentation rate may cause false-positive results.
- Tap water or soap residue may cause false-positive results.

TEST YOUR KNOWLEDGE OF CHAPTER 36

1. What are the components of the UA, and what information does the test provide?
2. When are a microscopic analysis of urine sediment and urine culture indicated?
3. What are the interfering factors for a urine culture?
4. Why is an early morning urine specimen required for a qualitative urine hCG test?
5. What information does a quantitative urine hCG test provide that a qualitative urine hCG test does not?

 ## BIBLIOGRAPHY

Diagnostics. An A-Z Guide to Laboratory Tests. (2000). Springhouse, PA: Springhouse.

Ewald, G. A., & McKenzie, C. R. (Eds.). (1999). *Manual of medical therapeutics* (32nd ed.). Boston: Little, Brown & Co.

Fischbach, F. (1999). *A manual of laboratory & diagnostic tests* (6th ed.). New York: J. B. Lippincott.

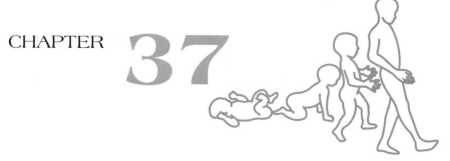

Culture, Antibiotic Sensitivity, and Skin Testing

MARGARET R. COLYAR

OBJECTIVES
- Become familiar with culture, antibiotic sensitivity, and skin testing commonly used in children.
- Identify interfering factors for common cultures and skin tests.

 CPT Codes

- 95004: Allergy skin tests
- 87186: Antibiotic sensitivity assay
- 87070: Aerobic wound culture
- 87075: Anaerobic wound culture
- 87070F: Ear culture
- 87070E: Eye culture
- 87070H: Nose culture
- 87880: Rapid strep A
- 87070G: Throat culture

Cultures can be taken from any body orifice, the blood, or open wounds.

 PURPOSE

- To confirm the etiology of the infecting organism
- To confirm eradication of the infecting organism

548

☽ WHAT TEST RESULTS INDICATE

- Normal: No organism is seen.
- Abnormal: Usually only a single organism is causing an infection. When two or more types of organisms are reported, it usually indicates that the specimen was contaminated during collection.

☽ PROCEDURE

- Equipment needed: Culture tubes and medium (Table 37–1)
  - Wound cultures: Aerobic or anaerobic tubes
    - Aerobic: Use for an organism in a *superficial* wound site: Express wound and swab.
    - Anaerobic: Use for areas of *poor perfusion.*
    - Insert tube deeply into wound or aspirate using a needle and syringe.
  - Throat: Sterile rayon swab with plastic shaft (no wooden shafts)
    - Swab tonsils and posterior pharynx vigorously (avoid teeth, gums, tongue, and cheek surfaces).
  - Nasopharyngeal: Flexible wire swab: Rotate and remove
  - Sputum: Sterile collection container
    - Early morning specimen is best.
    - If the patient is unable to produce a specimen, try heated saline neb-ulizer to induce a specimen.
  - Urine: Sterile collection container
    - Midstream or clean catch
    - Bagged urine or catheterized urine if child is not potty trained
  - Stool: Sterile collection container
    - Put collection pan under the commode lid. Make sure that no urine or tissue paper gets into the sample.
  - Blood: Two inoculated culture media in bottles
    - Cleanse the site with alcohol swab.
    - Cleanse the site with 10% povidone-iodine (Betadine) swab in circu-lar motion from the center outward in concentric circles. Let dry for 1 minute.
    - Draw the blood specimen.
    - Change the needle on the syringe.
    - Inject appropriate amount of blood in each of two inoculated culture medium bottles.
  - Vaginal: Culture swab specific for organism: gonococci/chlamydiae.
    - Insert swab in vaginal canal and swab the lateral vaginal walls for *Trichomonas* spp., *Candida* spp., and bacterial vaginosis cultures.
    - Insert the swab into the cervix for gonorrhea and chlamydial cul-tures.
  - Urethral: Flexible wire culture swab
    - Insert the swab gently into urethra approximately 1 to 2 cm.

TABLE 37-1. CULTURE MEDIA AND AMOUNT OF SPECIMEN NEEDED

Type of Culture	Culture Medium	Amount Needed
Wound	Aerobic: Superficial wound	Small amount
	Anaerobic: deep wound	Small amount
Throat	Sterile rayon swab with plastic shaft (no wooden shafts)	Small amount
Nasopharyngeal	Flexible wire swab	Small amount
Sputum	Sterile collection container	3 mL
Urine	Sterile collection container	3 mL
Stool	Sterile collection container	3 mL
Blood	Two inoculated culture medium bottles	Age-specific bottle ● Neonates: 1 to 2 mL ● Infants: 2 to 3 mL ● Children: 3 to 5 mL ● Adolescents: 10 to 20 mL
Vaginal	Sterile rayon swab with plastic shaft	Small amount
Cervical	Sterile rayon swab with plastic shaft	Small amount (collection media required by laboratory for *Neisseria gonorrhea* and *Chlamydia*)
Urethral	Flexible wire culture swab	Small amount

- Amount needed
  - Wound, throat, nasopharyngeal, vaginal, and urethral: Small amount of secretions on culture swab
  - Sputum, urine, stool: 3 mL
  - Blood per bottle
    - Neonates: 1 to 2 mL
    - Infants: 2 to 3 mL
    - Children: 3 to 5 mL
    - Adolescents 10 to 20 mL
- Special treatment of sample: Storage
  - Wound, throat, nasal pharyngeal, vaginal, and urethral: Crush ampule. Not all cervical or vaginal cultures use this type of medium. The instructions are specific to the medium used.
  - Sputum, urine, and stool: Refrigerate if unable to culture immediately.
  - Blood: Do not refrigerate.

INTERFERING FACTORS

- Improper storage or collection
- Patient use of antibiotics before collection
- Contamination during specimen collection

TABLE 37–2. READING THE ANTIBIOTIC SENSITIVITY ASSAY		
Result	Decision	Interpretation
Sensitive (S)	Use	Smallest MIC is the best
Resistant (R)	Do not use	Organism is resistant to the antibiotic

MIC = minimum inhibitory concentration.

 # ANTIBIOTIC SENSITIVITY ASSAY

Cultures can be taken from any body orifice, the blood, or open wounds. Antibiotic sensitivity assays are used to study inhibition of the organism cultured. They are used by healthcare providers to select appropriate antibiotics for treatment.

PURPOSE

- To determine the antibiotic that will best inhibit the organism
- To confirm eradication of the infecting organism

WHAT TEST RESULTS INDICATE

The laboratory results will have either an S, which indicates the organism is sensitive to a particular antibiotic, or an R, which indicates the organism is resistant to a particular antibiotic (Table 37–2).

PROCEDURE

- Technique (usually done by laboratory technician)
    - Agar plates are inoculated with the organism in question. Paper disks containing various antibiotics are placed onto the surface, and the plate is incubated. This helps to determine the smallest amount of antibiotic needed to inhibit the growth of the organism. This is known as the minimum inhibitory concentration (MIC). The smaller the MIC, the better the antibiotic is at controlling the organism.
- Amount needed: One rayon culture swab saturated with the organism
- Special treatment of sample: Store at room temperature

INTERFERING FACTORS

- Medications: Antibiotics
- Food: None

 # WOUND CULTURES

PURPOSE

- Diagnosis: To confirm the etiology of an infecting organism

TABLE 37–3. ABNORMAL WOUND CULTURE TEST RESULTS	
Aerobic	**Anaerobic**
Staphylococus aureus	*Clostridium* spp.
Group A beta-hemolytic streptococci	*Proteus* spp.
Escherichia coli	*Bacteroides*
Enterobacteriaceae	
Group D streptococci	
Enterococci	
Streptococcus bovis	
Pseudomonas spp.	

- Symptoms of infection: Wound is red, swollen, warm, and has drainage of green or yellow exudates.
- Follow-up: To determine eradication of the infecting organism

WHAT TEST RESULTS INDICATE

- Normal test result: No organism is seen.
- Abnormal test result: Table 37–3 lists possible abnormal results and what they indicate.

PROCEDURE

- Amount needed: 1 to 5 mL of aspirate or saturated swab
- Nonfasting
- Type of swab: Aerobic or anaerobic swabs as needed
- Special treatment of swab
  - Storage: To laboratory within 15 minutes
  - Store at room temperature

INTERFERING FACTORS

- Medications: Antibiotics
- Foods: None
- Improper storage: Wrong culture medium
- Improper collection technique

ⓢ RAPID *STREPTOCOCCUS*: GROUP A BETA-HEMOLYTIC

The rapid strep test does not differentiate between the carrier state and acute infection. Although carriers are usually asymptomatic, those with acute infection are symptomatic.

PURPOSE

- Diagnosis
  - Symptoms
    - Sore throat: Hurts to swallow
    - Swollen, beefy red tonsils with purulent exudate; however, presentation may vary
    - Petechiae on the soft palate
    - Headache
    - Abdominal pain
    - Vomiting
    - Fever
    - Sandpaper-like rash with pastia lines
  - Qualitative detection of group A streptococcal antigen
  - To decrease severity of symptoms
  - To prevent rheumatic fever and glomerulonephritis

PROCEDURE

- Amount needed: Small amount of exudates or pharyngeal secretions on the swab
- Nonfasting
- Type of swab
  - Sterile rayon tube with plastic shaft (no wooden shafts).
  - Use two swabs so that one can be use for culture if rapid strep test result is negative.
- Special treatment of sample: Use as soon as possible. If this is not possible, store at room temperature or refrigerate for up to 24 hours.

INTERFERING FACTORS

- Medications: Antibiotics.
- Food: None.
- Improper storage: Failure to use proper transport medium will cause the specimen to dry out and the bacteria to die.
- Inadequate sample.
- Not swabbing the pharyngeal area thoroughly.

THROAT CULTURE

The throat culture does not differentiate between the carrier state and acute infection, but carriers are usually asymptomatic.

PURPOSE

- Diagnosis
  - To detect group A streptococcal antigen

TABLE 37–4. ABNORMAL WOUND CULTURE TEST RESULTS

Normal Organisms	Abnormal Organisms
Nonhemolytic streptococci	*Neisseria meningitidis*
Alpha-hemolytic streptococci	*Corynebacterium*
Staphylococci	*Bordetella pertussis*
Diphtheroids	*Corynebacterium diphtheriae*
Some *Haemophilus* organisms	*Haemophilus influenzae*
Pneumococci	*Candida albicans*
Enteric gram-negative rods	

- To detect other infectious organisms
- To decrease the severity of symptoms
- To detect group A beta-hemolytic streptococci not detected on the rapid strep test; all negative rapid strep test results should have back-up culture done
- Symptoms
  - Sore throat: Hurts to swallow
  - Swollen, red tonsils with purulent exudates; however, presentation can vary
  - Fever
  - Vomiting
  - Headache
  - Abdominal pain
  - Sandpaper-like rash: If strep is causative agent

WHAT TEST RESULTS INDICATE

- Table 37–4 lists possible results and what they indicate.
- Results: Within 1 to 3 days.

PROCEDURE

- Amount needed: Small amount on swab.
- Nonfasting.
- Type of swab: Sterile rayon tube with plastic shaft (no wooden shafts).
- Special treatment of sample: Streak on plate as soon as possible.
  - To plate specimen, streak the culture medium from side to side and then turn the culture dish 90 degrees and streak the culture plate from side to side again. Repeat this procedure until all four quadrants of the culture plate are streaked (Fig. 37–1).
  - Storage: Room temperature or refrigerate for up to 24 hours.

INTERFERING FACTORS

- Medications: Antibiotics.
- Food: None.

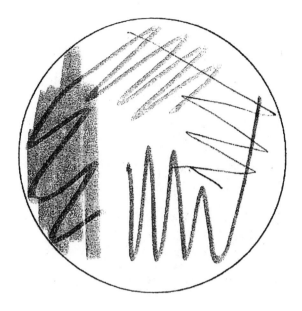

FIG. 37–1. Streak the culture medium on one side of the dish from side to side. Turn the dish 90 degrees and streak again. Repeat until all four quadrants of the dish are streaked.

- Improper storage: Failure to use proper transport medium will cause the specimen to dry out and the bacteria to die.
- Not swabbing pharyngeal area thoroughly.

⑤ RADIOALLERGOSORBENT TEST (RAST): SKIN TESTING

Use with children who have asthma, hay fever, atopic eczema, food allergies, and drug reactions.

PURPOSE

- To test for reaction to certain environmental and food allergy stimulants
- To determine allergy-specific IgE antibody, which indicates an immediate hypersensitivity to an allergen

RESULTS

- Positive RAST results indicate diagnosis of allergy irrespective of the level of total IgE: > 400% of control
- Negative RAST: < 150% of control
- Borderline RAST: 150 to 400% of control

PROCEDURE

- Amount needed: 7 mL; 1 mL is usually enough for five allergen assays.
- Nonfasting.

- Type of tube: Red-top tube.
- Special treatment of sample: None.
- Other: Make sure to note if there are specific allergens that need to be tested.

INTERFERING FACTORS

- Medications: Antihistamines, steroids.
- Food: None.
- Improper storage: Radioactive scan within 1 week of sample collection may alter the test results.

TEST YOUR KNOWLEDGE OF CHAPTER 37

1. Where is a culture taken from?
2. What is the difference between an aerobic and an anaerobic culture? How does the procedure of obtaining the specimen differ?
3. Describe the technique of obtaining a blood culture.
4. What is the significance of the MIC?
5. What are the normal organisms found on a throat culture?
6. What do the results of a radioallergosorbent test (RAST) indicate?

BIBLIOGRAPHY

Diagnostics. An A-Z Guide to Laboratory Tests. (2000). Springhouse, PA: Springhouse.

Ewald, G. A., & McKenzie, C. R. (Eds.). (1999). *Manual of medical therapeutics* (32nd ed.). Boston: Little, Brown & Co.

Fischbach, F. (1999). *A manual of laboratory & diagnostic tests* (6th ed.). New York: J. B. Lippincott.

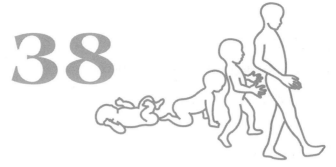

Stool Diagnostic Tests

Margaret R. Colyar

Objectives
- *Become familiar with stool diagnostic tests commonly used in children.*
- *Ascertain the correct procedure and storage for common stool diagnostic tests.*
- *Identify interfering factors for common stool diagnostic tests.*

 ## CPT Codes

- 87045A: Stool culture
- 87177: Ova and parasites
- 87205A: Stool for white blood cells
- 82270: Guaiac (occult blood)

Stool testing is the standard procedure for children with unexplained diarrhea for several days and with nonspecific symptoms such as abdominal pain and bloating or rectal bleeding. Examination of the feces is valuable for identification of pathogens. The most common pathogens are *Shigella* spp., *Salmonella* spp., *Giardia lamblia*, and *Campylobacter fetus*. Commonly used tests are culture and sensitivity, ova and parasites, leukocytes, and guaiac (Hemoccult).

PURPOSE

- Diagnosis: To identify and isolate pathogenic organisms
- To identify a carrier state

557

TABLE 38–1. STOOL SPECIMEN RESULTS		
Normal Organism	Abnormal Organism	Problem
	ANAEROBES: 96–99%	
Bacteroides	*Shigella* spp.	Shigellosis, bacillary dysentery
Anaerobic lactobacilli	*Salmonella* spp.	Enterocolitis, typhoid fever, salmonellosis
Clostridia	*Campylobacter fetus*	Gastroenteritis
Anaerobic streptococci	*Vibrio cholerae*	Cholera
	OTHER: 1–4%	
	Clostridium	***Pseudomembranous***
	Difficile	***Enterocolitis***
Escherichia coli	*Yersinia enterocolitica*	Enterocolitis, ileitis, mesenteric adenitis
Pseudomonas spp.	*Staphylococcus aureus*	Food poisoning
Proteus spp.	*Bacillus cereus*	Food poisoning
Enterococci	*Clostridium perfringens*	Food poisoning
Lactobacilli	*Clostridium botulinum*	Food poisoning
Candida spp.	*Aeromonas hydrophila*	Gastroenteritis

- To determine if gastrointestinal bleeding is occurring
  - Symptoms
    - Abdominal pain, diarrhea, bloating of unexplained origin

WHAT TEST RESULTS INDICATE

- Culture: Normal
  - *Bacteroides*, anaerobic lactobacilli, *Clostridium* spp., anaerobic strepto-cocci, *Escherichia coli*, small amounts of *Pseudomonas* and *Proteus* organ-isms., lactobacilli, *Candida* spp., and enterococci
- Culture: Abnormal: Must request tests for *Listeria, Yersinia, Salmonella, Giardia*, and *Campylobacter* spp., if desired
  - Positive for pathogenic organisms (Table 38–1)
- Ova and parasites
  - Normal: None
  - Abnormal: Positive for organisms; serial stool specimens have been found to be more effective in determining the problem (Table 38–2)
- Leukocytes: Helpful in determining the etiology of diarrhea
  - Normal: Negative
  - Abnormal: Positive (Table 38–3)
- Guaiac
  - Normal: Negative
  - Abnormal: Positive; do further testing (serial stool specimens have been found to be more effective; consider colonoscopy or sigmoi-doscopy)

TABLE 38–2. OVA AND PARASITE TEST RESULTS

Normal	Abnormal

None	**PROTOZOA (SINGLE-CELL ORGANISMS)**
	● Sarcodina (amebae)
	  ○ *Entamoeba histolytica:* Causes significant disease
	  ○ Zoomastigophora (flagellates)
	  ○ *Giardia lamblia*
	  ○ *Trichomonas* spp.
	HELMINTHS
	● Flatworms
	  ○ Tapeworms
	  ○ Leaf-shaped flukes
	  ○ Roundworms

 PROCEDURE

- Amount needed: 1 to 3 mL of fresh stool
- Nonfasting
- Airtight stool specimen container
- Special treatment of sample
  - Temperature: For all tests except culture, specimen may be refrigerated in an airtight container.

TABLE 38–3. LEUKOCYTES IN STOOL: CLINICAL IMPLICATIONS FOR DIARRHEA

Disease	Mononuclear	Polymorphonuclear	Absent
BACTERIA: TOXIGENIC			
● *Clostridium* cholera			X
● Staphylococci			X
COLITIS			
● Amebic			X
● Ulcerative		X	
DIARRHEA			
● *Escherichia coli:* Invasive		X	
● *Escherichia coli:* Noninvasive			X
● Nonspecific			X
PARASITES			
● Salmonellosis		X	
● Shigellosis		X	
● Typhoid	X		
● *Yersinia* spp.			X
● *Campylobacter* spp.			X
● *Giardia* spp.			X

INTERFERING FACTORS

- Medications
  - Antibiotics within preceding 7 to 10 days
  - Ova and parasites
  - Mineral oil, bismuth, magnesium, antidiarrheals, and barium
- Contamination: Urine, toilet paper, or stool passed into a toilet bowl
- Food: None
- Improper storage or collection: Ova and parasites: Freezing
- Delayed processing

TEST YOUR KNOWLEDGE OF CHAPTER 38

1. What normal and abnormal microorganisms are determined by stool cultures?
2. Which stool tests help to determine the etiology of diarrhea?
3. Testing for what microorganisms must be requested on a stool culture?
4. Describe how to ensure that a stool sample for ova and parasites is managed properly.
5. What medications interfere with stool testing?

 BIBLIOGRAPHY

Alcamo, I. E. (1987). *Fundamentals of microbiology* (2nd ed.). Menlo Park, CA: Benjamin/Cummins Publishing Co, Inc.
Diagnostics. An A-Z Guide to Laboratory Tests. (2000). Springhouse, PA: Springhouse.
Ewald, G. A., & McKenzie, C. R. (Eds.). (1999). *Manual of medical therapeutics* (32nd ed.). Boston: Little, Brown & Co.
Fischbach, F. (1999). *A manual of laboratory and diagnostic tests* (6th ed.). New York: J. B. Lippincott.

39

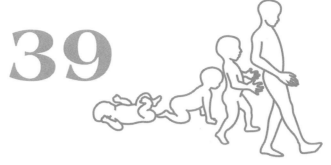

Vaginal Cultures

MARGARET R. COLYAR

OBJECTIVES
- *Become familiar with vaginal diagnostic tests commonly used in children.*
- *Ascertain the correct procedure and storage for common vaginal diagnostic tests.*
- *Identify interfering factors for common vaginal diagnostic tests.*

 ## CPT Codes

- 87201: Wet mount
- 87220: KOH
- 88164: Pap smear
- 88142: Thin prep Pap smear

- 87070C: Genital culture
- 87591: Culture: Gonorrhea
- 87320: Culture: *Chlamydia*

Vaginal cultures are obtained to identify specific organisms. To prevent vaginal, uterine, tubal, and ovarian infections, the use of condoms is suggested.

 ## PURPOSE

- Diagnosis: To identify infectious microbes in the vaginal vault
  - Symptoms
    - Low abdominal pain
    - Low back pain

561

    ○ Vaginal drainage
    ○ Vaginal symptoms: Discomfort, burning, pain

🎴 PROCEDURE

- Amount needed: Culture swab saturated
- Nonfasting
- Type of swab: Rayon culture swab
- Special treatment of sample: Make sure swab is crushed

🎴 INTERFERING FACTORS

- Douching within 24 hours of test
- For urethral swabs, the patient should not have voided 1 hour before the test
- Intercourse
- Lubricating jelly
- Vaginal medication

🎴 WET MOUNT: WET PREP AND POTASSIUM HYDROXIDE

The wet mount (wet prep or wet smear) is a tool used to evaluate the etiology of abnormal vaginal secretions. Saline and 10% potassium hydroxide (KOH) preparations are used. The saline preparation can detect the presence of white blood cells, bacteria, trichomonads, hyphae, budding yeasts, and clue cells. The 10% KOH preparation is used to test for the presence of amines (also known as a "whiff test") and can more easily detect hyphae and budding yeasts. Saline and KOH wet smears and Gram stains are indicated in all suspected vaginal infections.

PURPOSE

- Diagnosis: To assist in determination of disease etiology
  - Symptoms
    - ○ Unusual foul-smelling vaginal discharge
    - ○ Lower abdominal or low back pain
    - ○ Vulvar or vaginal itching or irritation
    - ○ Dysuria
    - ○ Perineal irritation and discomfort

RESULTS

- Normal values: Few white blood cells (WBCs), normal epithelial cells, and lactobacilli; otherwise, negative

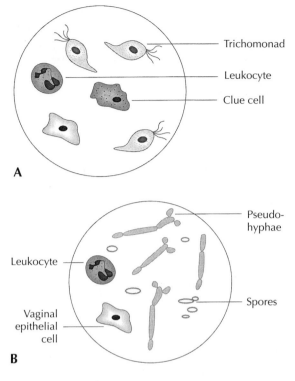

A

B

FIG. 39–1. *(A)* Saline preparation. *(B)* KOH preparation.

WHAT TEST RESULTS INDICATE

- Figure 39–1 shows results on saline and KOH preparations.
- Wet prep: Presence of clue cells in conjunction with other signs of bacterial vaginosis and trichomonads indicates disease.
- Clue cells (i.e., large epithelial cells with indistinct borders with multiple cocci clinging to them) are often described as appearing like "pepper on a fried egg." Clue cells in conjunction with other signs (e.g., elevated pH, positive whiff test result, homogeneous vaginal discharge) indicate bacterial vaginosis. A threshold of more than 20% clue cells is typically used.
- Trichomonads: Oval shaped with thin, whiplike tail (flagellum). Trichomonads are typically motile, but are occasionally seen not moving or "dead." They are typically seen in conjunction with many WBCs.
- KOH prep
  - Yeasts: Hyphae, spores (buds, candidiasis)

PROCEDURE

- Amount needed: Culture swab saturated
- Nonfasting

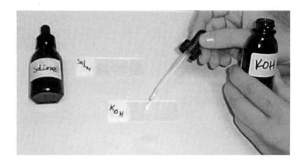

FIG. 39–2. Slide preparation. Saline on one slide and KOH on the other.

- Type of swab: Rayon culture swab
- Using cotton-tipped applicators, collect specimen of vaginal secretions from the lateral vaginal walls. Do not collect from the vaginal pool, which may contain cervical contaminants.
- Place one cotton-tipped applicator in the test tube with 1 mL 0.9% sodium chloride and mix well.
- With the cotton-tipped applicator, place a smear on each slide (Fig. 39–2).
    - On one slide, add 1 to 2 drops of saline and cover with the coverslip.
    - On the second slide, add 1 to 2 drops of 10% KOH and cover with the coverslip.
    - Gently heat the KOH slide for 2 to 3 seconds. Just rest the slide on the microscope light and the slide is easily heated.
    - Allow the KOH slide to sit for 15 to 20 minutes at room temperature if time permits, but this is not necessary.

INTERFERING FACTORS

- Recent douching
- Menses (can be done during menses, but this interferes with pH determination)
- Intravaginal medications
- Recent intercourse

PAPANICOLAOU SMEAR

The Papanicolaou (Pap) smear is a part of the pelvic examination and is used to examine the cells of the cervix to screen for signs of pre-cancerous lesions and cancer. Pap smears may also identify cellular changes associated with infection. The Pap smear is not a specific test for human papillomavirus (HPV), although sometimes the results suggest that HPV may be present. HPV testing can now be done if using the thin prep method of collection.

564

PURPOSE

- Diagnosis
  - To screen for precancerous cervical lesions
  - To screen for cancerous lesions
  - To identify infection (incidental finding but not purpose of the test)
  - To determine maturation index (hormonal assessment)
- Follow-up: To determine eradication of precancerous and cancerous lesions

RESULTS

- Normal
  - No precancerous or cancerous lesions
  - No infection
  - Maturation index: Child 80/20/0 (ratio of parabasal, intermediate, and superficial cells in vagina)
  - Reactive or benign cellular changes
- Abnormal: Bethesda Classification System
  - Atypical squamous cells of undetermined significance
  - Atypical glandular cells of undetermined significance
  - Squamous intraepithelial lesions (SILs)
    - CIN 1: Mild dysplasia: Low-grade SIL/HPV
    - CIN 2: Moderate dysplasia
    - CIN 3: Severe dysplasia or carcinoma *in situ*; squamous cell carcinoma
  - Identification of infectious organisms
    - *Candida* spp.
    - Gonococci
    - *Chlamydia*
    - Trichomonads
    - HPV

PROCEDURE

- Amount needed: Small amount of endothelial cells
- Scraping of cells from cervix and transformation zone
- Nonfasting
- Several collection containers are available. Follow the manufacturer's suggestions for specimen collection. Most common collection containers are:
  - Slides
  - Thin prep bottles
- Special treatment of sample
  - Slides: Rub specimen from cytobrush on one half of the slide and cytology scraper on other half of the slide; apply fixative to slides within 15 seconds

- Thin prep: Detach head of cervical broom and deposit into fluid
- Temperature: Store at room temperature

INTERFERING FACTORS

- Medications
  - Tetracycline
  - Digitalis
  - Vaginal medication
- Food: None
- Other
  - Fixative is not applied to slide
  - Intercourse
  - Use of lubricating jelly
  - Douching within 48 to 72 hours
  - Menstruation
  - Entire transformation zone not sampled

GONORRHEA CULTURE

Gonorrhea, which is caused by the organism *Neisseria gonorrhoeae*, is the most prevalent sexually transmitted disease (STD). Culture sites include the urethra, endocervix, anal canal, oropharynx, and conjunctiva.

PURPOSE

- Diagnosis: To rule out infection by *N. gonorrhoeae*
  - Symptoms
    - Abnormal vaginal drainage
    - Painful urination
    - Lower abdominal pain
    - Pharyngitis

RESULTS

- Normal: A negative test indicates no infection with *N. gonorrhoeae*.
- Abnormal: A positive test indicates infection with *N. gonorrhoeae*.

PROCEDURE

- Endocervical: Use a female swab (plastic shaft with cotton tip).
  - Place the swab in the cervical orifice for several seconds.
  - Rotate the swab.
  - Place in culture tube and crush vial.
- Urethral: Use a male swab (flexible wire shaft with cotton tip).
  - Have patient milk the penis.

- Insert 1 to 2 cm into urethra.
- Rotate.
- Leave in place for several seconds.
- Place in culture tube.
- Rectal: Use a culture swab with a plastic shaft with cotton tip.
  - Insert 1 inch into the anus.
  - Rotate.
  - Leave in place for several seconds.
  - Place in culture.
  - Insert into tube and crush vial.
- Throat: Use a culture swab with a plastic shaft and cotton tip.
  - Culture tonsillar area over inflamed and purulent areas.
  - Place the swab in culture tube and crush vial.
- Conjunctiva: Use a culture swab with plastic shaft and cotton tip.
  - Culture discharge from conjunctiva.
  - Place the swab in culture tube and crush vial.
- Amount needed: End of swab saturated
- Nonfasting

INTERFERING FACTORS

- Douching within 48 to 72 hours of test
- For urethral swabs, the patient should not have voided 1 hour before the test

 CHLAMYDIA CULTURE

Chlamydial infection, which is caused by the organism *Chlamydia trachomatis*, is the second most prevalent STD. Culture sites include the urethra, endocervix, anal canal, and oropharynx.

PURPOSE

- Diagnosis: To rule out infection by *C. trachomatis*
  - Symptoms
    - ○ Abnormal vaginal drainage
    - ○ Painful urination
    - ○ Lower abdominal pain
    - ○ Pharyngitis
    - ○ Abnormal vaginal bleeding, including spotting

RESULTS

- Normal: A negative test indicates no infection with *C. trachomatis*.
- Abnormal: A positive test indicates infection with *C. trachomatis*.

PROCEDURE

- Endocervical: Use a female swab (plastic shaft with cotton tip).
  - Place the swab in the cervical orifice for several seconds.
  - Rotate the swab.
  - Place in the culture tube and crush vial.
- Urethral: Use a male swab (flexible wire shaft with cotton tip).
  - Have patient milk the penis
  - Insert 1 to 2 cm into the urethra.
  - Rotate.
  - Leave in place for several seconds.
  - Place in the culture tube.
- Rectal: Use a culture swab with plastic shaft and cotton tip.
  - Insert 1 inch into the anus.
  - Rotate.
  - Leave in place for several seconds.
  - Place in culture tube and crush vial.
- Throat: Use a culture swab with plastic shaft and cotton tip.
  - Culture tonsillar area over inflamed and purulent areas.
  - Place swab in culture tube and crush vial.
- Conjunctiva: Use a culture swab with plastic shaft and cotton tip.
  - Culture discharge from the conjunctiva.
  - Place the swab in the culture tube and crush vial.
- Amount needed: End of swab saturated
- Nonfasting

INTERFERING FACTORS

- Douching within 48 to 72 hours of test.
- For urethral swabs, the patient should not have voided 1 hour before the test.

TEST YOUR KNOWLEDGE OF CHAPTER 39

1. What are the interfering factors with vaginal testing?
2. Describe how to prepare a wet mount and KOH slide for viewing.
3. Describe the appearance of microorganisms commonly seen on vaginal wet mounts.
4. What are the components available from a Pap smear?
5. Explain the maturation index.
6. If you are preparing a Pap smear using the slide technique, when should you apply the fixative?
7. From what orifice are gonorrhea and *Chlamydia* cultures obtained?

🌀 BIBLIOGRAPHY

Alcamo, I. E. (1987). *Fundamentals of microbiology* (2nd ed.). Menlo Park, CA: Benjamin/Cummins Publishing Co, Inc.

Diagnostics. An A-Z Guide to Laboratory Tests. (2000). Springhouse, PA: Springhouse.

Ewald, G. A., & McKenzie, C. R. (Eds.). (1999). *Manual of medical therapeutics* (32nd ed.). Boston: Little, Brown & Co.

Fischbach, F. (1999). *A manual of laboratory & diagnostic tests* (6th ed.). New York: J. B. Lippincott.

Index

Page numbers followed by *b* indicate boxes; those followed by *f* indicate figures; and those followed by *t* indicate tables.

571